Fetal Echocardiography

System requirement:
- Operating System – Windows Vista or above
- Recommended Web Browser – Google Chrome & Mozilla Firefox
- Essential plugins – Java & Flash player
    - Facing problems in viewing content – it may be your system does not have java enabled.
    - If Videos don't show up – it may be the system requires Flash player or need to manage flash setting. To learn more about flash setting click on the link in the help section.
    - You can test java and flash by using the links from the help section of the CD/DVD.

Accompanying CD/DVD Rom is playable only in Computer and not in DVD player.

CD/DVD has Autorun function – it may take few seconds to load on your computer. If it does not works for you then follow the steps below to access the contents manually:
- Click on my computer
- Select the **CD/DVD** drive and click open/explore – this will show list of files in the CD/DVD
- Find and double click file – "launch.html"

For more information about troubleshoot of Autorun click on:
http://support.microsoft.com/kb/330135

CD CONTENTS

Just images and videos

Sejal Shah, Pradeep S

1. Fetal Echo Still Images
2. Fetal Echo Videos

Fetal Echocardiography

Editor
Sejal Shah MD
Consultant Pediatric and Fetal Cardiologist
Rx Dx Clinic, Rainbow Children's Hospital
MS Ramaiah Memorial Hospital
Bengaluru, Karnataka, India

Co-editors
Sunita Maheshwari ABP ABPC (USA)
Pediatric Cardiologist and E-Teacher
Teleradiology Solutions and Rx Dx Clinic
Bengaluru, Karnataka, India

PV Suresh MD DM
Senior Consultant and Head
Department of Pediatric Cardiology
Narayana Hrudayalaya
Bengaluru, Karnataka, India

Foreword
Colin John

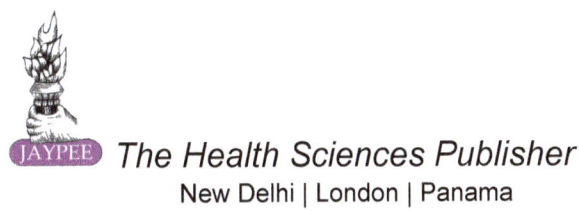

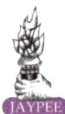 **Jaypee Brothers Medical Publishers (P) Ltd**

Headquarters
Jaypee Brothers Medical Publishers (P) Ltd
4838/24, Ansari Road, Daryaganj
New Delhi 110 002, India
Phone: +91-11-43574357
Fax: +91-11-43574314
Email: jaypee@jaypeebrothers.com

Overseas Offices

J.P. Medical Ltd
83 Victoria Street, London
SW1H 0HW (UK)
Phone: +44 20 3170 8910
Fax: +44 (0)20 3008 6180
Email: info@jpmedpub.com

Jaypee-Highlights Medical Publishers Inc.
City of Knowledge, Bld. 235, 2nd Floor, Clayton
Panama City, Panama
Phone: +1 507-301-0496
Fax: +1 507-301-0499
Email: cservice@jphmedical.com

Jaypee Brothers Medical Publishers (P) Ltd
17/1-B Babar Road, Block-B, Shaymali
Mohammadpur, Dhaka-1207
Bangladesh
Mobile: +08801912003485
Email: jaypeedhaka@gmail.com

Jaypee Brothers Medical Publishers (P) Ltd
Bhotahity, Kathmandu, Nepal
Phone: +977-9741283608
Email: kathmandu@jaypeebrothers.com

Website: www.jaypeebrothers.com
Website: www.jaypeedigital.com

© 2018, Jaypee Brothers Medical Publishers

The views and opinions expressed in this book are solely those of the original contributor(s)/author(s) and do not necessarily represent those of editor(s) of the book.

All rights reserved. No part of this publication and CD-ROM may be reproduced, stored or transmitted in any form or by any means, electronic, mechanical, photocopying, recording or otherwise, without the prior permission in writing of the publishers.

All brand names and product names used in this book are trade names, service marks, trademarks or registered trademarks of their respective owners. The publisher is not associated with any product or vendor mentioned in this book.

Medical knowledge and practice change constantly. This book is designed to provide accurate, authoritative information about the subject matter in question. However, readers are advised to check the most current information available on procedures included and check information from the manufacturer of each product to be administered, to verify the recommended dose, formula, method and duration of administration, adverse effects and contraindications. It is the responsibility of the practitioner to take all appropriate safety precautions. Neither the publisher nor the author(s)/editor(s) assume any liability for any injury and/or damage to persons or property arising from or related to use of material in this book.

This book is sold on the understanding that the publisher is not engaged in providing professional medical services. If such advice or services are required, the services of a competent medical professional should be sought.

Every effort has been made where necessary to contact holders of copyright to obtain permission to reproduce copyright material. If any have been inadvertently overlooked, the publisher will be pleased to make the necessary arrangements at the first opportunity.

Inquiries for bulk sales may be solicited at: jaypee@jaypeebrothers.com

Fetal Echocardiography

First Edition: **2018**

ISBN 978-93-5270-110-0

Dedicated to
All of you—my lovely readers
All inspiring children with heart diseases and their caretakers
All my teachers
All my students—who also have been teachers in many ways
and
My parents

CONTRIBUTORS

Anita Saxena MD DM FACC
Professor
Department of Cardiology
All India Institute of Medical Sciences
New Delhi, India

Balu Vaidyanathan MD DM FACC
Professor
Department of Pediatric Cardiology
Head
Department of Fetal Cardiology
Amrita Institute of Medical Sciences
Kochi, Kerala, India

BS Ramamurthy MBBS MD DMRD DNB
Consultant Radiologist and Fetal Medicine Specialist
Srinivasa Ultrasound Scanning Centre
Bengaluru, Karnataka, India

Meenakshi Bhat MD DCH DNB MRCP (Ire) CSST (Clinical Genetics, UK)
Consultant, Clinical Genetics
Professor
Centre for Human Genetics
Bengaluru, Karnataka, India

Nageswara Rao Koneti MD DM DNB FPC
Chief Pediatric Cardiologist
Department of Pediatric Cardiology
Care Hospitals
Hyderabad, Telangana, India

Pradeep S MBBS MD DNB (Radiology)
Head
Department of Radiology and Fetal Medicine
Fortis Hospital, Bannerghatta Road
Bengaluru, Karnataka, India

Prashant Bobhate MD (ped) FNB (Ped Card) FPVRI
Fellowship in Pulmonary Hypertension (Canada)
Consultant Pediatric Cardiologist
Kokilaben Dhirubhai Ambani Hospital
Mumbai, Maharashtra, India

Prathima Radhakrishnan FRCOG Diploma in Fetal Medicine (FMK, UK) Diploma in Advanced Obstetric Ultrasound (RCOG-RCR, UK)
Director and Consultant
Department of Fetal Medicine
Bangalore Fetal Medicine Centre
Bengaluru, Karnataka, India

PV Suresh MD DM
Senior Consultant and Head
Department of Pediatric Cardiology
Narayana Hrudayalaya
Bengaluru, Karnataka, India

R Saileela MD DNB FNB
Consultant Pediatric Cardiologist
Department of Pediatric Cardiology
Care Hospitals
Hyderabad, Telangana, India

Reeth Sahana DGO Fellowship in Fetal Medicine
Consultant
Department of Fetal Medicine
Bangalore Fetal Medicine Centre
Bengaluru, Karnataka, India

Sejal Shah MD
Consultant Pediatric and Fetal Cardiologist
Rx Dx Clinic, Rainbow Children's Hospital
MS Ramaiah Memorial Hospital
Bengaluru, Karnataka, India

Shardha Srinivasan MBBS
Director
Department of Fetal Cardiology
Co-Director
Department of Pediatric Echocardiography
American Family Children's Hospital
UW Madison WI, USA

SJ Patil MD (Ped) DM (Medical Genetics)
Consultant, Clinical Genetics
Narayana Hrudayalaya Hospitals/Masumdar-Shaw Medical Center,
Bengaluru, Karnataka, India

Snehal Kulkarni MD DNB (Card) FACC
Chief
Department of Pediatric Cardiology
Children's Heart Centre
Kokilaben Dhirubhai Ambani Hospital
Mumbai, Maharashtra, India

Sunita Maheshwari ABP ABPC (USA)
Pediatric Cardiologist and E-Teacher
Teleradiology Solutions and Rx Dx Clinic
Bengaluru, Karnataka, India

FOREWORD

As a pediatric cardiac surgeon, I see complex and difficult congenital cardiac anomalies. I have often felt if these babies were diagnosed prenatally, their outcome could be improved in many ways. This wonderful new book brought to you, by the scholarly experienced Dr Sejal Shah coupled with her clinical acumen and mastery over the art and science of echocardiography, along with the experience of all the well-known authors—sets out to do just that—change outcomes of babies with heart defects by educating and training concerned medical personnel to diagnose them during fetal life and thereafter offer appropriate counsel and direction to families with management options. It is a book that will help all those caring for children with heart defects from fetal life and beyond. Happy reading and learning!

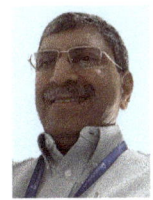

Colin John MS FRACS
Professor and Head
Department of Pediatric Cardiac Surgery
Narayana Hrudayalaya
Bengaluru, Karnataka, India

PREFACE

There has always been a great mismatch between the burden of congenital heart disease and the quantum of pediatric cardiac services available in our country. A lot of effort and finances are being put to bridge the gap. Diagnosing congenital heart diseases prior to birth may help in some ways supporting this effort by reducing morbidity and reducing the incidence of congenital heart disease. This book was conceived with an idea to enable the current and the future generation to suspect an abnormal heart in antenatal period and help in the management thereafter.

I sincerely hope that this book will fill the lacunae for the need for a standard book on fetal echocardiography in India. This book is meant for trainees and practitioners in the field of pediatric cardiology, radiology, obstetrics, fetal medicine, and sonography. A "Practical approach" has been taken while writing the Chapters. It covers the entire spectrum from "basics" to "diagnosis of abnormals". We have included lots of figures to ensure that the concept is well understood. Key points—learning messages have been provided with the Chapters along with suggested reading at the end of each chapter, in case the reader is keen on more information. A quiz which includes the basics and also interesting case scenarios, is in the CD format for the trainees. I have tried to minimize any overlap and keep consistency amongst Chapters.

It would be advisable to go systematically from the first chapter, for beginners. However, it can be used as a reference guide as and when needed in the echocardiography room. I hope this book comes handy to understand the subject and also serve as a guide to management protocols. I welcome suggestions, comments and feedback for the content of the book. I wish you all the very best and happy reading!

Sejal Shah

ACKNOWLEDGMENTS

This book is a product of combined efforts of the contributors and the publisher. I owe this book to the experience, knowledge and the hard work of all the contributors. I am thankful to all the authors for having devoted their valuable time and efforts.

I would like to acknowledge the informal assistance provided by the echocardiographers and my colleagues at Narayana Hrudayalaya during the time of getting the book ready.

I am thankful to my family, my husband and daughter for their patience, support and understanding, and allowing me to spend time getting this book ready. I would not forget at this stage, to thank our little children and their families for having taught us so much.

I am grateful to Shri Jitendar P Vij (Group Chairman) and Mr Ankit Vij (Group President) of M/s Jaypee Brothers Medical Publishers (P) Ltd, New Delhi, India, especially Mr Santosh Kumar (Commissioning Editor), and Mr Venugopal (Associate Director–South), Bengaluru Branch for entrusting me with the task of editing.

CONTENTS

1. Basics of Fetal Echocardiography 1-18
   PV Suresh, Sejal Shah
   A. Embryology of fetal heart 1-13
   B. Physiology of fetal heart 13-17
   C. Pathogenesis of congenital heart disease 17

2. General Guidelines for Performing Fetal Echocardiogram 19-32
   Prashant Bobhate, Snehal Kulkarni
   A. Equipment and fine tuning 19-20
   B. Image optimization 20-22
   C. Right-left orientation 22-24
   D. How to aim for comprehensive cardiac evaluation 24-31

3. Indications and Timing of Fetal Echocardiography 33-38
   Anita Saxena
   A. Risk factors for congenital heart disease 34-37
   B. Timing of fetal echocardiography 37-38

4. How to Perform a Normal Fetal Echocardiogram: A Practical Guide 39-50
   Balu Vaidyanathan
   A. Steps in fetal heart screening 40-47
   B. Color Doppler imaging 48
   C. Heart rate and rhythm 48
   D. Cardiac biometry 48-49
   E. Cardiac function assessment 49

5. Fetal Cardiac Defects 51-84
   BS Ramamurthy
   A. Situs 52-54
   B. Cardiac size, axis, position 55
   C. Four chamber view 55-71
   D. Outflow tracts 71-80
   E. Three vessel view 80-83

6. **Pitfalls in Fetal Echocardiography** 85-94
   Reeth Sahana, Prathima Radhakrishnan
   - A. Technical limitations 86-88
   - B. Commonly missed/incorrect diagnosis 88-90
   - C. Progression of lesions in utero 91-92
   - D. Conditions evident after birth 92

7. **Fetal Arrhythmias: Evaluation and Management** 95-119
   Shardha Srinivasan
   - A. Diagnosis and monitoring 96-102
   - B. Types of arrhythmia: Evaluation and basic management 103-116

8. **Fetal Heart Failure** 120-137
   Sejal Shah
   - A. Pathophysiology 121-122
   - B. Diagnosis 122-133
   - C. Management and prognosis 133-135

9. **Fetal Cardiac Interventions** 138-146
   Nageswara Rao Koneti, R Saileela
   - A. Procedure 140-144
   - B. Complications 144-145

10. **Genetics and Congenital Heart Disease** 147-199
    Pradeep S, SJ Patil, Meenakshi Bhat
    - A. Approach: To evaluate for extracardiac malformations and chromosome anomalies after diagnosis of fetal congenital heart disease 147-179
    - B. Genetic contribution to the origin of congenital heart disease ... 180-190
    - C. Genetic counseling after diagnosis of fetal congenital heart disease ... 191-199

11. **Management of Pregnancy after Prenatal Diagnosis of Congenital Heart Disease** 200-203
    Sunita Maheshwari
    - A. Mother and baby 200-201
    - B. Family counseling 201-203

12. **Does Prenatal Detection of Heart Disease Improve the Outcome?** ... 204-210
    Sejal Shah
    - A. Counseling 205-206
    - B. Perinatal interventions 206-210

Index *211*

CHAPTER 1

Basics of Fetal Echocardiography

PV Suresh, Sejal Shah

ABSTRACT

The aim of this Chapter is to provide a basic understanding of the fetal heart in terms of embryology, physiology, and pathogenesis, which is crucial to grasp the facts in the further Chapters. In addition; this would help practically handling the normal and abnormal hearts. Fetal heart is unique and different in many ways compared to the adult heart. This Chapter provides an insight into the fetal heart development which is a complicated process with multiple events happening simultaneously. The cardiovascular system originates from the mesoderm germ layer and the development starts from day 21–22 and continues till day 56. In addition to the structural differences, the physiological differences in fetal heart are responsible for the impact of a cardiac defect. The fetal heart is having a parallel circuit with ventricular output being combined and the placenta functions as the respiratory center. The basic etiology of congenital heart disease is proposed to be multifactorial and largely remains unknown.

Congenital heart disease is the most frequent congenital defect and accounts for significant morbidity and mortality. The responsibility to reduce this human suffering and the financial burden cannot be underestimated. This can be effectively achieved if we could reduce the incidence of congenital heart disease, which would need further advances in the understanding of the etiology and pathogenesis of heart disease.

CARDIAC EMBRYOLOGY

To understand the etiology and pathogenesis of congenital heart disease, it is imperative to have an understanding of cardiac embryology and physiology. Fetal cardiovascular system is the first major system to start functioning.

During the first 20 days of life after fertilization, the human embryo has no cardiovascular structure. During the development of cardiovascular system, angiogenic cell islets that appear to begin with transform into a complex four-chambered structure. Understanding this complex development is a difficult task. Readers should refer to animated movies available in the internet to understand the embryonic folding, heart tube looping and development of vascular system.

Embryonic Folding

During the third week of development, the germ disk has the appearance of a flat oval disk and is composed of two layers: The epiblast facing amniotic cavity and the hypoblast facing the yolk sac (Figs 1.1A and B). A primitive groove, ending caudally with the primitive pit surrounded by a node, first appears at approximately 16 days. Some epiblast cells detach from the edge of the groove and migrate inwards toward the hypoblast and replace it to form the endoderm. After the endoderm is formed, cells from the epiblast continue to migrate inwards to infiltrate the space between the epiblast and the endoderm to form the intraembryonic mesoderm. After this process is complete, the epiblast is termed the ectoderm.

The flat germ disk transforms into a tubular structure during the fourth week of development. There is differential growth causing the embryo to fold in two different dimensions:
1. Craniocaudal axis due to the more rapid growth of the neural tube forming the brain at its cephalic end.
2. Lateral folding, causing the two lateral edges of the germ disk to fold forming a tube-like structure.

Angiogenic cell clusters appearing on either side of the neural crest coalesce to form capillaries in the mesoderm of the germ disk. These capillaries then join to form a pair of blood vessels on each side of the neural crest (total of four blood vessels). The blood vessels on either side of the neural tube join at their cranial end.

As the embryo folds in its lateral dimension, it causes the lateral edges of the germ disk to approach each other until they meet, causing the embryo to acquire a tubular form. The two outer endocardial tubes will come close to each other in the median of the embryo, ventral to the primitive gut, and start fusing cranially to caudally, thus forming a single median tube—the primitive heart tube (Fig. 1.2).

The Primitive Heart

By 20th day, the formation of the single median heart tube is complete. The heart starts to beat on day 22, but the circulation

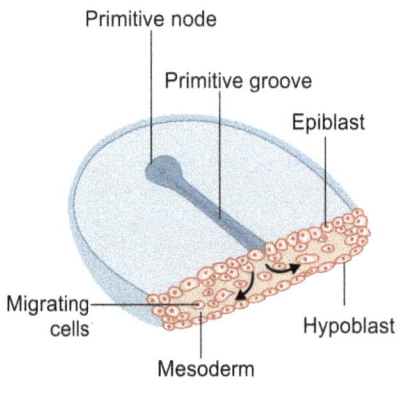

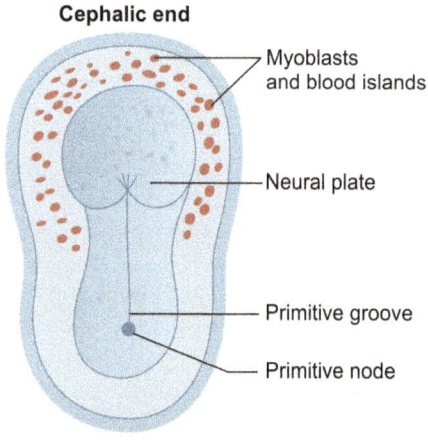

Figs 1.1A and B: (A) Transverse section of an embryo in the third week showing the epiblast and the hypoblast. Epiblast cells are shown to be migrating towards hypoblast, in order to form endoderm and mesoderm; (B) Dorsal view of a 3 week old embryo showing the neural plate, the primitive groove and the position of the myoblasts and blood islands in the splanchnic mesoderm

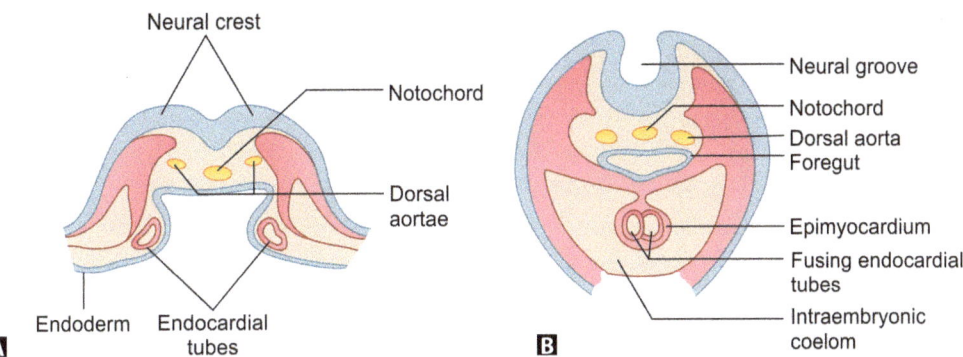

Figs 1.2A and B: Transverse sections through embryos at different stages, showing fusion of paired endocardial tubes to form a single heart tube: (A) 18 days old embryo; (B) 22 days old embryo

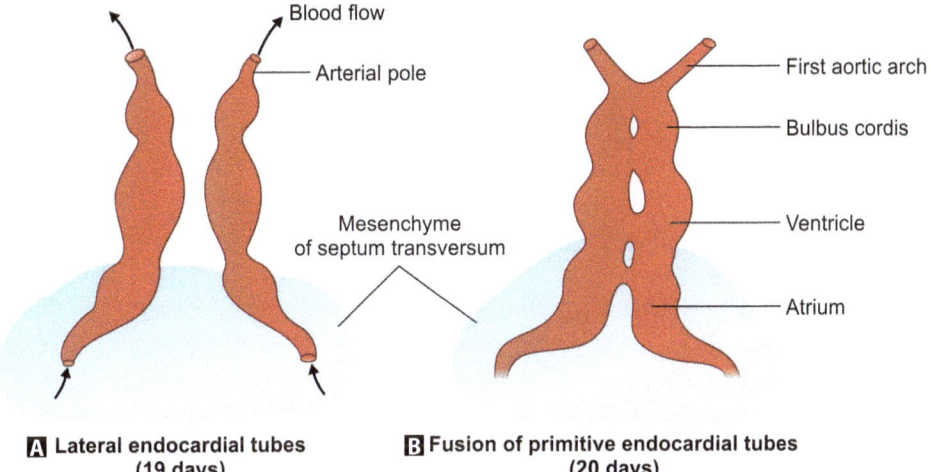

Figs 1.3A and B: (A) Dorsal view of paired endocardial tubes in a 19 day old embryo. The caudal poles are embedded in septum transversum. The direction of blood flow is caudocranial; (B) Fusion of the endocardial tubes, in a 20 day old embryo, beginning caudally. The primitive atrium, primitive ventricle and bulbus cordis are beginning to be identified

does not start until days 27–29. The single tubular heart develops many constrictions outlining future structures (Figs 1.3A and B). The cranial most area is the bulbus cordis, which extends cranially into the truncus arteriosus. This, in turn, is connected to the aortic sac and through the aortic arches to the dorsal aorta. The primitive ventricle is caudal to the bulbus cordis and the primitive atrium is the caudal-most structure of the tubular heart (Fig. 1.4A). The atrium connects to the sinus venosus, which receives the vitelline veins (from the yolk sac), common cardinal (from the embryo) and umbilical (from primitive placenta) veins. The primitive atrium and sinus venosus lay outside the caudal end of the pericardial sac, and the truncus arteriosus is outside the cranial end of the pericardial sac (Fig. 1.4B).

Looping of the primitive heart occurs on approximately day 23 of development. As the heart tube loops, the cephalic end of the heart tube bends ventrally, caudally, and slightly to the right (Figs 1.5A and B). The bulboventricular sulcus becomes visible from the outside, and from the inside a primitive interventricular foramen forms. The internal fold formed by the bulboventricular sulcus

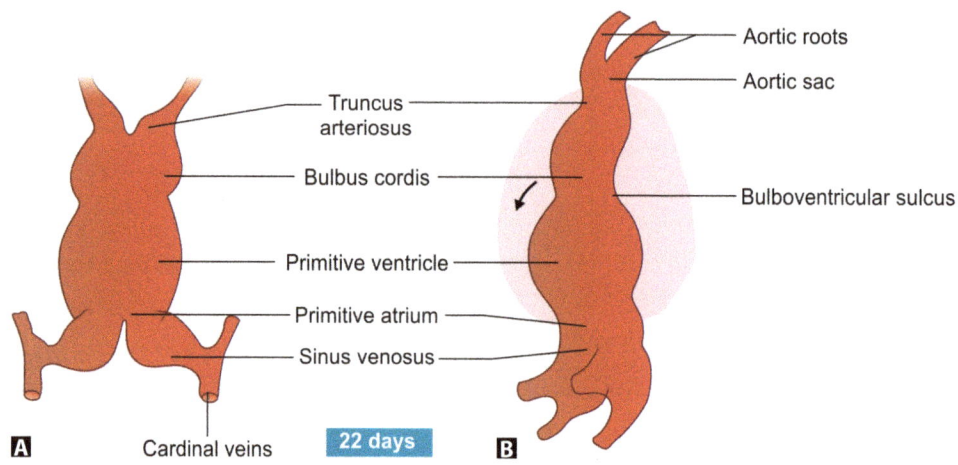

Figs 1.4A and B: The primitive heart of the 22 day old embryo in (A) dorsal; and (B) lateral views, after fusion of endocardial tubes. Precursors of cardiac structures and vessels are identified

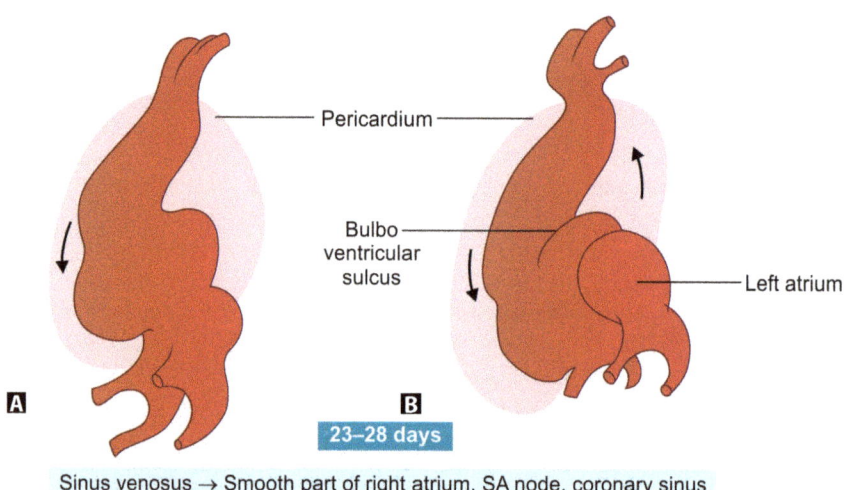

Sinus venosus → Smooth part of right atrium, SA node, coronary sinus
Primitive atrium → Rough part of right and left atria and auricles
Primitive ventricle → Left ventricle
Proximal bulbus cordis → Right ventricle
Distal bulbus cordis → Outflow tract of both ventricles
Truncus arteriosus → Roots of great vessels

Figs 1.5A and B: Cardiac looping. (A) 22 days; (B) 23 days. During cardiac looping, the straight and short cardiac tube lengthens and bends ventrally, caudally and to the right. This brings the atrial region dorsal to the heart loop. The bulboventricular foramen is visible

is known as the bulboventricular fold. The bulboventricular segment forms the right arm of the U-shaped heart tube and the primitive ventricle forms the left arm (Fig. 1.6). The looping of the bulboventricular segment of the heart will cause the atrium and sinus venosus to become dorsal to the heart loop. At this stage, the paired sinus venosus extends laterally and gives rise to the sinus horns.

As the cardiac looping progresses, the paired atria form a common chamber and move into the pericardial sac. The atrium now occupies a more dorsal and cranial position and the common atrioventricular junction becomes the atrioventricular canal, connecting the left side of the common atrium to the primitive ventricle. At this stage, the heart has a smooth lining except for the area just proximal and just distal to the bulboventricular foramen, where trabeculations form. The primitive ventricle will eventually develop into the left ventricle and the proximal portion of the bulbus cordis will form the right ventricle. The distal part of the bulbus cordis, an elongated structure, will form the outflow tract of both ventricles, and the truncus arteriosus will form the roots of both great vessels. The bulbus cordis gradually acquires a more medial position due to the growth of the right atrium, forcing the bulbus to be in the sulcus in between the two atria.

Systemic Venous System

On day 21, there is a common atrium as a result of fusion of the two endocardial tubes. The common atrium communicates with two sinus horns, a left and a right horn, representing the unfused ends of the endocardial tubes. These two horns will form the sinus venosus.

The sinus venosus is located dorsal to the atria. The following veins drain into the sinus venosus on each side: The common cardinal vein, which drains from the anterior cardinal vein (draining the cranial part of the embryo); the posterior cardinal vein (draining the caudal part of the embryo); the umbilical vein (connecting the heart to the primitive placenta); and the vitelline vein (draining the yolk sac, gastrointestinal system and the portal circulation).

On week 4, the sinus venosus communicates with the common atrium. During week 7, the sinoatrial communication becomes more right sided, connecting it to the right atrium. At 8 weeks, the distal end of the left cardinal vein degenerates, and the more proximal portion of it now connects through the anastomosing vein (left brachiocephalic vein) to the right anterior cardinal vein (right brachiocephalic vein), thus forming the superior vena cava. The left posterior

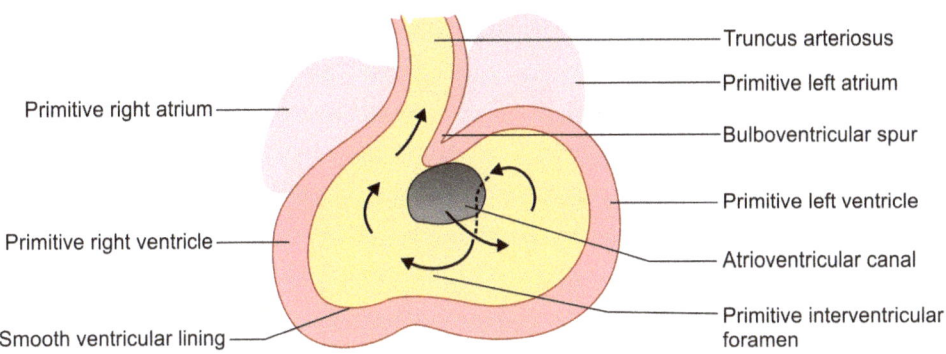

Fig. 1.6: Frontal section through the heart of a 30-day embryo showing the primitive atria and ventricles, the atrioventricular canal, and the primitive interventricular foramen. The bulboventricular spur is noted

cardinal vein also degenerates, and the left sinus horn receiving venous blood from the heart becomes the coronary sinus. The right vitelline vein becomes the inferior vena cava, and the right posterior cardinal vein becomes the azygos vein (Figs 1.7A and B). All this is completed in week 8 of development. The left umbilical vein degenerates and the right umbilical vein connects to the vitelline system through the ductus venosus (which is derived from the vitelline veins)(Fig. 1.7C).

Pulmonary Circulation

Airways, lung parenchyma and distal pulmonary arteries.

On day 21 of development, a groove forms in the floor of the foregut just dorsal to the heart. This is termed the pharyngeal groove, which develops to form the pharynx. On day 23, the laryngotracheal groove, a median structure in the pharyngeal region, develops. The edges of the laryngotracheal tube fuse to form the

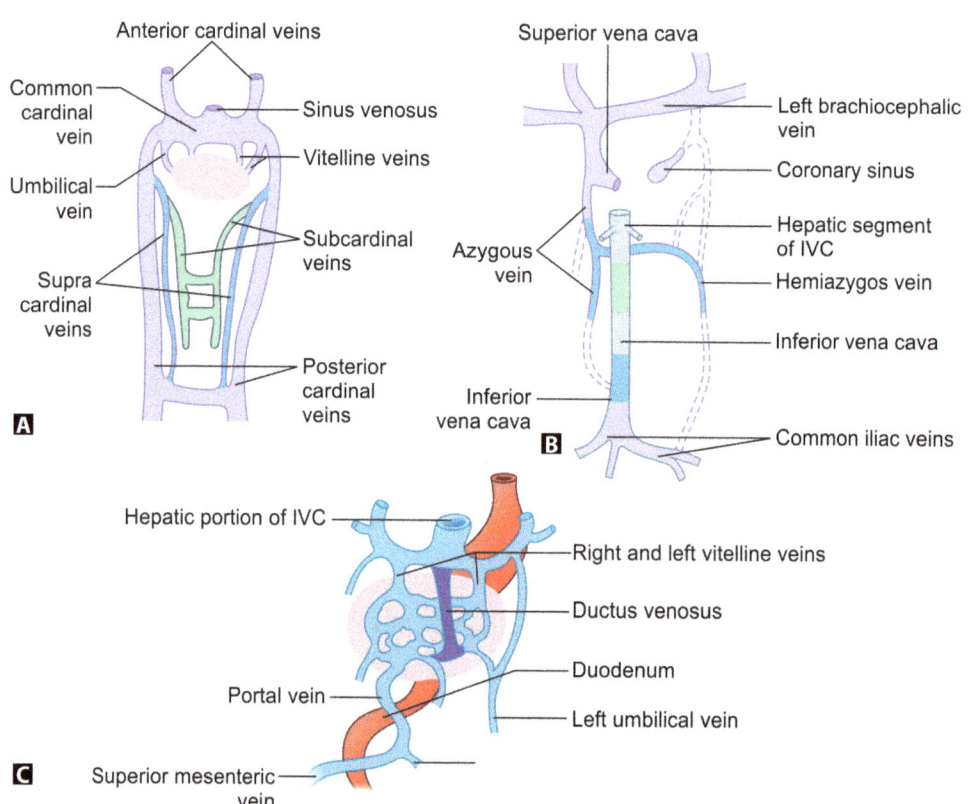

Figs 1.7A to C: Development of the systemic venous system. (A) The embryonic venous system in the seventh week shows the anastomosis between the subcardinal, supracardinal and anterior cardinal veins; (B) The venous system at birth. The left cardinal and left posterior cardinal veins have degenerated in the eighth week, thus giving rise to a predominantly right sided venous system; (C) Development of vitelline and umbilical veins in the second month. The portal vein and the left umbilical vein are seen joining the hepatic sinusoidal system. The vitelline veins are seen joining the hepatic portion of the IVC, along with ductus venosus

larynx and trachea cranially and the right and left main bronchi and right and left lung buds distally. The growth and branching of the lung buds, together with the surrounding mesoderm, form the distal airways, lung parenchyma, and pulmonary blood vessels. By week 16 of gestation, a full complement of preacinar airways and blood vessels have formed. The pulmonary arteries in utero are muscular, similar to that of the aorta. The thick, muscular walls of pulmonary arteries extend much further into distal arteries than what is seen in adults. Thinning of distal pulmonary arteries occurs postnatally as the pulmonary vascular resistance decreases after the onset of breathing and improved oxygenation.

Proximal Pulmonary Arteries

The proximal main pulmonary artery develops from the truncus arteriosus. The left arch of the sixth pair of aortic arch contributes to the formation of the distal main pulmonary artery and the proximal left pulmonary artery. The right sixth arch contributes to the formation of the proximal right pulmonary artery. The distal right pulmonary artery and the left pulmonary arteries form from the postbranchial arteries, which develop from the lung buds and surrounding mesoderm. The ductus arteriosus develops from the distal left sixth aortic arch artery.

Pulmonary Venous System

Initially, a single pulmonary vein opens into the left atrium which then bifurcates twice to give four pulmonary veins that grow toward the developing lungs. The lung buds develop from the foregut. A plexus of veins is formed in the mesoderm enveloping the bronchial buds; these veins will meet with the developing pulmonary veins out of the left atrium to establish a connection during week 5 of gestation. As the left atrium develops, it progressively incorporates the common pulmonary vein into the left atrial wall until all four pulmonary veins enter the posterior wall of the left atrium separately. The incorporated pulmonary veins form the smooth posterior wall of the left atrium, whereas the trabeculated portion of the left atrium comes to occupy a more ventral aspect.

Atrioventricular Canal

The atrioventricular valves form during the fifth to eighth week of development. Initially, endocardial cushion tissue forms bulges at the atrioventricular junction (Figs 1.8 A to E). These bulges have the appearance of valves, and although such tissue may play an important role in the eventual formation of the atrioventricular valves, endocardial cushion tissues are not the precursors of the mitral and tricuspid valves.

The formation of the atrioventricular valve starts when the atria and inlet portion of the ventricle enlarge; the atrioventricular junction (or canal) lags behind. Such a process causes the sulcus tissue to invaginate into the ventricular cavity, forming a hanging flap. The endocardial cushion tissue is located at the tip of this flap, which is formed from three layers—the outer layer from atrial tissue, the inner layer from ventricular tissue and the middle layer from invaginated sulcus tissue. The inlet portion of the ventricles then becomes undermined, forming the tethering cords holding the newly formed valve leaflets. The inner sulcus tissue will eventually come in contact with the cushion tissue at the tip of valve leaflets, thus interrupting the muscular continuity between the atria and ventricles.

The Atria and Atrial Septum

The atria of the mature heart have more than one origin. The trabeculated portions (appendages) of the right and left atria are from the primitive atria. The posterior aspect of the left atrium is formed by the incorporation of the pulmonary veins, whereas the posterior

Fetal Echocardiography

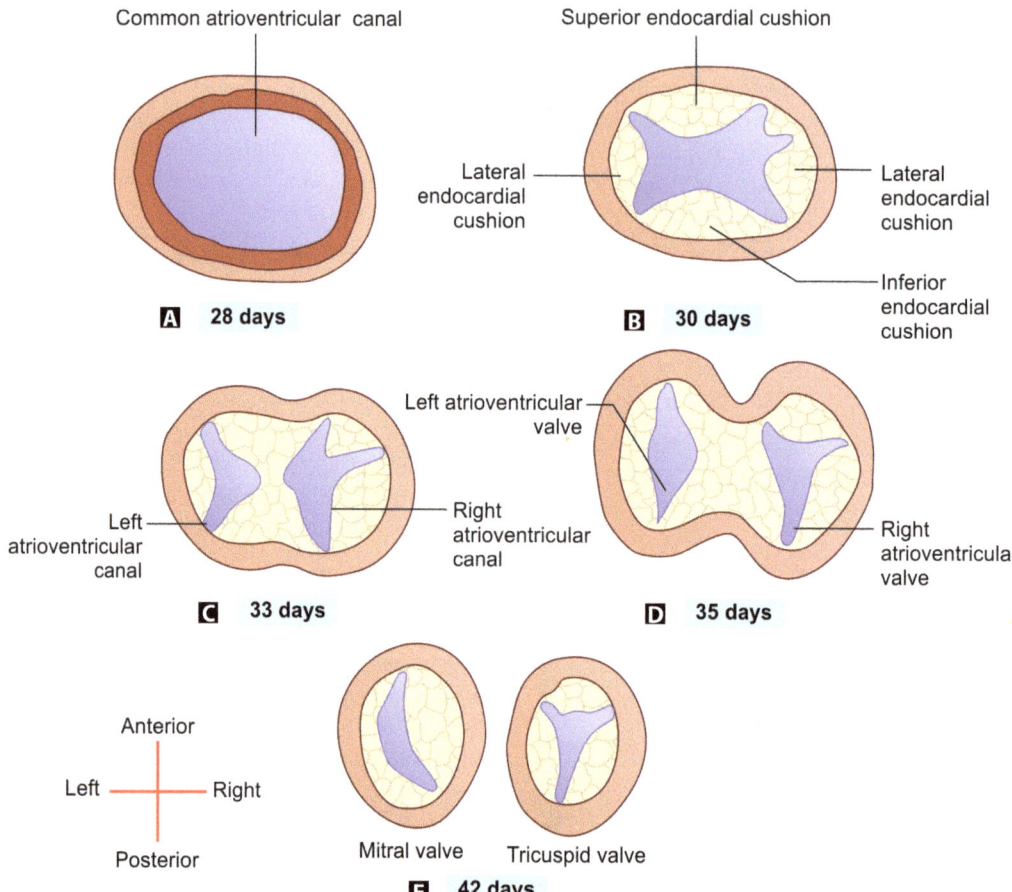

Figs 1.8A to E: (A) 28 days; (B) 30 days; (C) 33 days; (D) 35 days; and (E) 42 days. Formation of the septum in the atrioventricular canal and subsequent development of atrioventricular valves: The initial circular opening widens transversely, showing growth and fusion of the superior and inferior endocardial cushions in the atrioventricular canal. The right and left atrioventricular canals are thus formed. The atrioventricular valves begin to form between the fifth and eighth weeks of development. The left atrioventricular valve has anterior and posterior leaflets and is termed the bicuspid or mitral valve. The right atrioventricular valve has a third, small septal cusp and thus is called the tricuspid valve

smooth portion of the right atrium is derived from the sinus venosus.

The two sinus horns are initially paired structures; later, they fuse to give a transverse sinus venosus. The entrance of the sinus venosus shifts rightward to eventually enter into the right atrium exclusively. The veins draining into the left sinus venosus (left common cardinal, umbilical and vitelline veins) eventually degenerate. The left sinus venosus will become smaller because it will drain only the venous circulation of the heart, becoming the coronary sinus.

The sinus venosus orifice of the right atrium is slit-like and to the right of the undeveloped septum primum. The sinus venosus now connecting to the right atrium will assume a more vertical position. The sinoatrial junction will become guarded by two valve-like structures, resulting from the invagination of the atrial wall at the right and left sinoatrial junction. This orifice enlarges, with the superior and inferior venae cavae and the coronary sinus opening separately and directly into the right atrium. The right and left sinoatrial valves join at the top, forming the septum spurium. This septum and the two sinoatrial valve-like structures obliterate and are not appreciated in the mature heart.

Atrial septation starts when the common atrium becomes indented externally by the bulbus cordis and truncus arteriosus. This indentation will correspond internally with a thin sickle-shaped membrane developing in the common atrium on day 35. This membrane divides the atrium into right and left chambers. It grows from the posterosuperior wall and extends toward the endocardial cushion of the atrioventricular canal. This is the septum primum (Figs 1.9A and D). The septum primum initially has a concave-shaped edge growing toward the atrioventricular canal. This orifice connecting the two atria is called the ostium primum. As the superior and inferior endocardial cushions fuse, thus dividing the atrioventricular canal into a right and left orifice, the concave lower edge of the septum primum fuses with it, obliterating the ostium primum. However, just before this happens fenestrations appear in the posterosuperior part of the septum forming the ostium secundum, thus maintaining a communication between the two atria. The ostium secundum and superior vena cava later acquire a more anterosuperior position, although they maintain their relationship with each other; this is achieved through the growth of the atria.

These fenestrations then coalesce and form a larger fenestration. Meanwhile, another sickle-shaped membrane develops on the anterosuperior wall of the right atrium, just right of the septum primum and left of the sinus venosus valve. It grows and covers the ostium secundum, which continues to allow blood passage since the two membranes do not fuse. The septum secundum grows toward the endocardial cushion, leaving only an area at the posterosuperior part of the interatrial septum where the septum primum continues to exist as the foramen ovale membrane (Figs 1.9B, C and E). The septum primum disappears from the posterosuperior portion of interatrial septation and the edge of the septum secundum forms the rim of the fossa ovalis on approximately day 42 of development.

Ventricular Septation

Ventricular septation is a complex process involving different septal structures from various origins and positioned at various planes. These structures eventually meet to complete the separation of the right and left ventricles.

Muscular Interventricular Septum

During the fifth week, on approximately day 30, a muscular fold extending from the anterior wall of the ventricles to the floor appears at the middle of the ventricle near the apex and grows toward the atrioventricular valves with a concave ridge (Figs 1.10A to C). Most of the initial growth is achieved by growth of the two ventricles on either side of the ventricular septum. In addition, trabeculations from the inlet region coalesce to form a septum, which grows into the ventricular cavity at a slightly different plane than that of the primary septum; this is the inlet interventricular septum, which is in the same plane of that of the atrial septum. The point of contact between these two septa will cause the edge of the primary septum to protrude slightly into the right ventricular cavity, forming the trabecular septomarginalis. The fusion of these two septa forms the bulk of the muscular interventricular septum. This septum will then come into contact with the outflow septum.

The interventricular foramen, which is bordered by the concave upper ridge of the

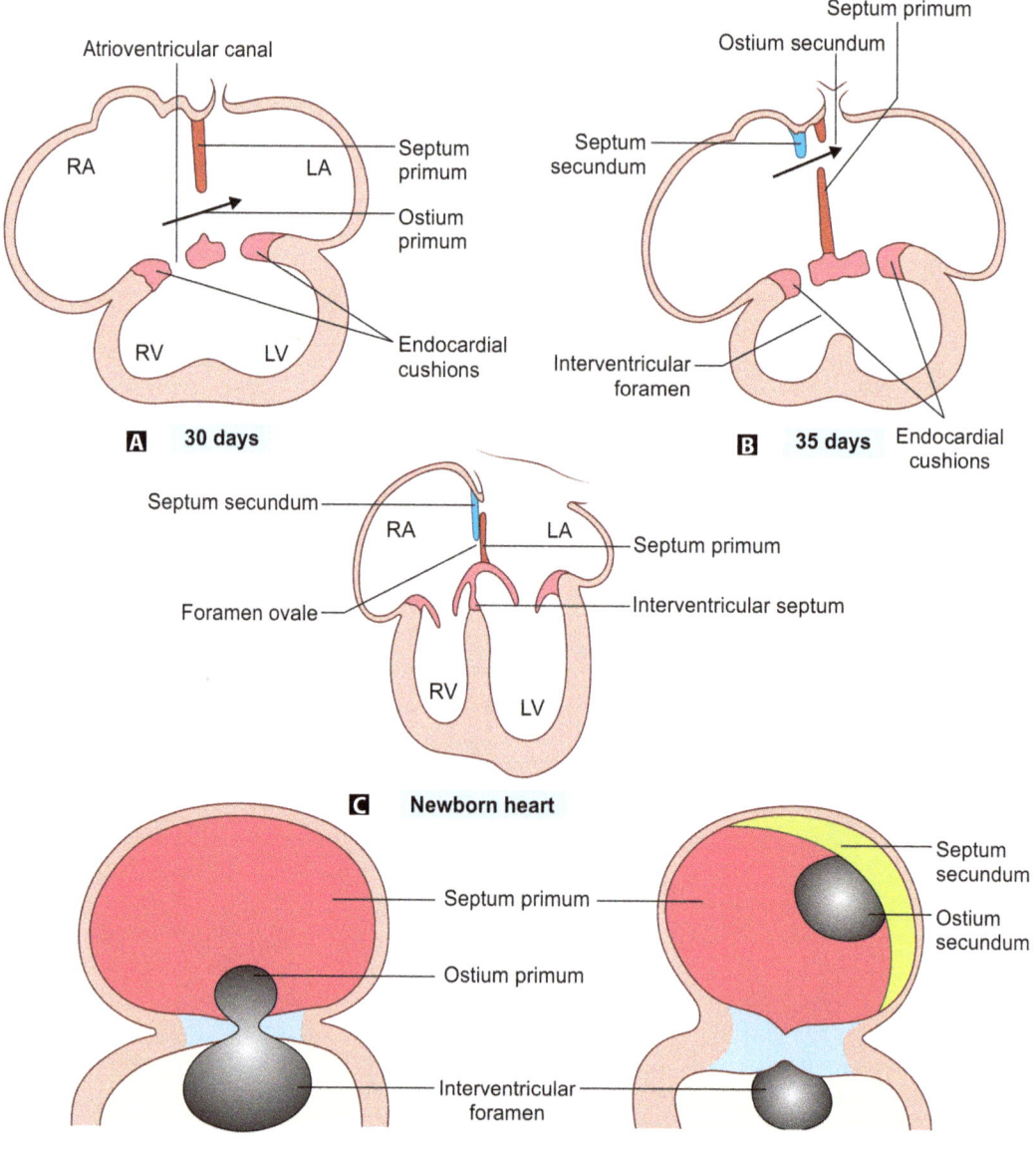

Figs 1.9A to E: Normal atrial septum formation. (A) Fetal heart at 30 days, frontal view, showing formation of septum primum; (B) Fetal heart at 35 days, frontal view, showing formation of septum secundum, ostium secundum identified; (C) Newborn heart showing completion of atrial septation, formation ovale identified; (D) Fetal heart at 30 days, viewed from right atrium, corresponding to Figure 1.9A. Note the crescentic shape of septum primum; (E) Fetal heart at 35 days, viewed from right atrium, corresponding to Figure 1.9B: septum secundum appears

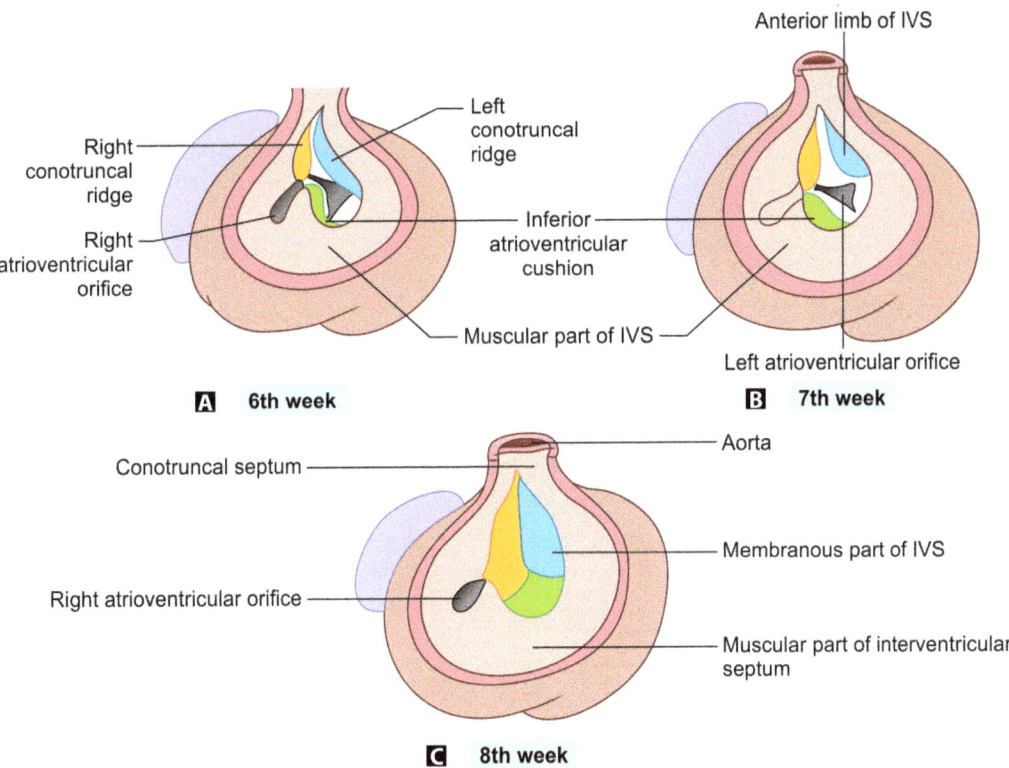

Figs 1.10A to C: Development of the conotruncal ridges and closure of the interventricular foramen. The right and left conotruncal ridges, combined with the inferior atrioventricular cushion, proliferate and close the interventricular foramen and form the membranous portion of the interventricular septum. (A) 6 weeks; (B) 7 weeks; (C) 8 weeks

muscular interventricular septum, the fused atrioventricular canal endocardial tissue, and the outflow tract septation ridges, never actually closes. Instead, communication between the left ventricle and the right ventricle is closed at the end of week 7 by growth of three structures—the right and left bulbar ridges and the posterior endocardial cushion tissue—that baffle the left ventricular output through a newly formed left ventricular outflow tract (LVOT). The LVOT is posterior to a right ventricular outflow tract, connecting the right ventricle to the pulmonary trunk.

Outflow Tract Septum

The cardiac outflow tract includes the ventricular outflow tract and the aorto-pulmonary septum. There has been much debate regarding this process. This section provides a summary of various theories.

In 1942, Kramer suggested that there are three embryological areas: The conus, the truncus and the pulmonary arterial segments. Each segment develops two opposing ridges of endocardial tissue; the opposing pairs of ridges and those from various segments meet to form a septum separating two outflow tracts and aortopulmonary trunks (Fig. 1.11). The aortopulmonary septum is formed by ridges separating the fourth (future aortic arch) and the sixth (future pulmonary arteries) aortic arches. The truncus ridges are formed in the area where the semilunar valves are destined to be formed, thus forming the septum between the ascending aorta and the main pulmonary artery. The conus ridges form just below the semilunar valves and form the septation between the right and left ventricular outflow tracts.

In 1989, Bartlings et al. stated that the septation process of the ventricular outflow tracts, pulmonary and aortic valves, and the great vessels is mostly caused by a single septation complex, which they termed aortopulmonary septum. The ventricular outflow septation is formed by condensed mesenchyme, embedded in the endocardial cushion tissue just proximal to the level of the aortopulmonary valves. The condensed mesenchyme will come in close contact with the outflow tract myocardium, from the area just above the bulboventricular fold, and participate in the septation of the outflow tract by providing an analog to muscle tissue.

Conduction System

Primary myocardium, found in the early heart tube, gives rise to the contracting myocardium (of the atria and ventricles) and the conducting myocardium (nodal and ventricular conducting tissue). Conducting myocardial tissue is frequently referred to as being highly specialized tissue, implying that it has a homogenous function. In reality,

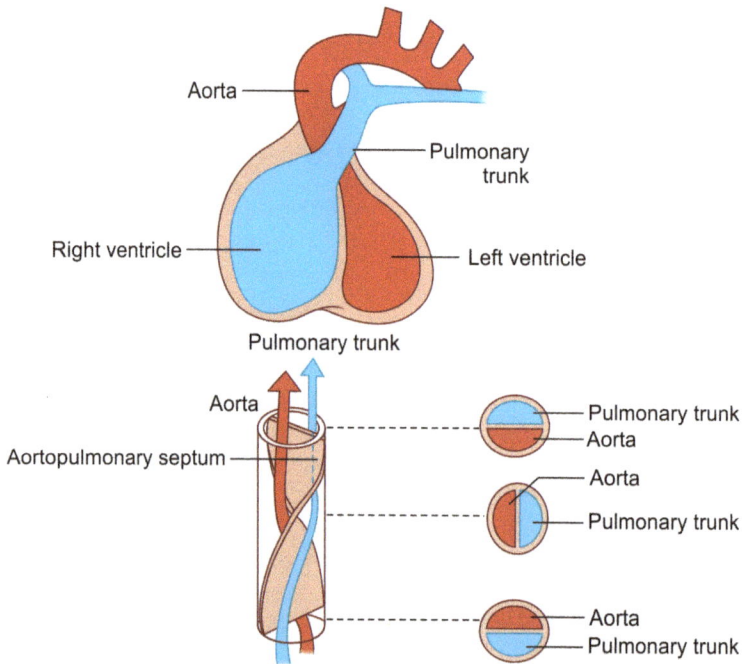

Fig. 1.11: Formation of aortopulmonary septum. The spiral aortopulmonary septum separates the truncal outflow tract into aortic and pulmonary channels. It defines the relationship of the great vessels to each other, so that, normally the aorta lies anterior and to the right of pulmonary artery

some portions, such as nodal tissue, are slow conducting and resemble less developed primary myocardium, whereas other portions, such as ventricular conduction tissue, are fast conducting.

The embryological origin and formation of the sinus and atrioventricular nodal tissue is not clear. The ventricular conduction system formation is better known. The latter starts with the formation of an encircling ring of conducting myocardial tissue around the bulboventricular foramen. The dorsal portion of the ring will become the bundle of His. The portion of the ring covering the septum will become the left and right bundle branches.

Aortic Arches

The first pair of aortic arches is formed by the curving of the ventral aorta to meet the dorsal aorta; these will eventually contribute to the external carotid arteries. The second pair of aortic arch arteries appears in week 4. These regress rapidly and only a portion remains, which forms the stapedial and hyoid arteries. The third pair of the aortic arch arteries appears at approximately the end of the fourth week; these will give rise to the common carotid arteries and the proximal portion of the internal carotid arteries. The distal portion of the internal carotid arteries is formed by the cranial portions of the dorsal aorta. The fourth aortic arch arteries develop soon after the third arch arteries. Their development differs on the left from that on the right. On the left side, they persist, connecting the ventral aorta to the dorsal aorta and forming the aortic arch. On the right, they form the proximal portion of the right subclavian artery. The fifth pair of aortic arch arteries is rudimentary and does not develop into any known vessels; this pair of aortic arch arteries is not seen in many embryo specimens. The sixth aortic arch, on the right side proximally forms the proximal part of the right pulmonary artery and distally it regresses completely. The sixth arch, on the left side proximally persists as the proximal part of the left pulmonary artery, whereas the distal portion of the left aortic arch artery develops into the ductus arteriosus (Figs 1.12A to C).

PHYSIOLOGY OF FETAL HEART

Fetal heart is different that the adult mature heart in many ways. These differences are related to the structure as well as the physiology. Understanding the fetal circulation enables us to understand the cardiac defects that would influence the circulation in fetal life and neonatal life.

While we know that the postnatal heart circulation is in series, i.e. the right ventricle provides full cardiac output to the lungs and the left ventricle provides the same full cardiac output to the body, prenatally the circulation is parallel, i.e. the organs receive blood from both the ventricles and there is a concept of "combined ventricular output". Primarily, this happens as lungs do not do the function of gas exchange. Instead, the placenta functions not only as the respiratory center, but also does the filtration for plasma nutrients and wastes. The low resistance in the placenta promotes blood flow to the placenta. Hence, the fetal circulation is often understood as fetoplacental circulation which includes the umbilical cord and the blood vessels within the placenta carrying fetal blood. The fetal circulation has number of features to divert most of the blood away from lungs. There are three sites of intercommunication: the ductus venosus, the foramen ovale and the ductus arteriosus. Hence, fetal circulation is a shunt dependent circulation. An additional important fact is that, the pressure in the right system is higher than that in the left system.

Fetal Echocardiography

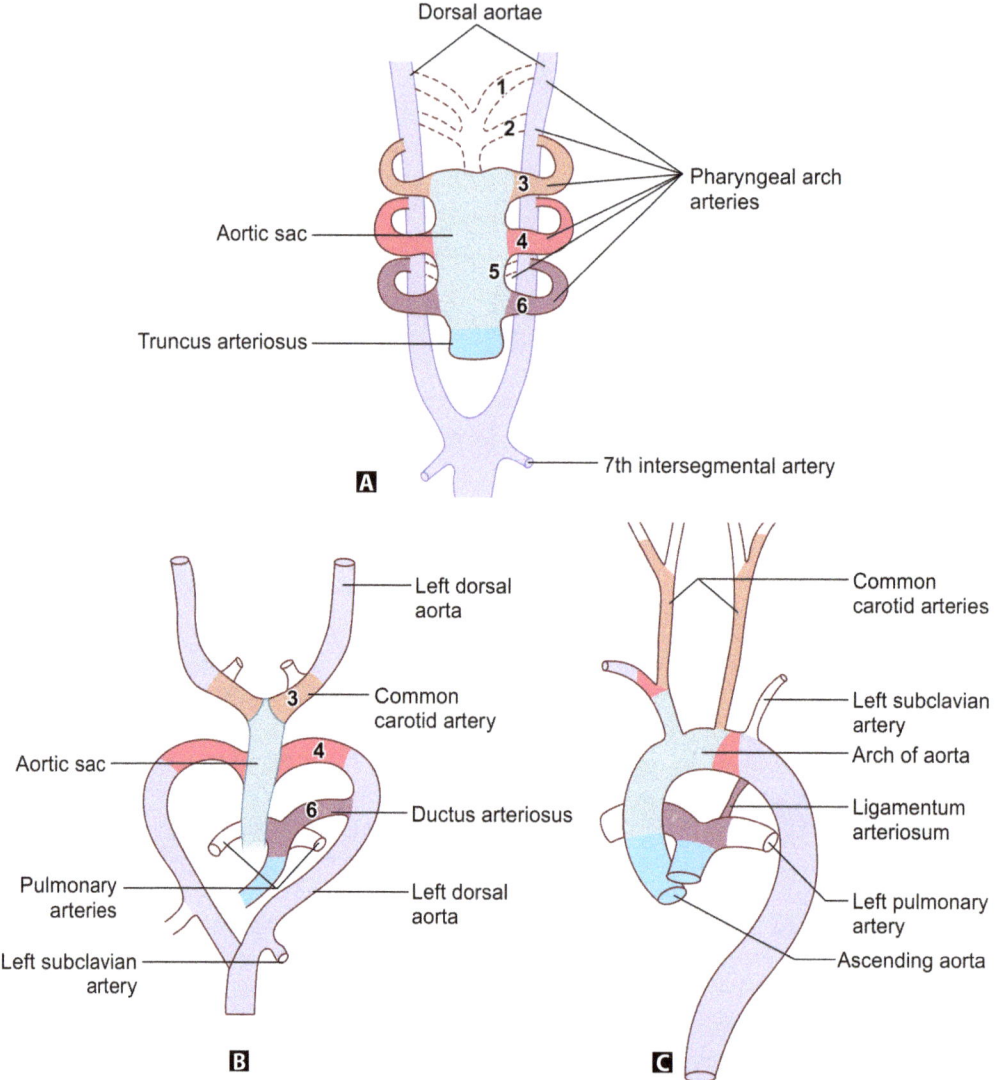

Figs 1.12A to C: (A) Primitive aortic arches and dorsal aortae; regression of the first, second and fifth arches represented; (B) Aortic arches and dorsal aortae giving rise to the carotid arteries, ductus arteriosus and aortic arch and descending aorta; (C) The great arteries in the adult

The oxygenated blood from the placenta is carried through the umbilical vein (Fig. 1.13). Out of two umbilical veins, the right umbilical vein regresses completely early in fetal life. Twenty to thirty percent of the blood flows through the ductus venosus into the IVC and is diverted away from entering the liver (Fig. 1.14). The remainder enters the liver sinusoids and mixes with the portal circulation. The ductus venosus sphincter near the umbilical vein regulates the umbilical blood flow through the liver sinusoids. The more oxygenated blood from the ductus venosus usually streams separately and does not get

Basics of Fetal Echocardiography

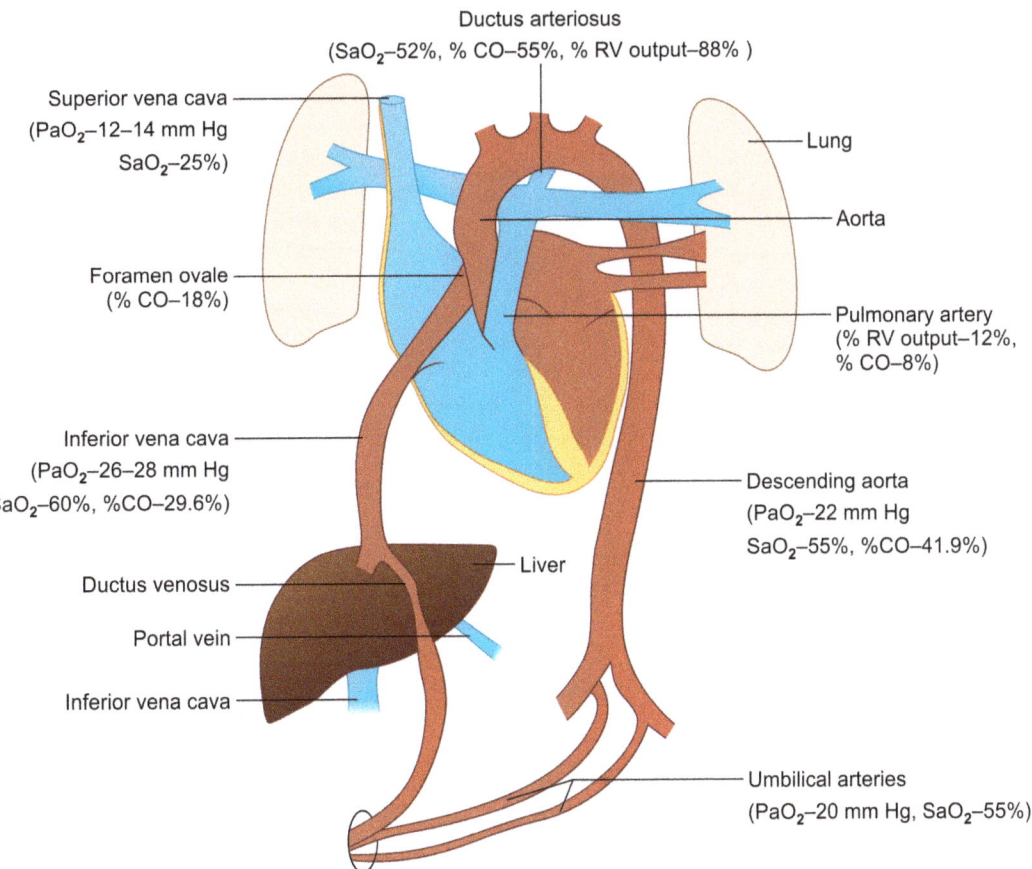

Fig. 1.13: Fetal circulation. Mixing of oxygenated blood with deoxygenated blood occurs in the liver, in the inferior vena cava, in the right atrium, in the left atrium and at the entrance of the ductus arteriosus into the descending aorta.
The partial pressure of oxygen (PaO_2), oxygen saturation (SaO_2) and percentage cardiac output (% CO) received is indicated at various sites. About 60–65% of cardiac output is ejected by right ventricle and 35–40% by the left ventricle, corresponding to a ratio of right to left cardiac output of 1.5 to 1.85

mixed with the deoxygenated blood returning from the lower parts of the body. Most of the blood that enters the IVC through ductus venosus is shunted through the foramen ovale to the left atrium. Small amount is prevented to enter into the left atrium by the lower edge of septum secundum. This saturated blood then mixes in the right atrium with the deoxygenated blood coming from the superior vena cava and the slow moving blood coming from the IVC through the hepatic veins, and then enters the right ventricle into the main pulmonary artery. Due to high pulmonary vascular resistance, the blood from the main pulmonary artery is predominantly shunted through the ductus arteriosus (57% of the combined output) into the descending aorta. Only 8% of the combined cardiac output goes to the lungs. The oxygenated blood which has been shunted from the right atrium to the left atrium then mixes with the small amount of desaturated blood coming from the

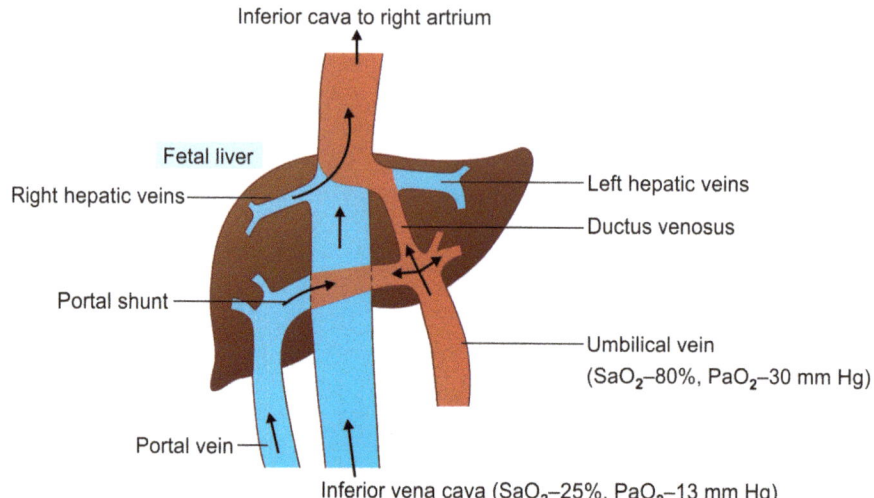

Fig. 1.14: Development of the hepatic venous system. The liver receives blood from both portal vein and umbilical vein. The ductus venosus, carrying oxygenated blood from the umbilical vein, drains into the IVC, thus bypassing the hepatic sinusoids. This channel gets obliterated after birth

pulmonary veins, which then enters the left ventricle into the ascending aorta. Most of this blood (21% of the total output) is supplied to the head and the upper arms. The remaining (10% of the total output) then passes into the descending aorta mixing with the blood coming from ductus arteriosus. From here on, the blood is taken by two umbilical arteries to the placenta. The placenta receives 50% of the combined ventricular output.

As we have seen, the circulation in fetus is parallel and the stroke volume of both the ventricles is not the same. Though both the ventricles have near equal pressures, the right ventricle handles approximately 55% of the combined ventricular output. The combined ventricular output varies from 210 mL/min at 20 weeks of gestation to 1900 mL/min at 38 weeks of gestation.

Fetal hemoglobin enables greater adaptability to the lower oxygen saturations/partial pressure of oxygen available in the fetus than that in neonates. The fetal cardiovascular system is designed in such a way that highly saturated blood is delivered to the myocardium and the brain. The highest saturation is found in the umbilical vein (85%) and the lowest in the IVC (abdominal) and SVC. However, due to mixing at the foramen ovale level, the saturations in the blood leaving both the ventricles are only 10%. Saturation in the returning blood in the umbilical artery is 58%.

Transition at Birth

Multiple synchronized events happen at birth. The transition of fetal circulation to neonatal circulation is due to two major events. One is the cessation of placental blood flow and the second is the beginning of the pulmonary respiration. This leads to multiple changes in the cardiovascular system. The inflated lungs release a vasoactive peptide—bradykinin which causes muscular contraction of the ductus arteriosus. Ductus arteriosus closes almost completely after birth. Functional ductal closure happens by 96 hours of life, which is followed by anatomical closure by 2-3 weeks. Once closed, it forms ligamentum arteriosum. Closure of ductus arteriosus results in increased pressure in the left atrium.

At the same time the right atrial pressure reduces due to cessation of placental blood flow. This results in functional closure of foramen ovale within minutes to hours of birth. Anatomical closure of foramen ovale may take up to 1 year of age by tissue proliferation. Umbilical arteries though close immediately after birth; complete anatomical closure may take 2–3 months wherein the distal portions form the medial umbilical ligaments. Proximal part of the umbilical arteries remains open and become superior vesical arteries. Umbilical vein and ductus venosus close after the closure of umbilical arteries. Ductus venosus is expected to close by 3–10 days after birth. The umbilical vein forms ligamentum teres and obliterated ductus venosus forms ligamentum venosum. The pulmonary vascular resistance falls to less than 20% of the fetal value once the lungs are expanded. Fetal shunts are unnecessary after birth; on the contrary their persistence may cause hemodynamic compromise.

PATHOGENESIS OF CONGENITAL HEART DISEASE

The known causes of congenital heart disease which include chromosomal abnormalities, single gene defect and teratogens account only for about 15% of cases. The basic etiology of majority of congenital heart diseases remains unknown. Congenital heart disease is a multifactorial disease where genetic and environmental factors play an important role. Different pathogenic mechanisms are expected in different congenital heart diseases. The insult has to happen during the 14 to 60 days of gestation to produce congenital heart disease.

Following are the proposed pathogenetic mechanisms to cause congenital heart disease.

- *Abnormal migration of ectomesenchymal tissue:* The tissue that forms the outflow tracts in the heart originates in the neural crest and branchial cell mesenchyme. Interference in the migration of these cells cause conotruncal malformations, e.g. Double outlet right ventricle, tetralogy of Fallot, ventricular septal defect, aorto-pulmonary window.
- *Abnormal intracardiac blood flow:* The volume of the blood and force of cardiac contraction are considered essential in growth and development of heart structures. Reduction in the amount of flow can cause left and right sided heart defects, e.g. Hypoplastic left and right heart.
- *Abnormal cellular death:* Selective resorption of certain areas of the ventricular myocardium is a mechanism involved in formation of atrioventricular valves. Cell death can impede this process and cause congenital heart diseases like muscular ventricular septal defect, Ebstein's anomaly.
- *Abnormalities of the extracellular matrix:* The endocardial cushions fuse to form the mitral and tricuspid orifices at atrioventricular level, and aortic and pulmonary orifices at semilunar level. This happens as endocardial cells are transformed into mesenchymal cells that migrate and cause them to fuse to each other. Failure of this process can cause endocardial cushion defects.
- *Abnormal targeted growth:* This involves impedance in the process by which pulmonary veins get absorbed into the left atrium.
- *Abnormalities of situs and looping:* The heart tube which should normally bend to the right, bends to the left can cause L looped ventricles. Situs abnormalities are related to absence of controlled gene mapped to chromosome 12.

ACKNOWLEDGMENT

We thank Dr Monica Madvariya for the contribution of the pictures in this Chapter.

KEY MESSAGES

1. Fetal heart develops from the splanchnic mesoderm.
2. Fetal cardiovascular system starts functioning by 4th week of gestation.
3. Fetal circulation is "Shunt dependent".
4. Placenta is the fetal lung.
5. The cardiac output in fetus is defined as "combined ventricular output".
6. The transition from fetal to neonatal life is a dynamic process with multiple events happening in a coordinated fashion.
7. Genetic, environmental and unknown causes through different proposed pathogenic mechanisms cause congenital heart disease.

SUGGESTED READING

1. Angelini P. Embryology and congenital heart disease. Tex Heart Inst J. 1995;22:1-12.
2. Clark EB. Pathogenetic mechanisms of congenital cardiovascular malformations revisited. Semin Perinatol. 1996;20:465-72.
3. De Smedt MC, Visser GH, Meijboom EJ. Fetal cardiac output estimated by Doppler echocardiography during mid-and late gestation. Am J Cardiol. 1987;60:338-42.
4. Drose JA. Embryology and physiology of fetal heart. In: Drose JA, (Ed). Fetal echocardiography. Philadelphia: Saunders. 2010.p.1-12.
5. Layton WM JR. The biology of asymmetry and the development of the cardiac loop. In: Ferrans VJ, Rosenquist GC, Weinstein C (Eds). Cardiac morphogenesis. New York Elsevier, 1985;134-40.
6. Murphy PJ. The fetal circulation. Contin Educ in Anaesth Crit Care Pain. 2005;5:107-12.
7. Nora JJ, Nora AH. The environmental contribution to congenital heart disease. In: Nora JJ, Takao A (Eds). Congenital heart disease: causes and processes, Mount Kisko. New York: Future Publishing Co. 1984;15-27.
8. Pexieder T. Cell death in morphogenesis and teratogenesis of the heart. Adv Anat Embyol Cell Biol. 1975;51:1-100.
9. Rudolph AM. Fetal and neonatal pulmonary circulation. Ann Rev Physiol. 1979;41:83-95.
10. Rudolph AM. The changes in the circulation at birth. Their importance in congenital heart disease. Circulation. 1970;41:343-59.
11. Sadler TW. Cardiovascular system. In Langman's medical embryology, 12th ed. Philadelphia: Lippincott Williams & Wilkins; 2012.p.162-200.

CHAPTER 2

General Guidelines for Performing Fetal Echocardiogram

Prashant Bobhate, Snehal Kulkarni

ABSTRACT

Prenatal detection is essential for improving perinatal outcomes of neonates with critical congenital heart disease. Through knowledge of the sonographic machine is essential for the accurate diagnosis of complex congenital heart diseases. Comprehensive evaluation of the fetal heart includes evaluation of the situs, sagittal and transverse plane imaging, evaluation the fetal cardiac rate and rhythm and Doppler assessment. Once the mechanism to obtain the cardiac views is understood and practiced; a comprehensive and detailed assessment of the fetal heart can be easily performed in every case. Use of machine controls for fine-tuning of the images is essential for minimizing the errors in diagnosis.

INTRODUCTION

Congenital heart defect (CHD) is the most common structural anomaly in the fetus accounting for 1% of all live born neonates. However, it is most frequently missed anomaly in the prenatal ultrasound. Prenatal detection can significantly improve perinatal outcomes in neonates with critical CHD. Various technical advances in ultrasound and imaging have vastly improved the imaging of the fetal heart. However, operator training and expertise is essential for accurate diagnosis of CHD in the fetus. This Chapter attempts to give an overview of the basic views and technical advances, which could help image optimization, and thus improve the detection of fetal cardiac anomalies.

EQUIPMENT AND FINE-TUNING OF THE IMAGES

Thorough knowledge of the equipment including the probes, machine and the various presets available is essential part of image acquisition by ultrasonography.

Transducer

Electronic Focusing and 2D Matrix Array Transducers

Proper selection of probe is the key to acquiring good images during imaging of the fetal heart. Usually curvilinear probes are used for image acquisition in the prenatal period. These are array transducers in which each transducer is divided into very large number of small transducers. Pulse is transmitted from each of these small parts beginning at the edge and coming towards the center thus, producing a spherical wave front.

With the current two dimension matrix array transducers electronic focus can be achieved not only in the plane of ultrasound elements but also perpendicular to it. Artifacts are reduced and a crisper picture is generated.

Image Optimization: Machine Controls

Gray Scale Optimization

Various machine controls used for optimization of gray scale and imaging are mentioned in Table 2.1. One can use default presets; which are available with each machine. However, it should be remembered that presets are generated for an average population and fine adjustments are needed for individual patients. Certain simple maneuvers like use of appropriate depth, narrow field of imaging, use of zoom and single focus can greatly improve image quality (Figs 2.1 to 2.3).

Advanced Machine Controls

Tissue Harmonic Imaging

Tissue penetration of ultrasound waves depends upon the frequency of transducer

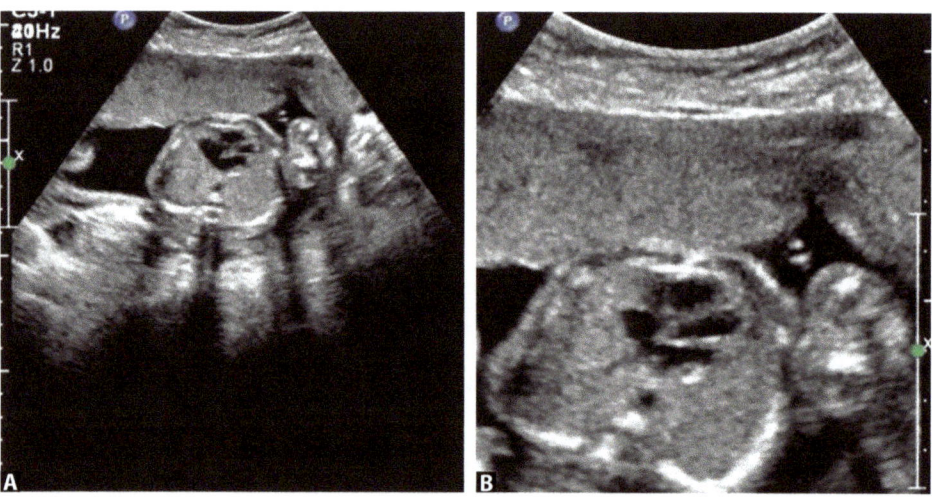

Figs 2.1A and B: For improving image quality depth of the ultrasound image should be adjusted so that the field of interest occupies at least ¾th of the surface area of the monitor

Table 2.1: Gray scale machine controls

Machine control	Effect
Gain	Optimizing the gains helps visualize weak echoes. However, it saturates strong echo signals
Compress	Helps sharpen image and visualize small structures
Time gain compensation	Optimizes gain throughout the depth of the image
Frequency	Increasing frequency helps detailed evaluation of near structures at the cost of penetrance and vice versa
Field of image	Limiting the field of image to the targeted structure of interest vastly improves image quality as well as frame rates
Focus	Optimizes image quality for the field of interest

General Guidelines for Performing Fetal Echocardiogram

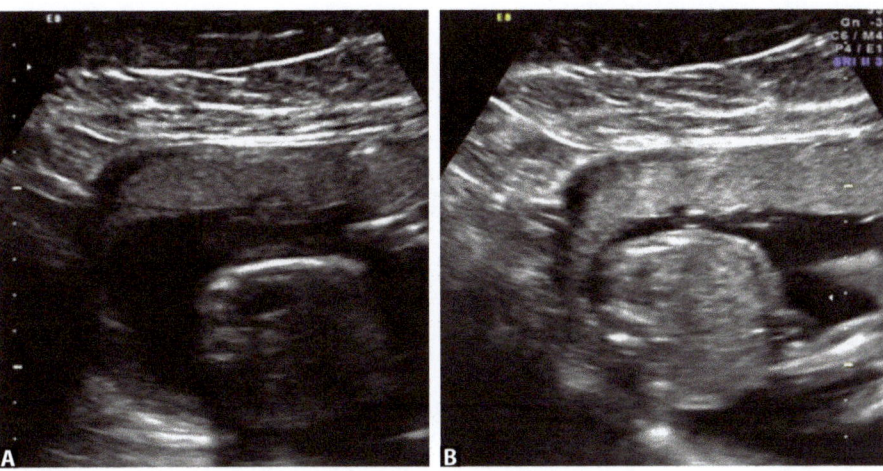

Figs 2.2A and B: 'Focus' in an ultrasound imaging determines the area where maximal sampling is performed by the transducer. Adjusting the focus to the area on interest greatly improves the image quality

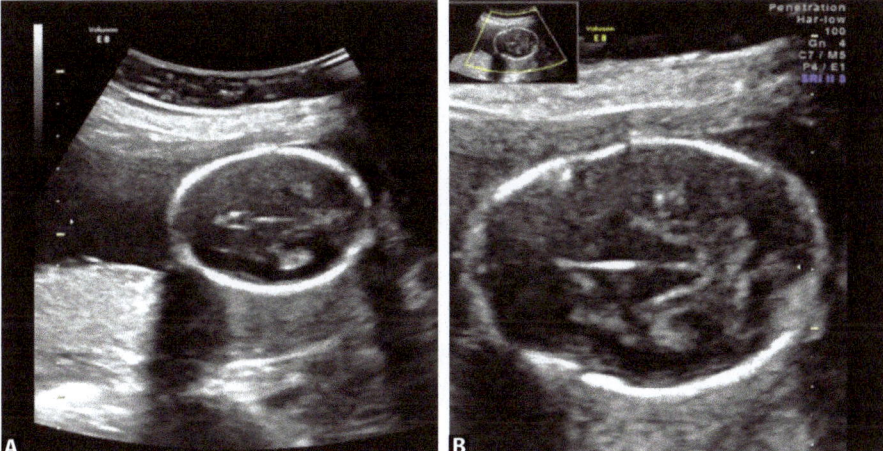

Figs 2.3A and B: (A) Use of zoom leads to increase in frame rates with better resolution and allows detailed assessment; (B) Demonstrates the effect on image quality by use of zoom as compared to standard resolution

used as well as tissue properties like density, pressure, and temperature. Lower frequency transducers have better penetration but poor resolution. As the ultrasound waves penetrate tissue, there is change in their properties from a pure sinus waveform to a compound waveform consisting of additional waves with higher frequency but lower amplitude. These lower amplitude and higher frequency wave are known as harmonic frequencies. Tissue harmonic imaging significantly improves gray scale images especially in difficult scanning conditions like in obese patients.

Real Time Compound Imaging

Ultrasound waves are transmitted perpendicular to the transducer, if these transmitted waves hit the reflector surface at 90° most of the waves are reflected.

However, if they hit at different angles, the waves get scattered which are reflected away from the transducer, thus reducing the signal received. Electronic beam steering is used in real time compound imaging (CI)(Fig. 2.4) in which several overlapping scans of the object from different angles are obtained thus reducing artifacts such as speckle, improving contrast resolution and tissue differentiation. CI is available marketed under various names (e.g. Philips: Sono CT, GE healthcare: Cross X beam imaging). However, there is loss of frame rate as the beams are acquired from various angles and then compounded before display.

Speckle Reduction

Speckles are artifactual ultrasound signals secondary to interference of reflected ultrasound energy from scatters that are too small and too close to be resolved by the frequency used. Speckle reduction can be obtained by using higher frequency transducers, matrix array transducers, harmonic imaging, temporal averaging and post-processing approaches using different filters. Post-processing algorithms are available under various names (e.g. Philips: Xres, GE: Speckle reduction imaging).

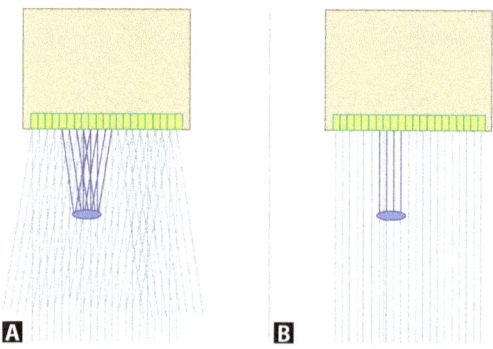

Figs 2.4A and B: By using real time compound imaging (A), artifacts can be significantly reduced as compared to the conventional single line of sight (B). By electronically steering the ultrasound beams to image objects from different angles, true reflectors can be differentiated from artifacts

B-Flow Imaging and Power Doppler

Conventional color Doppler techniques tend to exaggerate the size of vessel in ultrasound (Bleeding of color). B-Flow imaging can be used to detect direction of flow. With use of two separate beams for assessing cross-sectional imaging and moving particles; B-Flow allows better frame rate and resolution as compared to conventional color Doppler. This is particularly helpful to demonstrate small structures like the pulmonary veins and aortopulmonary collaterals in complex congenital heart disease.

Conventional color Doppler is used to demonstrate the direction of blood flow. The amplitude component is displayed by power Doppler. Combination of both, advanced dynamic flow (ADF), has been demonstrated to provide higher resolution, good lateral discrimination and higher sensitivity as compared to conventional color Doppler imaging.

Comprehensive cardiac evaluation, major planes of the body and heart and probe manipulation:

For a complete and comprehensive evaluation of the fetal heart, the following points should be investigated:
1. Visceral situs.
2. Structural evaluation of the fetal heart in transverse and sagittal planes.
3. Assessment of heart rate and cardiac rhythm.
4. Doppler assessment of the fetal heart.

Determination of Visceral Situs and Right-Left Orientation

Determination of the visceral situs is the first and the most important step in evaluation of the fetal heart. Accurate determination of the visceral situs would help the operator to accurately determine the atrial situs. This has to be done taking into consideration the orientation of the fetus and its relative position in the maternal abdomen. One cannot establish right-left orientation on the basis of position of internal organs, such as the stomach and the heart. There could be normal variations in this position and moreover their position varies in abnormalities of the situs. Thus, the position of the stomach and the cardiac apex on the same side in no way guarantees that both are normally positioned on the left.

Various methods have been described for accurate determination of the visceral situs.

Method 1

Step 1: Locate the fetal head within the uterus to determine the presenting part (cephalic or breech).

Step 2: Determine whether the part of the fetus which is anterior (spine or abdomen).

Step 3: Determine the fetal lie depending on the relation of the fetal spine to maternal spine by obtaining a sagittal view of the fetus. (Longitudinal lie: Fetal spine is parallel to maternal spine, Transverse lie: Fetal spine is perpendicular to the maternal spine, Oblique lie: Fetal spine is oblique to the maternal spine).

Step 4: After successful completion of the first three steps determine the location of the fetal left side with respect to the position of the transducer and maternal abdomen, e.g. Left is closer to the transducer, fetal left would be anterior and vice versa.

Method 2

Described by Cordes, et al. (Figs 2.5A to C).

In the sagittal view, the head is positioned to the right side of the screen and the transducer is rotated by 90° in the clockwise manner to obtain the transverse view. In this view, the spine of the fetus is located and the right to left is traced in a clockwise manner.

Method 3

Described by Bronshtein, et al. right hand thumb rule for abdominal scanning and the left hand thumb rule for vaginal scanning (Fig. 2.6).

The examiner hold the hand according to the side of the fetal face, the palm of the hand corresponds to the fetal face and the heart and the stomach are shown by the thumb of the examiner.

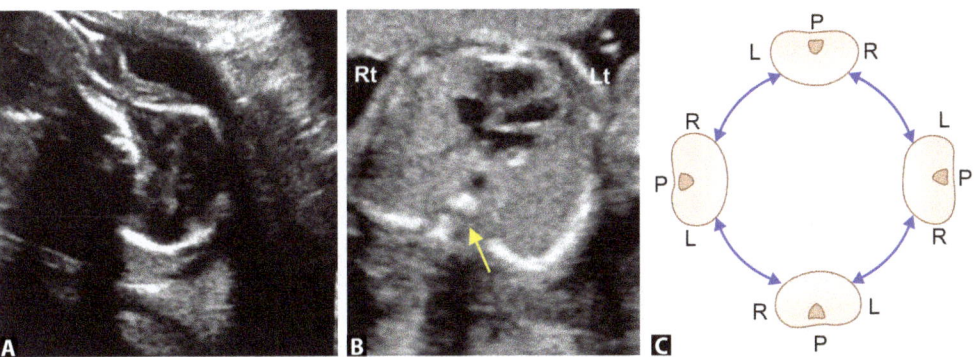

Figs 2.5A to C: Determination of the fetal right and left side by use of method described by Cordes et al. The fetal head is aligned to the right of the screen (A) The transducer is then rotated clockwise by 90° to obtain an image in the transverse plane at the level of the abdomen; (B) The spine is identified (yellow arrow), going clockwise from the spine is the right side followed by the left; (C) Showing diagrammatic representation that demonstrates the right and left sidedness according to the position of the spine in the transverse plane

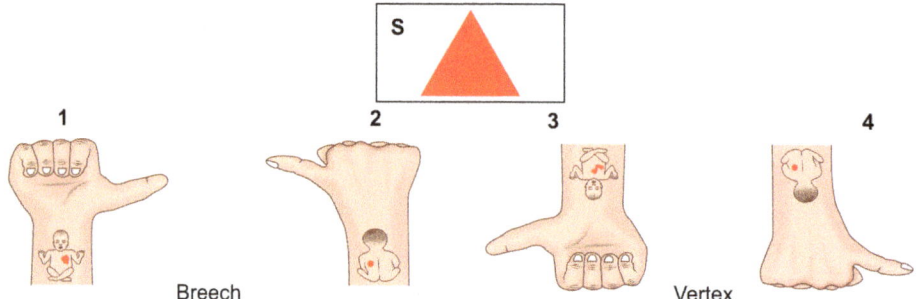

Fig. 2.6: Right hand thumb rule for transabdominal scanning and left hand thumb rule for transvaginal scanning as described by Bronshtein, et al. The palm represents the fetal face and the thumb represents the fetal heart and aorta
Reproduced with permission from: Bronshtein et al.

Structural Evaluation of the Fetal Heart in Transverse and Sagittal Planes

Once the situs of the fetus is accurately determined; detailed morphological assessment of the fetal heart should be carried out.

Transverse Planes

Aligning the transducer at the level of the fetal abdomen, a slow cephalad sweep up to the thoracic inlet maintaining more or less horizontal cut would reveal the cross section of the abdomen, the four chamber view, the left ventricular outflow tract view, the right ventricular outflow tract view and three vessel tracheal view in succession.

The cross section of the abdomen, in a fetus with situs solitus demonstrates the stomach to the left, the major liver mass to the right, the aorta lies anterior and to the left of the spine while the inferior vena cava lies right and anterior to the aorta (Fig. 2.7).

The Four-chamber View

Cephalad sweep from the transverse abdominal view would reveal the four-chamber view. Correct technique of obtaining the four-chamber view is vital prior to its accurate interpretation. The ultrasound beam must be placed in the correct orthogonal plane at right level of the fetal heart. The correct plane is a completely transverse plane with at least one rib seen completely. Appearance of multiple ribs would suggest that the ultrasound beam is not exactly perpendicular to the transverse

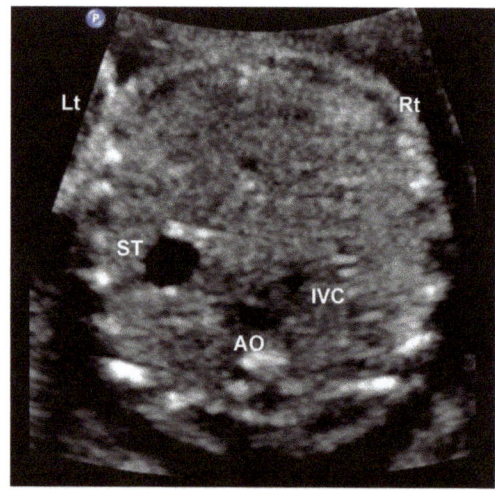

Fig. 2.7: Transverse plane of the abdomen at the level of the diaphragm, demonstrates that the aorta (Ao) is left and anterior to the spine, the inferior vena cava (IVC) is on the right and anterior to the aorta and the stomach (ST) lies on the left side

plane (Figs 2.8A and B). The correct level reveals the crux of the heart in the center, if the plane is too low the coronary sinus (Fig. 2.9) is seen, and if the plane is too high the aortic valve is seen. Detailed evaluation of the four-chamber view with the assessment of morphology, size, axis and function is described in detail in the following Chapters (Figs 2.10 to 2.12). Checklist for the four-chamber view is as mentioned in Box 2.1.

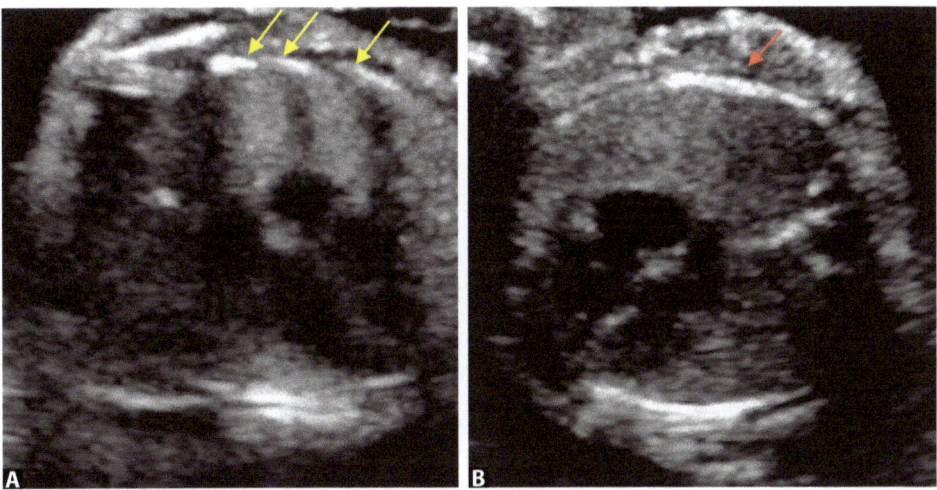

Figs 2.8A and B: For accurate assessment of the four-chamber view; the ultrasound beam must cut perpendicular to the body (B), presence of multiple ribs (A) suggests that the ultrasound beam is not exactly perpendicular to the transverse plane

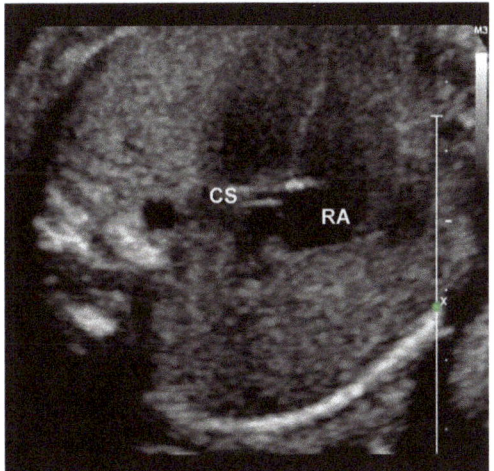

Fig. 2.9: If the transverse plane is slightly below the apical four-chamber view the coronary sinus (CS) can be seen entering the right atrium (RA)

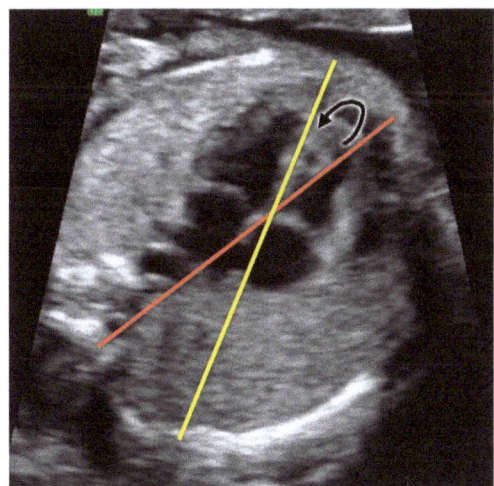

Fig. 2.10: The axis of the fetal heart can be determined by drawing two imaginary lines. One passing through the anterior chest wall and the spine (red) and another passing through the interventricular septum (yellow). The normal cardiac axis is between 25–65°

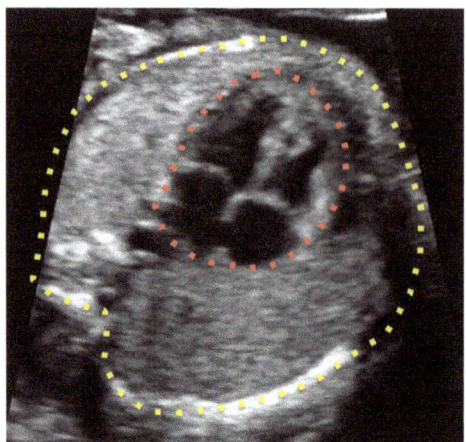

Fig. 2.11: Cardiac size can be determined by calculating the cardiothoracic ratio. It is the ratio of the area covered by the heart (red) to the entire thoracic area (yellow)

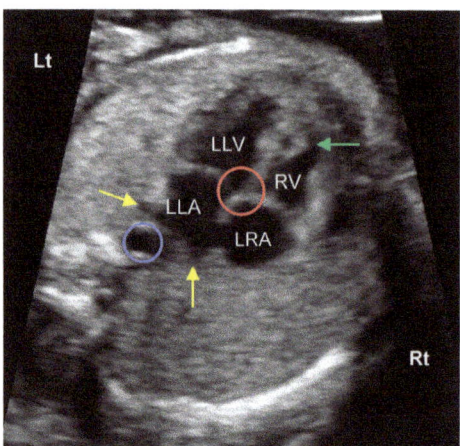

Fig. 2.12: The cardiac chambers can be identified in the four-chamber view. The left atrium (LA), receives the pulmonary veins (yellow arrow) and the flap of the foramen ovale opens in the left atrium in normal fetal cardiac anatomy as well as most of the disease conditions. The right atrium (RA) receives the coronary sinus demonstrated in Figure 2.9. The atrioventricular valves and the ventricles go together. The tricuspid valve is apically displaced which can be seen at the crux of the heart (red circle) as well as it is septophilic while the mitral valve is septophobic. A moderator band (green arrow) can be identified in the right ventricle (RV). The left ventricle (LV) is smooth walled

> **Box 2.1: Checklist for four-chamber view**
> - Cardiac position
> - Cardiac size
> - Cardiac axis
> - Identification of the cardiac chambers
> - Position and form of the foramen ovale
> - Pulmonary venous connections
> - Atrioventricular connection
> - Cardiac function
> - Cardiac rhythm
> - Septal defects
> - Atrioventricular valve functions

The Left Ventricular Outflow Tract View

Cephalad sweep with slight rotation towards the right shoulder of the baby; from the four-chamber view would reveal the left ventricular outflow tract. The aorta is wedged between the two atrioventricular valves (Fig. 2.13). Aorto-mitral and aortoseptal continuity seen in this view is essential to rule out perimembranous VSD.

The Right Ventricular Outflow Tract View

Cephalad sweep from the left ventricular outflow tract view would reveal the right ventricular outflow which in a fetus with normal cardiac morphology, crosses the left ventricular outflow tract at a right angle (Fig. 2.14). The great vessels are identified by their morphologic criteria rather than their connections to the ventricles. Morphologically, the aorta gives rise to the coronary arteries, which in normal circumstances cannot be seen in fetal echo. Hence, the first branches of the aorta, which can be seen, are the head and neck vessels that originate at a fair distance from the aortic valve. The pulmonary artery on the other hand gives three branches, the right and left pulmonary arteries and the ductus arteriosus at a very short distance form the pulmonary valve. Additionally, a short axis view of the RVOT can be obtained which shows branching of the pulmonary artery (Trousseau sign)(Figs 2.15A and B).

General Guidelines for Performing Fetal Echocardiogram

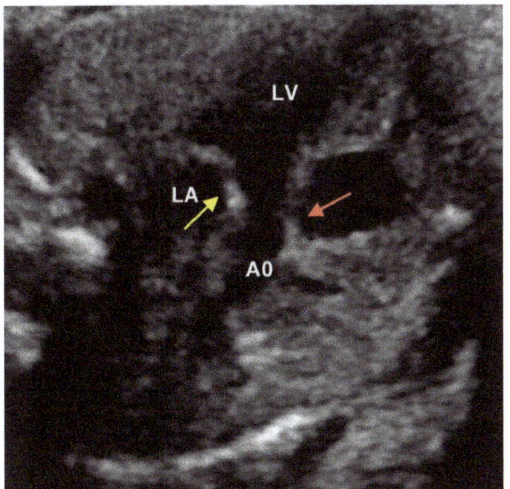

Fig. 2.13: The left ventricular outflow tract can be opened up by slight rotation towards the right shoulder and cephalad sweep from the four-chamber view. Demonstration of aortomitral (yellow arrow) and aortospetal continuity is prudent to rule out perimembranous ventricular septal defect, which is the most common congenital heart disease

The Three Vessel and Three Vessel Tracheal View

Cephalad sweep from the right ventricular outflow tract reveals the aortic and the ductal arches which meet together in a 'V' shape, and cross posteriorly on the left side of the trachea (Fig. 2.16). Thymic shadow can be seen anterior to these vessels and its absence would indicate presence of DiGeorge syndrome in certain congenital heart disease. Checklist for the three vessel tracheal view is as mentioned in Box 2.2.

> **Box 2.2: Checklist for three vessel tracheal view**
>
> - Identification of the superior vena cava, ductal arch and the aortic arch
> - Size of the ductal arch vs size of the aortic arch. (Isthmus to duct ratio >0.75)
> - Arch sidedness (The aortic arch should pass to the left of the trachea in a left aortic arch)
> - Flow in the ductal and aortic arch
> - Abnormalities of number, size and position of the three vessels
> - Thymus: Presence and its size.

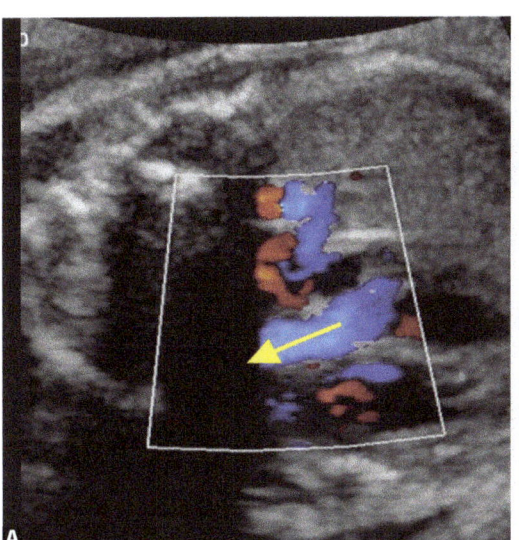
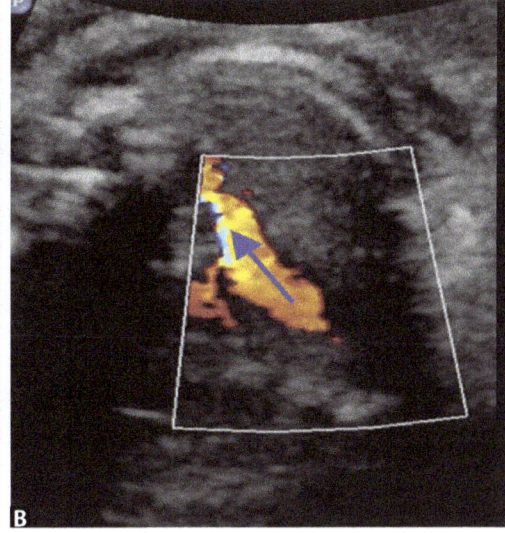

Figs 2.14A and B: Cephalad sweep from the left ventricular outflow tract view would reveal the right ventricular outflow (blue arrow), which in a fetus with normal cardiac morphology crosses the left ventricular outflow tract (yellow arrow) at a right angle

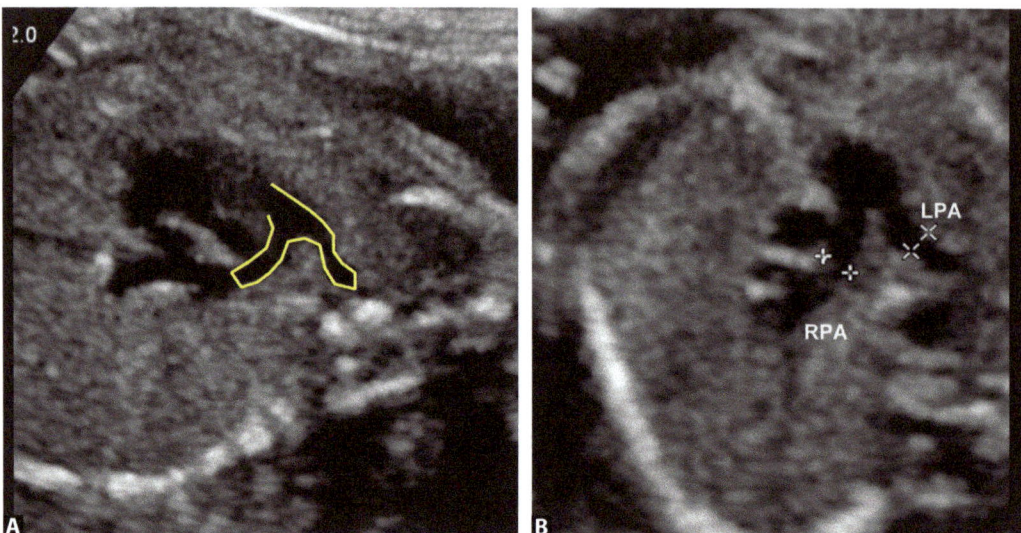

Figs 2.15A and B: The right ventricular outflow tract (RVOT) can be demonstrated by rotating the transducer by 90° from the four-chamber view. In this view (A) the RVOT is seen (Trosseau's sign), and (B) the bifurcation of the pulmonary arteries (PA) can be demonstrated
Abbreviations: LPA, left pulmonary artery; RPA, right pulmonary artery

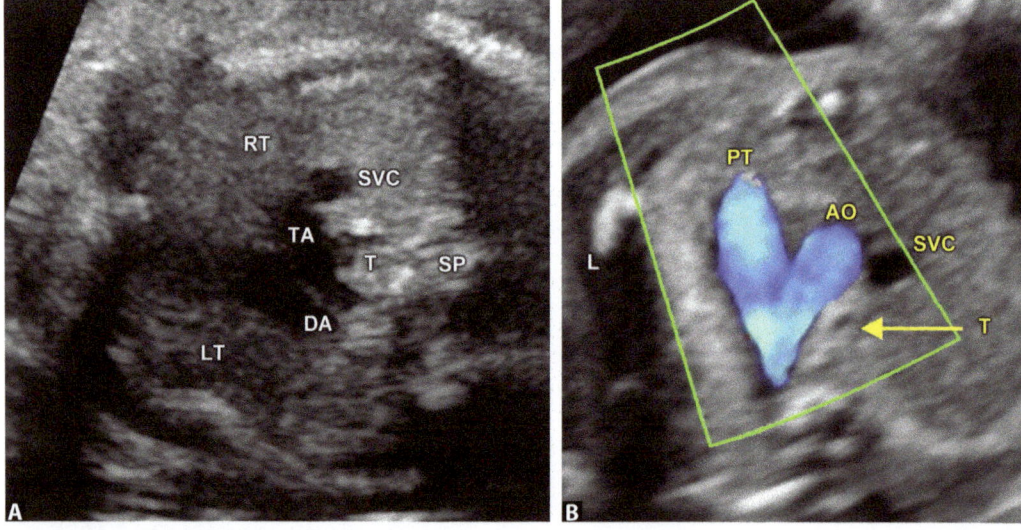

Figs 2.16A and B: Cephalad sweep from the right ventricular outflow tract reveals the TA and the DA, which meet together in a 'V' shape, and cross posteriorly on the left side of the T. From right to left and anterior to posterior the three vessels in this view are SVC
Abbreviations: TA, transverse aortic; DA, ductal arches; T, trachea; SVC, superior vena cava, SP, spine

Thus, a slow cephalad sweep in the transverse plane would in majority of the cases is enough to identify normal features of the fetal heart and exclude cardiac malformations. However, the sagittal views are a good adjunct to diagnosis especially in disease states. A 90° rotation and slow sweep from the left to the right of the fetus would reveal the short axis of the left ventricle, the long axis of the aortic arch, the long axis of the ductal arch and the bicaval view in succession (Figs 2.17A to C).

Doppler Assessment of the Fetal Heart

After a detailed morphologic assessment of the fetal heart by transverse and sagittal sweeps, it is extremely important to use both color and pulsed wave Doppler for functional assessment of the fetal heart.

Color Doppler

Color Doppler interrogation is used for functional assessment of the atrioventricular and semilunar valves as well as to detect presence of septal defects. A few practical points need to be considered while using the color Doppler.

- Reduce the size of the box for color Doppler to the area on B mode which one wants to interrogate.
- Increase the velocity scales and optimize the gains sufficiently to visualize the blood flow and at the same time to avoid excessive spill of color.

Pulse Wave Doppler Assessment

Use of pulse wave Doppler at cardiac and extracardiac sites can provide valuable information regarding the cardiac function as well as general well-being of the fetus. In normal fetal echo, if color flow is normal, it is not absolutely necessary to use pulsed Doppler. To estimate abnormally increased velocity, continuous wave Doppler with cardiac probes need to be used. Following are few tips to be considered while doing pulsed Doppler:

1. Place the sample volume distal to the respective valve.
2. Insonating angle should be in 15–20° of the direction of the blood flow.
3. Place the sample volume at the brightest colors of the blood flow segment.
4. Multiple measurements should be taken.

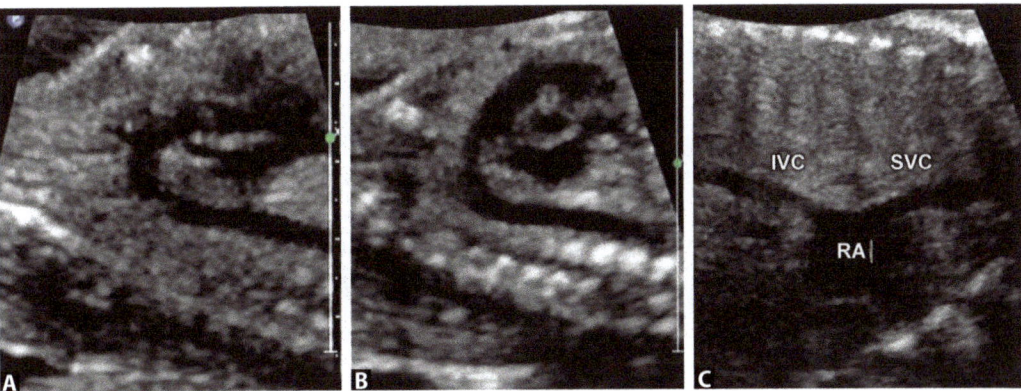

Figs 2.17A to C: A 90° rotation from the four-chamber view and slow sweep from the left to the right of the fetus would reveal the short axis of the left ventricle, the long axis of the aortic arch (A), the long axis of the ductal arch (B) and the Bicaval view (C) in succession.
Abbreviations: IVC, inferior vena cava; SVC, superior vena cava; RA, right atrium

Fetal Echocardiography

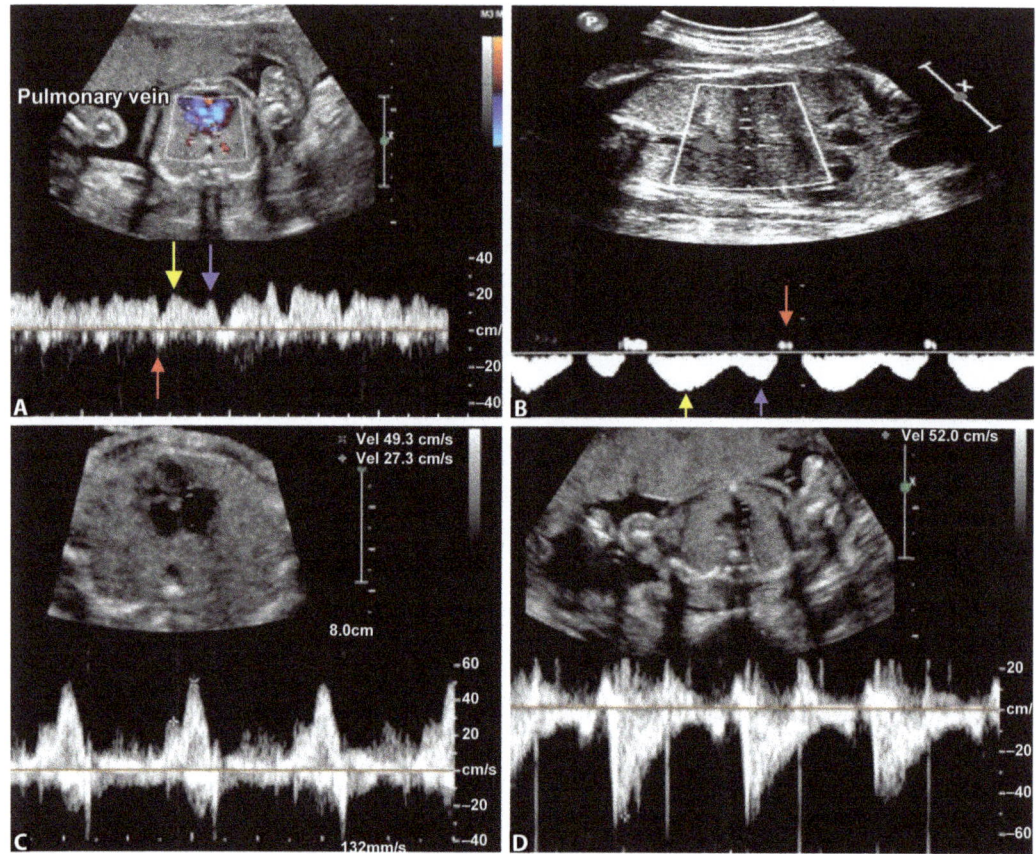

Figs 2.18A to D: Pulse wave Doppler signal at the pulmonary veins (A), inferior vena cava (B), Atrioventricular valve (C) and the right ventricular outflow tract (D). The venous Doppler demonstrate the S (yellow arrow), D (blue arrow) and the A (red arrow) waves. The atrioventricular valve Doppler demonstrates the early filling (E) wave and late filling (A) wave. In a fetus, the A wave velocity is more that the E wave velocity. Peak velocity and time to peak velocities at the semilunar valve Doppler can be plotted against the available normograms

Pulse wave Doppler should be obtained at each of the valves (Figs 2.18A to D). Standard wave formats and their assessment is described in the following Chapters.

Assessment of Heart Rate and Cardiac Rhythm

The last step of comprehensive fetal echocardiography is calculation of the fetal heart rate and demonstration of 1:1 atrioventricular conduction using M mode or pulse wave Doppler (Figs 2.19A to C).

CONCLUSION

Once the mechanism to obtain the cardiac views is understood and practiced, a comprehensive and detailed assessment of the fetal heart can be easily performed in every case. Use of machine controls for fine-tuning of the images is essential for minimizing the

General Guidelines for Performing Fetal Echocardiogram

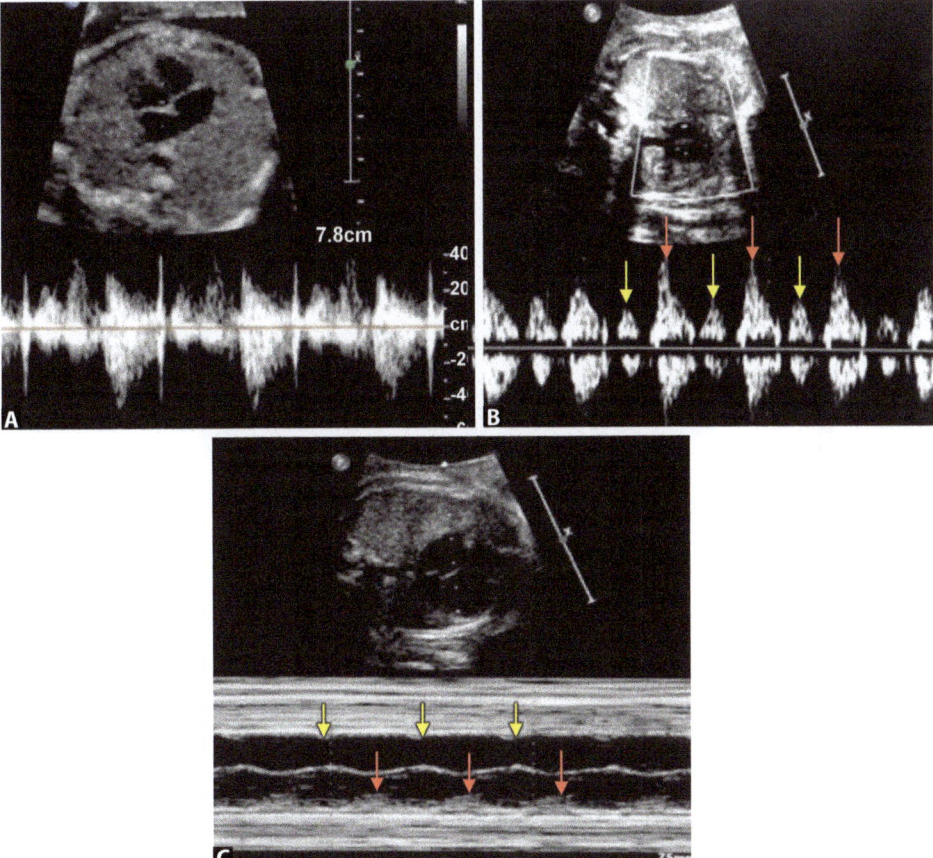

Figs 2.19A to C: The heart rate and the 1:1 AV conduction can be determined using the pulse wave Doppler at the aorto mitral continuity (A) or by the simultaneous Doppler of the SVC and the aorta; (B) M Mode through an atria and ventricle; (C) can also be used for determining the heart rate as well as the AV conduction. The Yellow arrows indicate atrial contraction and the Red arrows indicate ventricular contraction

errors in diagnosis. The details of normal and abnormal of each view are described in the following Chapters.

KEY MESSAGES

1. Appropriate use of the advanced imaging tools available is key to obtaining a high quality image.
2. Detailed and stepwise assessment of the fetal heart is essential to suspect and diagnose congenital heart disease.

SUGGESTED READING

1. Bronshtein M, Gover A, Zimmer EZ. Sonographic definition of the fetal situs. Obstet Gynecol. 2002;99(6):1129-30.
2. Brown DW, Cohen KE, O'Brien P, Gauvreau K, Klitzner TS, Beekman RH3rd, et al. Impact of prenatal diagnosis in survivors of initial palliation of single ventricle heart disease: analysis of the national pediatric cardiology quality improvement collaborative database. Pediatr Cardiol. 2015;36(2): 314-21.

3. Chawengsettakul S, Russameecharoen K, Wanitpongpan P. Fetal cardiac function measured by myocardial performance index of small-for-gestational age fetuses. J Obstet Gynaecol Res. 2015;41(2):222-8.
4. Entrekin RR, Porter BA, Sillesen HH, Wong AD, Cooperberg PL, Fix CH. Real-time spatial compound imaging: Application to breast, vascular, and musculoskeletal ultrasound. Semin Ultrasound CT MR. 2001;22(1):50-64.
5. Heling KS, Chaoui R, Bollmann R. Advanced dynamic flow—a new method of vascular imaging in prenatal medicine. A pilot study of its applicability. Ultraschall Med. 2004;25(4):280-4.
6. Hoffman JI, Kaplan S. The incidence of congenital heart disease. J Am Coll Cardiol. 2002;39(12):1890-900.
7. Ozkutlu S, Bostan OM, Deren O, Onderoglu L, Kale G, Güçer S, Orhan D. Prenatal echocardiographic diagnosis of cardiac right/left axis and malpositions according to standardized Cordes technique. Anadolu Kardiyol Derg. 2011;11(2):131-6.
8. Volpe P, Campobasso G, Stanziano A, De Robertis V, Di Paolo S, Caruso G, Volpe N, Gentile M. Novel application of 4D sonography with B-flow imaging and spatio-temporal image correlation (STIC) in the assessment of the anatomy of pulmonary arteries in fetuses with pulmonary atresia and ventricular septal defect. Ultrasound Obstet Gynecol. 2006;28(1):40-6.
9. von Kaisenberg CS, Kuhling-von Kaisenberg H, Fritzer E, Schemm S, Meinhold-Heerlein I, Jonat W. Fetal transabdominal anatomy scanning using standard views at 11 to 14 weeks' gestation. Am J Obstet Gynecol. 2005; 192(2):535-42.
10. Wunsch R, Dudwiesus H, Reinehr T. Prospective comparison of different ultrasound modalities to measure thicknesses less than 1 mm. Rofo. 2007;179(1):65-71.

CHAPTER 3

Indications and Timing of Fetal Echocardiography

Anita Saxena

ABSTRACT

Examination of fetal heart by echocardiography is best reserved for high-risk pregnancies. A number of factors are known which increase the risk of development of cardiac abnormality in the fetus several folds. These include a family history of CHD, metabolic diseases in the mother such as diabetes mellitus, maternal exposure to teratogenic substances and drugs in early pregnancy, maternal infections and others. All these would constitute indications for a detailed fetal heart scan. However, the most common indication for fetal echocardiography is detection of fetal cardiac or extra cardiac abnormality on a screening obstetric ultrasound. The risk of CHD in fetus is very high in such cases. Fetal echocardiography is best done at 18–22 weeks of gestation when the details of fetal heart are easier to discern. An earlier scan may be indicated in special situations, but it should be repeated at 18–22 weeks. Those detected to have an abnormality of fetal heart may require repeat or serial scans to see the progress of the cardiac abnormality and to detect complications early, should they occur.

INTRODUCTION

Congenital heart disease (CHD) is a common abnormality in neonates, occurring in 6–12/1000 live births. It accounts for half of all deaths from lethal malformations in children. The estimates of CHD for fetuses are not well-documented but are likely to be higher since spontaneous and elective terminations of pregnancies do happen in some cases. In one of the studies, CHD was seen in 23/1000 high risk fetuses screened by echocardiography. Availability of echocardiography has enabled prenatal detection of CHD. With early diagnosis, optimal care can be offered to a newborn with CHD. Prenatal diagnosis of CHD has been shown to have a significant impact on postnatal management and outcomes. Ideal would be to screen all pregnancies for CHD, but the yield is likely to be quite low with this strategy. This strategy has not been found to be feasible even in countries with much lower rates of pregnancy and better resources as compared to those in India. An approach of screening those who are considered high risk seems more reasonable and practical. High risk may be due to maternal disease, history of CHD in the previous siblings, increased nuchal translucency or other maternal, fetal or familial factors. A common cause for performing fetal echocardiography is the suspicion of CHD or presence of some congenital abnormality on an obstetric ultrasound. The basal risk of CHD is considered to be <1%. Fetal echocardiography is best performed in cases where the risk exceeds 2-3%. So, the indications for fetal echocardiography may vary from region to region according to the health care system of that region as this diagnostic tool is likely to require extra resources.

RISK FACTORS FOR CONGENITAL HEART DISEASE IN THE FETUS

The list of risk factors is a moving target as scientific knowledge and experience expand. Several risk factors have been described where likelihood of CHD increases several folds, though the exact reason for higher CHD rates remains elusive. Some of these risk factors have been found to have special predilection for specific types of CHD.

Fetal echocardiography is also indicated in those referred due to an abnormality of the heart picked up on screening ultrasound, irrespective of the presence or absence of known risk factors. Some of the known risk factors with their degree of risk for CHD and the specific type of CHD (if known) are described in the Table 3.1.

INDICATIONS FOR FETAL ECHOCARDIOGRAPHY

It must be pointed out that nearly 90% of heart defects detected in utero occur in otherwise low risk pregnancies. It is also well known that detection rate for CHD will be much better with fetal echocardiography as compared to screening by obstetric ultrasound. Women with one or more risk factors, as detailed above, should be recommended for a detailed fetal echocardiography by a qualified sonographer, cardiologist or any other trained personnel. However, those referred for suspected CHD on screening ultrasound have the highest

Table 3.1: Risk factors for occurrence of congenital heart disease in fetus

Condition			Risk of CHD (%)	Type of CHD
A	Family history condition of CHD			
	A1	Mother with CHD	4–6	Overall for any CHD
			15	AS
			10	AVSD
			3	TOF, TGA
			<3	Others (?CHDs other than the above list)
	A2	Father with CHD	2–3	VSD, AS, other CHD
	A3	Sibling with CHD:		HLHS (8%), other CHD
		One sibling with CHD	2–6	
		Two or more siblings with CHD	5–10	
	A4	Second degree relative with CHD	<2	Left sided obstructive lesions, other CHD
	A5	Relative with syndrome (e.g. Marfan, Ehlor-Danlos, HCM, etc.)	50	MVP, MR, AR, LVOTO
B	Increased nuchal thickness at 10–12 weeks (mm)			25% of CHD are major and complex (AVSD, TOF, DORV, CoA, HLHS)
	B1	3.0–3.4	3	
	B2	>3.5	6	
	B3	>6	24	
	B4	>8.5	>60	

Contd...

Contd...

Condition			Risk of CHD (%)	Type of CHD
C	Maternal infections			
	C1	Rubella	50	PDA, peripheral PS
	C2	Parvovirus, Coxsackie, Adenovirus, cytomegalovirus	2–3	Fetal myocarditis
D	Diabetes Mellitus in mother			
	D1	Pre-gestational	3–5	Heterotaxy, truncus arteriosus, TGA, single ventricle
	D2	Gestational well controlled	1–2	
	D3	Gestational uncontrolled	>5 (in 3rd trimester)	Ventricular hypertrophy
E	Systemic lupus, Sjogren syndrome		3–5	CHB, myocarditis
	E1	Previous child with CHB/ neonatal lupus	20	CHB, myocarditis
F	Maternal teratogens exposure			
	F1	ACE inhibitors	3	Any CHD
	F2	Anticonvulsants	2	ASD, VSD, TOF, PDA
	F3	Lithium	5–8	Ebstein's anomaly
	F4	Retinoic acid	10–20	Conotruncal abnormalities: TOF, TGA
	F5	Vitamin K antagonists (Warfarin dose > 5 mg)	2–5	PDA, ASD
G	Miscellaneous			
	G1	In vitro fertilization	2–3	VSD, ASD, other CHD
	G2	Cardiac abnormality on screening ultrasound	60	Any CHD
	G3	Non-cardiac abnormality on ultrasound	20–30	Any CHD
	G4	Chromosomal abnormality	60	AVSD, PS, CoA, conotruncal abnormality
	G5	Hydrops fetalis	15–20	SVT, CHB, myocardits

Abbreviations: AR, aortic regurgitation; AS, aortic stenosis; ASD, atrial septal defect; AVSD, atrioventricular septal defect; CHB, complete heart block; CHD, congenital heart disease; CoA, coarctation of aorta; DORV, double outlet right ventricle; HCM, hypertrophic cardiomyopathy; HLHS, hypoplastic left heart syndrome; LVOTO, left ventricular outflow tract obstruction; MR, mitral regurgitation; MVP, mitral valve prolapse; PDA, patent ductus arteriosus; PS, pulmonary stenosis; SVT, supraventricular tachycardia; TGA, transposition of great arteries; TOF, tetralogy of Fallot; VSD, ventricular septal defect.

prevalence of CHD. The next group with a high yield is those in whom the obstetric ultrasound has shown an extracardiac abnormality or a chromosomal abnormality. In a study from USA, 99% of mothers of babies born with serious CHD had undergone screening obstetric ultrasound; only about 30% of the CHD were identified prenatally. The Figures are going to be perhaps even lower for India. It is believed that an abnormal four chamber view on screening ultrasound is likely to show CHD on fetal echocardiography in >40% of fetuses. If outflow views could be added to the screening ultrasound, the detection of CHD is likely to be even better. Addition of three vessel view with trachea will further

Table 3.2: Indications for fetal echocardiography

Fetal indications	Maternal indications
Suspicion of or detection of CHD on screening anomaly scan	Metabolic disorders like diabetes mellitus, phenylketonuria
Increased nuchal translucency thickness*	History of CHD in mother (father or siblings, first degree relatives)
Major extra cardiac abnormalities, e.g. diaphragmatic hernia, duodenal atresia	Exposure to teratogens, drugs like anticonvulsants, lithium, ACE inhibitors, etc.
Fetal hydrops fetalis	Maternal infections such as rubella and other viruses
Fetal arrhythmias: tachyarrhythmia, complete heart block	Autoimmune disorders like Lupus, Sjogren syndrome or positive anti-Ro or anti-La antibodies
Chromosomal abnormality in fetus such as trisomy 13, 18, 21, Turner syndrome	Exposure to prostaglandin synthetase inhibitors, e.g. Ibuprofen, salicylic acid, indomethacin
Multiple gestation due to risk of CHD and twin to twin transfusion syndrome	Familial inherited disorders like Marfan's syndrome, Ellis-van Creveld syndrome, Noonan's syndrome, etc.
Abnormal ductus venosus waveform	Assisted conception or in vitro fertilization

*Increased nuchal thickness has been an important indication and the cut-off values for indication has varied between centers. In general, values >99th centile according to crown-rump length may be taken as an indication for fetal echocardiography. Others have used a cut-off of 3.5 mm, some other as 3.0 mm for recommending fetal echocardiography.
Abbreviation: CHD, congenital heart disease.

improve detection rates. The indications for fetal echocardiography are shown in Table 3.2. These can be divided primarily into fetal and maternal indications.

Significance of Intracardiac Echogenic Focus on Fetal Echocardiography

Intracardiac echogenic focus (ICEF) has been observed in 1.5–2% of all fetal ultrasound examinations (Fig. 3.1). In the past, its presence has been considered as a marker of fetal aneuploidy. Several studies have been published since then but the jury is still out on the significance of ICEF and its association with fetal chromosomal anomalies. Some of the recent studies have considered ICEF as a soft marker that may be of interest only in high risk pregnancies for chromosomal anomalies. The ICEF has been graded into grade 1 to 3 depending on the brightness as compared to fetal thoracic spine and only those which were equal to or more than the echogenicity of fetal spine were associated with chromosomal

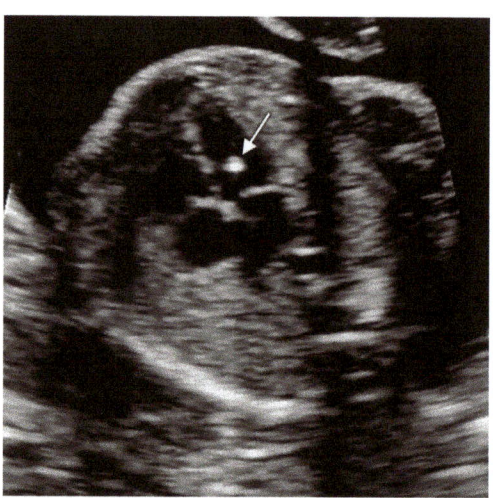

Fig. 3.1: Four-chamber view of a fetus showing an echogenic focus in left ventricle (arrow)

abnormality in the fetus. It is also believed that multiple ICEF are more likely to be associated with increased risk of Trisomy 21 when compared with a single ICEF. 8.5% of fetuses with multiple ICEF had Trisomy 21 as compared to 0.6% with single ICEF and 0.4% with no ICEF. Current consensus seems to be that a single ICEF may be considered as an incidental finding, especially in those with normal serum aneuploidy screening results. Fetal echocardiography and other studies for chromosomal abnormalities may be advised to those with multiple ICEF.

Timing of Fetal Echocardiography

Conventionally fetal echocardiography for screening of high risk pregnancies for assessment of fetal heart should be performed at 18-22 weeks of gestation. Most obstetric units recommend a screening ultrasound scan for fetal anomaly around the same time. The timing of fetal echocardiography is also dependent on several other factors, such as the reason for referral and the age at which a cardiac or extracardiac abnormality is detected by the anomaly scan. A single scan at 18-22 weeks may also miss some of the CHDs where the abnormality is very subtle or absent in mid-pregnancy period and the evolution of abnormality occurs in late part of second trimester, e.g. supraventricular tachycardia, congenital complete heart block or even hypoplasia of a cardiac chamber. Fetal echocardiography should be done as early as possible after the screening test if an abnormality has been detected on screening ultrasound. This would give sufficient time in case additional tests such as amniocentesis, etc. are required. Early diagnosis of a CHD will also allow the family to be counseled for the various options including delivery at a center equipped to deal with CHD. For very complex conditions such as heterotaxy syndrome with complex cardiac malformations, family may opt for termination of pregnancy and the timing becomes very important. After 28-30 weeks, it may be difficult to obtain images of the fetal heart because ratio of fetal body mass to amniotic fluid increases. Acoustic shadowing from fetal spine and sternum further compromise the image quality.

Early Fetal Echocardiography

Advances in image resolution and development of high frequency transducers have allowed assessment of fetal heart earlier than 18 weeks. Examination as early as 8-9 weeks of gestation by a transvaginal ultrasound transducer is possible, although a detailed cardiac anatomy cannot be ascertained at this stage of cardiac development. Transabdominal echo pictures are generally obtainable at about 14-16 weeks, especially in experienced fetal units, but performing a comprehensive assessment of fetal heart is difficult and often a repeat examination is required at 18-22 weeks. Recent report of performing the fetal echocardiography at 11-13 weeks by obtaining a four chamber view, 3 vessel view and their combination with color mapping has shown that most cases with complex CHD, such as univentricular hearts, atrioventricular septal defect, pulmonary atresia and conotruncal defects could be diagnosed.

The consensus for timing of fetal echocardiography continues to be at 18-22 weeks of gestation. Early fetal echocardiography should be reserved for:

- Detection of cardiac or extracardiac abnormality on an earlier screening ultrasound.
- Increased thickness of nuchal translucency at 10-12 weeks.
- Anxiety due to loss of a previous child with serious CHD.
- Fetus at a risk for chromosomal anomalies.
- Fetus with a very high risk for CHD (*refer to* Table 3.1 *for the list*).

It is recommended to repeat fetal echocardiography in high-risk pregnancies even though an earlier echo at 14-16 weeks has been reported as normal. Early fetal echocardiography may miss septal defects and lesions that are likely to be progressive.

Repeat Fetal Echocardiography

If a fetal cardiac abnormality is detected or suspected at mid-trimester fetal echocardiography, repeat examination is recommended. At times serial echocardiography may be required as pregnancy advances, to look for any complications and to guide therapy, antenatal or postnatal. The timing and frequency will be determined by the underlying type and severity of heart disease. Several abnormalities of fetal heart may progress with advancing pregnancy. These include atrioventricular valve regurgitation/stenosis, progressive ventricular, great artery or aortic arch hypoplasia secondary to an obstructive lesion, myocardial dysfunction. Some of the conditions cause complications over a period of time, e.g. left ventricular dysfunction developing due to severe aortic stenosis, fetal hydrops occurring due to either very fast fetal heart rate (supraventricular tachycardia/atrial flutter) or very slow heart rate secondary to complete heart block. Development of fetal hydrops is a very serious condition and unless taken care of (by drugs or by early delivery) can lead to intrauterine death of the fetus. Rarely foramen ovale may get restricted or patent ductus arteriosus constricts prematurely. Cardiac tumors, such as rhabdomyoma may progress or regress during fetal life. All conditions enumerated above will require repeat, at times serial fetal echocardiography.

CONCLUSION

Fetal echocardiography is the single most important tool for diagnosis of CHD in fetus. It should be offered to all high-risk pregnancies. Several factors are known to be associated with higher likelihood of CHD in the fetus, but highest number of fetuses with CHD is diagnosed in those who were found to have a cardiac or an extracardiac abnormality on screening obstetric ultrasound. Fetal echocardiography is best performed between 18–22 weeks of gestation. With advances in imaging technology, fetal echocardiography can be performed in first trimester with a reasonable degree of accuracy and it should be recommended in certain special situations.

SUGGESTED READING

1. Donofrio MT, Moon-Grady AJ, Hornberger LK, Copel JA, Sklansky MS, Abuhamad A, et al. Diagnosis and treatment of fetal cardiac disease. A scientific statement from the American Heart Association. Circulation. 2014;129:2183-242.
2. Hunter LE, Simpson JM. Prenatal screening for structural congenital heart disease. Nat Rev Cardiol. 2014;11:323-34.
3. Lee W, Allan L, Carvalho JS, Chaoui R, Copel J, Devore G, et al. The ISUOG Fetal Echocardiography Task Force. ISUOG consensus statement: What constitutes a fetal echocardiogram? Ultrasound Obstet Gynecol. 2008;32:239-42.
4. Murphy H, Phillippi JC. Isolated intracardiac echogenic focus on routine ultrasound: implications for practice. J Midwife Womens Health. 2015;60:83-8.
5. Pike JI, Krishnan A, Donofrio MT. Early fetal echocardiography: congenital heart disease detection and diagnostic accuracy in the hands of an experienced fetal cardiology program. Prenatal Diagnosis. 2014;34:790-6.
6. Saxena A, Shrivastava S, Kothari SS. Value of antenatal echocardiography in high risk patients to diagnose congenital cardiac defects in fetus. Indian J Pediatr. 1995;62:575-82.
7. Saxena A, Soni NR. Fetal echocardiography: Where are we? Ind J Ped. 2005;72:603-8.
8. Wiechec M, Knafel A, Nocun A. Prenatal detection of congenital heart defects at the 11- to 13-week scan using a simple color doppler protocol including the 4-chamber and 3-vessel and trachea views. J Ultrasound Med. 2015;34:585-94.

CHAPTER 4

How to Perform a Normal Fetal Echocardiogram: A Practical Guide

Balu Vaidyanathan

INTRODUCTION

Prenatal diagnosis of major forms of congenital heart disease (CHD) is eminently feasible in the modern context through ultrasound evaluation during pregnancy. Several approaches to prenatal screening for CHD have been proposed. It is extremely important to remember the fact that most forms of CHD, including the complex ones, occur in low-risk populations with no conventional risk factors for CHD. It is also important to realize that a detailed fetal echocardiography cannot be offered to all low-risk pregnancies on a mass community level. Hence, in the classic 'bottom-up approach', 'basic' or an 'extended basic' evaluation of the fetal heart needs to be performed as a part of the targeted anomaly scan during early to mid-trimester pregnancy evaluation. Referral for a detailed fetal echocardiography is indicated in situations where an anomaly is suspected in the screening or in situations where a detailed evaluation is indicated in view of risk factors (high-risk pregnancies).

This Chapter aims to familiarize the reader with the concept of an 'extended basic' scan in evaluating the fetal heart along with providing a preview into a more detailed approach of performing an exhaustive cardiac evaluation in the fetus. A list of references for further reading is provided at the end of the chapter for the more interested reader to pursue and further his/her knowledge.

The topic shall be discussed under the following headings:
1. Basic considerations, technical factors.
2. Components of the extended basic scan.
3. Views and identification of normal patterns (with illustrations).
4. Basics of Doppler evaluation.
5. Heart rate and rhythm.
6. Cardiac biometry.
7. A brief overview of evaluation of fetal cardiac function and advanced techniques.

BASIC CONSIDERATIONS AND TECHNICAL FACTORS

Timing

The optimal timing of the fetal heart examination needs to be decided considering downstream consequences of a situation where a complex CHD is diagnosed including the option of medical termination of pregnancy as a possible scenario. In our health care scenario, the initial fetal heart screen needs to be completed within the 16-18 weeks gestation window to exclude very complex anomalies (especially those involving the four-chamber view) so that a broad range of management options are made available for the expectant family. Follow-up scans maybe required to evaluate finer structures like pulmonary veins or for confirmation of findings at a later stage of gestation.

Technical Factors

It is a popular misconception amongst obstetric sonographers that imaging of the fetal heart is difficult and can be performed only by experts and using high end equipment. On the contrary, basic views for screening can be obtained under most circumstances once the sonographer is familiar with the protocol. Optimizing the machine settings can help to get the best possible images, even with difficult fetal position and maternal habitus. These include:
- Use of high frequency transducers, preferably curvilinear probes.
- High frame rates (<50 Hz): This may be achieved by a combination of narrowing the image depth and sector width and further enhanced by dynamic zoom capabilities. The image of the heart should fill one-third to one-half of the screen.
- Bring the focal zone to the point of interest to improve the image resolution.
- Cross-sectional gray scale imaging is the mainstay of the fetal cardiac scan. Settings should emphasize high resolution, increased contrast and low persistence.
- The cine-loop feature should be used to assist real-time evaluation of the heart, rather than still images.

COMPONENTS OF THE SCREENING: EXTENDED BASIC SCAN

Guidelines for ultrasound screening of the fetal heart have been laid down by various professional societies. For mass population screening, the four-chamber view was introduced as a 'basic scan' of the fetal heart. However, a substantial proportion of CHDs, especially those involving the outflows were missed by this approach. Hence, the 'extended basic approach' including the evaluation of the size and relationships of the outflow tracts also is recommended for screening in the current guidelines. Fetal echocardiography extends this evaluation further to a more comprehensive segment based evaluation of the heart including Doppler and functional assessment. It is expected that complimenting the four-chamber view with outflow tract evaluation in the cardiac screening will detect most forms of CHD thereby improving antenatal detection rates of CHD.

While performing the fetal heart screening, the transverse sweep with cephalad movement of the transducer from the fetal abdomen through the four-chamber view and towards the upper mediastinum provides the various views for assessment (Sweep technique). Sagittal plane imaging maybe performed in addition to evaluate the arches and get special views of the outflow tracts. The study is completed by performing basic color Doppler evaluation and assessment of the heart rate and rhythm.

STEPS IN FETAL HEART SCREENING

Identification of the Fetal Lie and Laterality

This constitutes the initial step and is particularly important in certain forms of CHD characterized by isomeric patterns. The fetal lie maybe identified easily with reference to the fetal head and spine. Once the lie is identified, the sidedness is best identified by imagining oneself as the fetus and identifying the right and the left sides of the fetus with reference to the maternal abdomen.

Visceral Situs

Once the laterality is identified, one proceeds to ascertaining the position of the stomach and the heart, which are normally on the left side of the fetus.

Recommended View

This is done by obtaining a transverse view of the fetal abdomen just below the diaphragm.

Interpretation

The fetal stomach is imaged on the left side of the abdomen, the descending aorta is to the left of the spine and the inferior vena cava is anterior to the aorta and on the right (Fig. 4.1). By sliding the transducer to the chest, the fetal heart can be imaged pointing to the left on the same side as the stomach. A normal situs is thus determined by locating the stomach, descending aorta and cardiac apex on the left side and the inferior vena cava on the right.

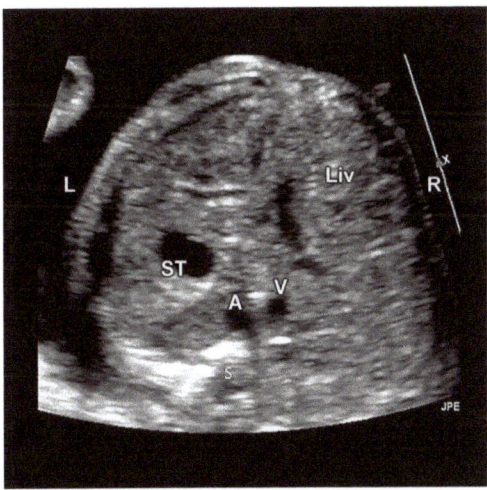

Fig. 4.1: Evaluation of situs: Transverse view of the abdominal situs. The stomach bubble (ST) is seen on the left side while the liver (Liv) on the right side. The aorta (A) is seen to the left of spine (S) while the IVC (V) is seen to the right and anterior to the aorta

Anomalies of the situs are often associated with complex forms of CHD characterized by cardiac and visceral isomerism.

Cardiac Position and Size

The heart is normally on the left size of the fetus and is usually no larger than one-third the area of the chest.

Recommended View

Fetal cardiac dimension can be assessed by measuring the ratio of cardiac circumference or area to the chest circumference or area measured at the level of the fours chamber view (Figs 4.2A and B).

Interpretation

Normal values for the CT circumference is 0.38–0.45 with a slight increase as gestation advances. Value of >0.5 at any stage is abnormal. CT area values are constant throughout pregnancy with normal values ranging from 0.25–0.35.

Cardiac Axis

The normal cardiac axis points to the left by about 45 ± 20 degrees.

Recommended view

This is obtained using a transverse view of the chest at the level of the four-chamber view.

Interpretation

A line is drawn from the spine to the anterior chest wall. The cardiac axis is the angle that the interventricular septum makes with this line (Figs 4.2A and B). Abnormal axis increases the risk of cardiac malformations, especially those involving outflow tracts. This may also be caused by extracardiac anomalies of the lung or diaphragmatic hernias.

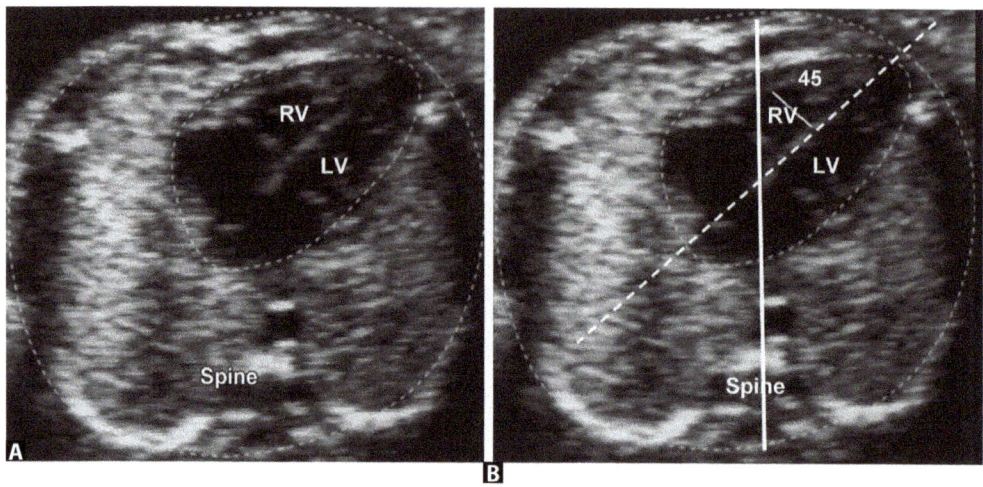

Figs 4.2A and B: Cardiac size and axis: (A) shows measurement of the cardiac size. The circumference of the heart shadow and the chest circumference are traced in the four-chamber view and their ratio gives the cardiac size; (B) Shows the method to measure the cardiac axis. A line is drawn in the plane of the interventricular septum (dotted line) and made to intersect with another drawn from the anterior chest wall to the spine (straight line). The angle subtended by the two lines gives the cardiac axis

Four-chamber View

This involves more than a simple chamber count and the sonographer should pay specific attention to a number of features which identify the normal heart. The four-chamber view is critical since it can identify all forms of complex CHD characterized by a single ventricle physiology.

How to Obtain the View

The view can be obtained in the transverse plane by a cut just above the level of the diaphragm. Three types of four-chamber view can be obtained according to the position of the fetus-apical, basal or long-axis or axial views (Figs 4.3A to C). In the first two views, the ultrasound beam will be parallel to the ventricular septum while in the third the beam will be perpendicular to the septum.

Interpretation

Components of the four-chamber view evaluation includes (Fig. 4.4):

- Assessment of the cardiac size and position as described above.
- Normal heart rate and rhythm.
- Presence of pericardial effusions.
- Identification of atrial chambers. This is best identified with reference to the flap of the fossa ovalis which points towards the left atrium. In addition, in normal hearts, the pulmonary veins can be traced towards joining the left atrium.
- Cardiac crux and atrioventricular junction: The cardiac crux is the point in the center of the heart where the lower rim of the atrial septum (called the septum primum) meets the upper part of the ventricular septum and where the atrioventricular valves insert. Two distinct valves can be imaged opening separately with the septal leaflet of the tricuspid valve (right sided) inserted into the septum closer to the apex compared to the mitral valve (normal offsetting). Abnormalities of the cardiac crux, atrioventricular valves and offsetting are a key sonographic finding

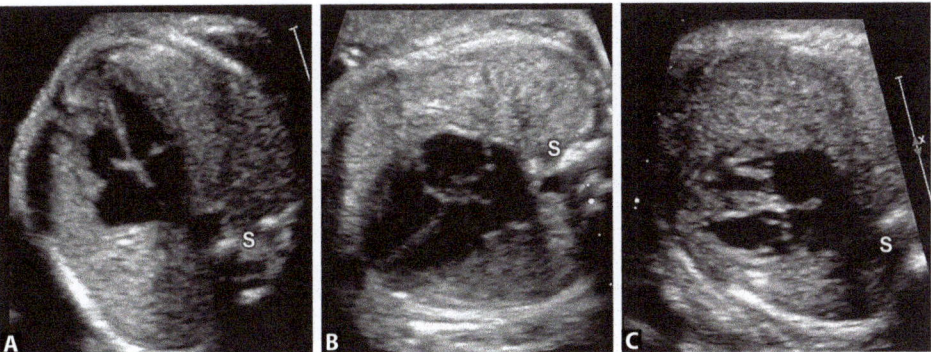

Figs 4.3A to C: The 3 types of four-chamber view: (A) Shows the classic apical four chamber view with the apex pointing upwards. (B) Shows the basal four-chamber view with the apex pointing downwards. (C) Shows the axial four-chamber view, typically seen with the more horizontal fetal lie. The spine position (S) is also depicted in each of these views

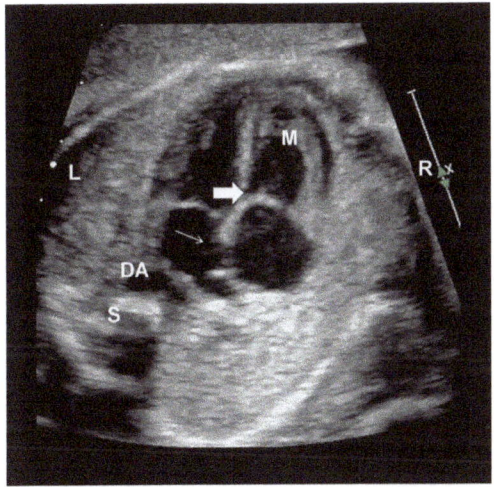

Fig. 4.4: The four-chamber view: Besides the symmetry of the four chambers and the heart size and axis, careful attention should be made to identify the flap of the fossa ovalis as pointing towards the left atrium (small arrow). The cardiac crux with the slightly more apical attachment of the tricuspid valve vis-à-vis the mitral valve (offsetting) is demonstrated (bold arrow). The right ventricle is more coarse and trabeculated and is identified by the moderator band (M). The left ventricle forms the cardiac apex and is smoother. The descending aorta (DA) and spine (S) are posterior to the left atrium and the pulmonary veins can be seen joining the left atrium. A thin rim of pericardial effusion is often found in normal hearts as seen in this picture (around the RV)

for anomalies like atrioventricular septal defect and anomalies associated with atrioventricular discordance like congenitally corrected transposition of great arteries.

- Ventricles: The moderator band, a distinct muscle bundle seen near the apex, helps to identify the morphological right ventricle. The left ventricle in contrast is smooth and forms the apex of the heart. The ventricles should be similar in size and the contractility (squeeze) should be evaluated. Mild asymmetry or disproportion in ventricular sizes may be a clue to obstructive lesions and needs careful evaluation and follow-up for further progression.
- Ventricular septum: This should be evaluated for defects from the apex to the crux. Small septal defects (<2 mm) can be very difficult to confirm during evaluation of the fetal heart and may not have major clinical significance. When the ultrasound beam is directly parallel to the ventricular wall, a false dropout is often imaged near the cardiac crux and this may be reassessed using a different plane of imaging (long axis views).

Outflow Tracts

Evaluation of the left and right ventricular outflow tracts are considered to be an integral part of the fetal heart screening. It is important to assess:

- Normality of the two vessels with connection to the appropriate ventricles.
- The normal "crossing" of the arteries at right angles.
- Relative size and position.
- Adequate opening of the semilunar valves.

How to Get the Views

The sweep technique in the transverse plane is the simplest method to evaluate the outflow tracts. Once the four-chamber view is completed, a further cephalad sweep will reveal the LV outflow and aorta (the five-chamber view) (Fig. 4.5A). A slight cephalad movement of the transducer will image the RV outflow coursing from anterior aspect of chest to the spine from right to left (Fig. 4.5B). In the sagittal plane, it is possible to obtain a short-axis view of the outflow tracts with the aorta in the center and the RV outflow wrapping around it before bifurcating into the branch pulmonary arteries (circle and sausage view) (Fig. 4.6).

Interpretation

In the LVOT view (5-chamber view), continuity should be established between the ventricular septum and the anterior wall of the aorta. The normal aorta courses from the left towards the right first before crossing over to the left again as the arch (Fig. 4.5A). It will be possible to trace the aorta into its arch with the arch vessels originating from it. Outlet VSDs and conotruncal anomalies are detected in this view. The RVOT view confirms the presence of a great vessel originating from the morphological RV and crossing the ascending aorta at right angles. The pulmonary artery can be identified by its bifurcation into the right and left branches on tracing it further (Fig. 4.5B).

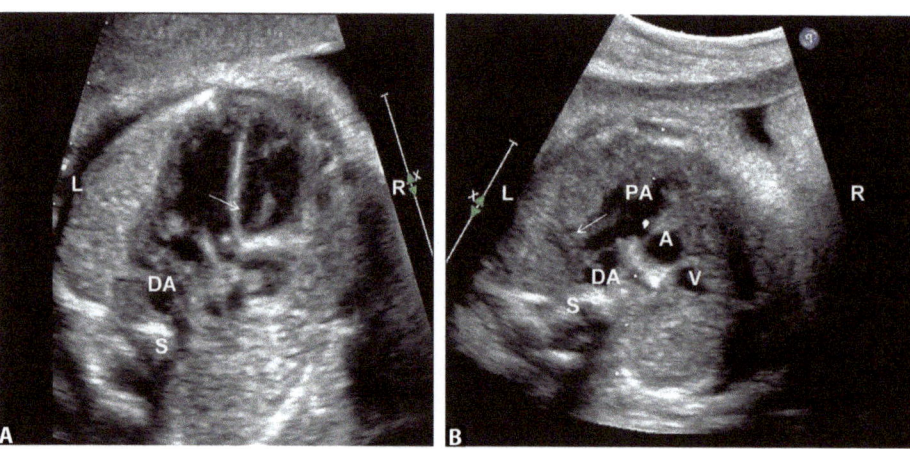

Figs 4.5A and B: The outflow tracts: (A) Shows the left ventricular outflow tract (LVOT) and aorta arising from the LV. The LVOT courses from the left towards the right and continues as the aorta which then courses down the left of spine in the normal left arch. Note the continuity of the ventricular septum with the anterior wall of the aorta (arrow); (B) Shows the right ventricular outflow tract (RVOT) culminating in the 3-vessel view. The RVOT courses from the right towards the left crossing the LVOT at right angles running from the anterior chest wall posteriorly in the direction of the descending aorta (DA) and spine (S). The RVOT is identified by its branching into the branch pulmonary arteries (arrow). The position of the aorta (A) and superior vena cava (V) relative to the main pulmonary artery (PA) are shown in B

How to Perform a Normal Fetal Echocardiogram: A Practical Guide

The Three-vessel and Three-vessel and Tracheal View

This is a view high up in the fetal mediastinum where the two great arteries, the superior vena cava and the trachea can be imaged and their relationships with each other can be defined. This view provides useful information about the number, size and arrangement of the outflow tracts and their spatial relationships and should be done as a part of the extended screening protocol.

How to Get the View

Once the crossing of the outflows are demonstrated, a further cephalad sweep in the transverse plane will show the 3-vessel view (Figs 4.7A and B). A further cephalad sweep will show the 3-vessel and trachea (3VT view) (Figs 4.8A and B).

Interpretation

In the normal 3-vessel view, from left to right, the 3 vessels seen are the pulmonary

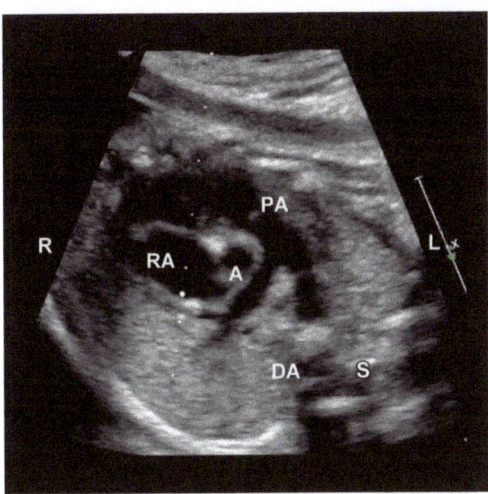

Fig. 4.6: The short axis view of the outflow tracts (Circle and sausage view): This is obtained in the sagittal plane at the level where the outflow tracts cross each other. In this view, the RVOT and main pulmonary artery (PA) wraps around the aorta (A) before bifurcating into the branch pulmonary arteries. The RVOT after bifurcation will continue into the ductal arch connecting with the descending aorta (DA) seen just anterior to the spine (S). RA depicts the right atrium

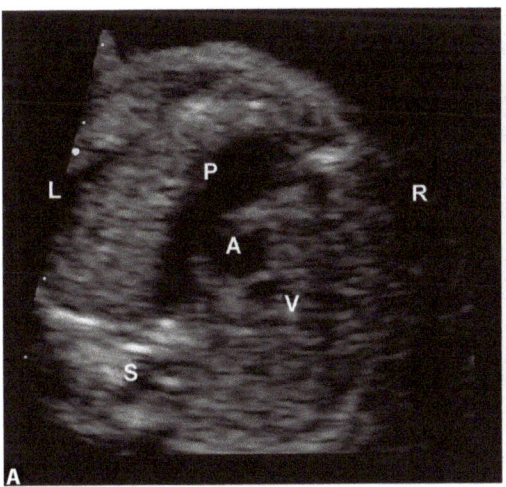
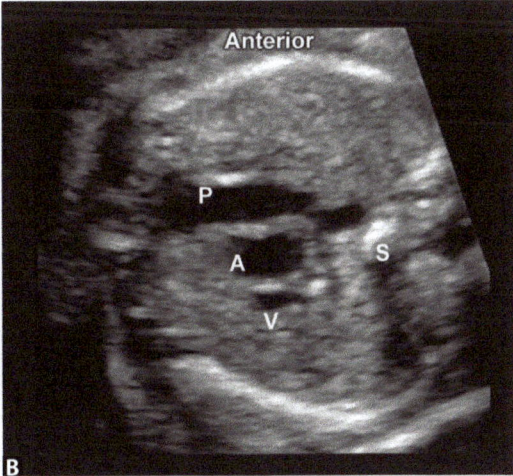

Figs 4.7A and B: The three-vessel view. In this view, one can identify the three vessels from left to right (A) or anterior to posterior (B) as pulmonary artery (PA), aorta (A) and superior vena cava (V). The sizes of the pulmonary artery and aorta can be compared with the PA slightly larger than the aorta

artery, aorta and the superior vena cava. The pulmonary artery is the most anterior and the SVC the most posterior (Figs 4.7A and B). The relative diameters decrease from anterior to posterior with the PA being the largest vessel. CHDs associated with normal four-chamber view like transposition of great arteries, tetralogy of Fallot and pulmonary atresia with VSD are likely to have an abnormal 3-vessel view. Discrepant sizes of the outflow tracts in the 3-vessel view (e.g. smaller aorta vis-á-vis pulmonary artery) provides a valuable clue to the possibility of outflow tract obstructions like coarctation of aorta.

In the 3-vessel tracheal view (3VT view), the relationship of the ductal and aortic arches with the trachea can be imaged. Normally the ductal and aortic arches are positioned to the left of the trachea and they form a 'V' shape as they both join the descending aorta (Fig. 4.8A). Color flow imaging will show this classical V shape with same direction of flow in both arches (Fig. 4.8B). The trachea is identified as a hyperechoic ring lying outside the V. The 3VT view is useful in identifying abnormalities of the arches like right or double aortic arch, aberrant right subclavian artery, etc. Measurement of the isthmus size and isthmus duct ratios may enable suspicion of coarctation of aorta especially in setting where there is associated ventricular disproportion as well. The isthmus to duct ratio should be more than 0.75.

Additional Views: The Sagittal Plane

The transverse sweep technique as described above provides a complete assessment of the situs and intracardiac anatomy and evaluation of the outflow tracts including the ductal and aortic arches. If feasible, additional information about the arches can be obtained in the sagittal plane. The ductal arch is typically seen as a 'hockeystick' shaped structure as the continuation of the main pulmonary artery into the descending aorta (Fig. 4.9). The aortic arch is the most cephalad structure and is identified by its more rounded contour like a 'cane handle' and by the origin of the neck vessels (Fig. 4.10).

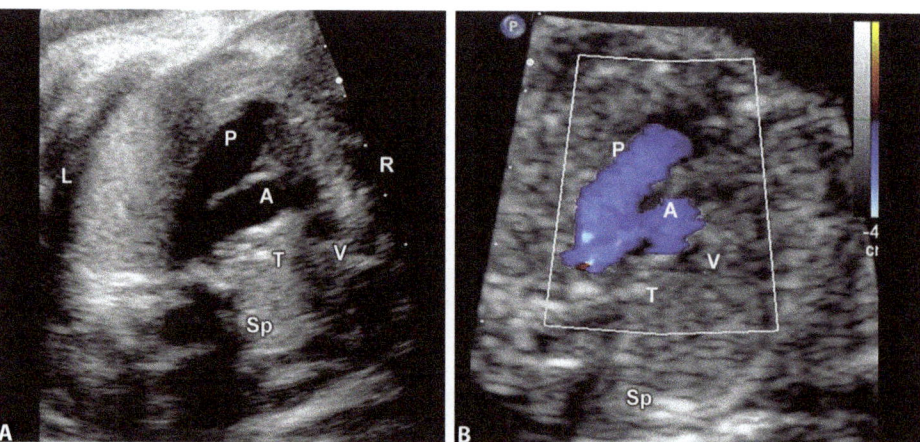

Figs 4.8A and B: Three-vessel tracheal view (3VT view): (A) Shows the 3VT view and the relation of the arch confluence in relation to the trachea (T) and spine (Sp). In the normal left arch, the confluence of the ductal (P) and aortic (A) arches form a V on the left side of the trachea. The SVC (V) will be seen on the right side. The trachea will lie outside the V. (B) Shows color flow in the 3VT view with the same flow direction in both the arches

How to Get the Views

From the 3-vessel view, align the pulmonary artery to the descending aorta vertically and then rotate the transducer through 90° to get the sagittal view of the ductal arch. In the same manner, aligning the ascending aorta to the descending aorta vertically with 90° rotation will show the aortic arch in the sagittal plane.

Sagittal plane imaging also is useful in evaluating the systemic veins, especially confirming the patency of the inferior vena cava. The bicaval or hammock view is obtained at the level of the abdominal situs by a 90° rotation from the transverse plane. Both the vena cava can be seen joining the right atrium in this view (Fig. 4.11) with the ductus venosus joining the inferior vena cava just prior to its joining the right atrium.

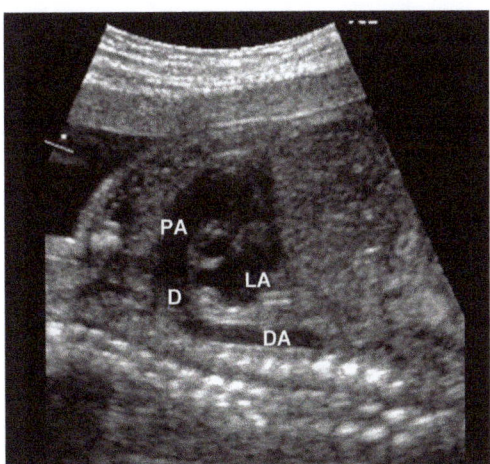

Fig. 4.9: Sagittal view of the ductal arch: The typical hockeystick appearance of the ductal arch is clearly seen. The pulmonary artery (PA) continues as the ductus arteriosus (D) and joins the descending aorta (DA). The left atrium (LA) is imaged between the PA and descending aorta

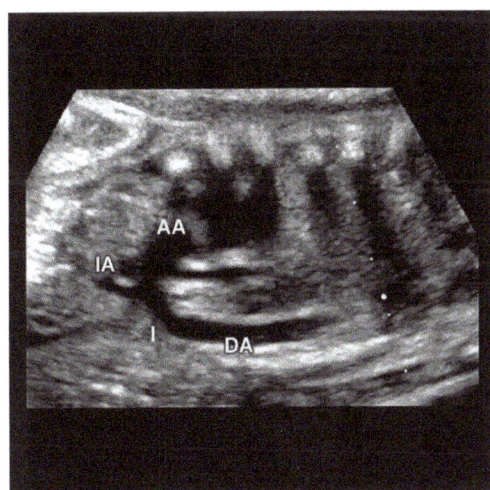

Fig. 4.10: Sagittal view of the aortic arch: The typical cane handle appearance of the aortic arch is seen. The ascending aorta continues as the isthmus (I) into the descending aorta. The innominate artery (IA) is seen as the first branch of the aortic arch. This will be followed by the left common carotid and left subclavian arteries in the normal arch

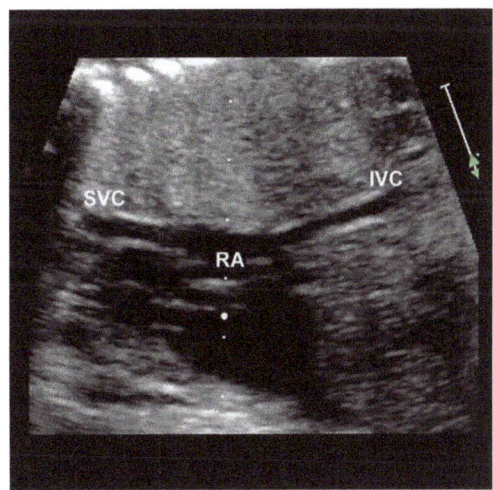

Fig. 4.11: The bicaval view: This is also referred to as the hammock view. This is obtained in the longitudinal plane of the abdominal situs where the inferior vena cava (IVC) and the superior vena cava (SVC) are seen joining the right atrium (RA). The ductus venosus can be seen joining the IVC in this view

COLOR DOPPLER IMAGING

Color flow mapping facilitates imaging of cardiac structures as well as highlighting abnormal blood flow patterns. It is a valuable tool in the evaluation of cardiac anatomy in situations of poor acoustic windows and may facilitate detection of major CHD in low-risk pregnancies. Optimal color settings include the use of narrow color box (region of interest), appropriate pulse repetition frequency, low color persistence and adequate gain settings.

Color Doppler imaging should evaluate flows through the systemic and pulmonary veins (including the ductus venosus), foramen ovale, atrioventricular valves, atrial and ventricular septa (Fig. 4.12A), semilunar valves and the ductal and aortic arches. Low-flow power Doppler color imaging is particularly useful in evaluating the pulmonary vein connections (Fig. 4.12B). An attempt should be made to see at least 2 pulmonary veins draining into the left atrium. Color flow imaging of the 3 vessel tracheal view is often very helpful in identifying normal arch patterns in first trimester pregnancy scans (Fig. 4.8B).

HEART RATE AND RHYTHM ASSESSMENT

This evaluation can be performed either by the Doppler technique or M-mode interrogation. A normal fetal heart rate at mid-gestation is 120 to 180 beats per minute. For the evaluation of the cardiac rhythm, simultaneous assessment of the atrial and ventricular contraction should be performed using either simultaneous Doppler sonography of the mitral inflow-aortic outflow (Fig. 4.13) or M-mode sonography of the atrium and ventricle (Fig. 4.14). Additional methods to evaluate the rhythm include simultaneous superior vena cava-ascending aorta Doppler or tissue Doppler sonography.

CARDIAC BIOMETRY

Normal ranges for fetal cardiac measurements have been published as percentiles and Z-scores based on gestational age or fetal biometry. Individual measurements can be determined from 2-dimensional or M-mode images and may include the following parameters:

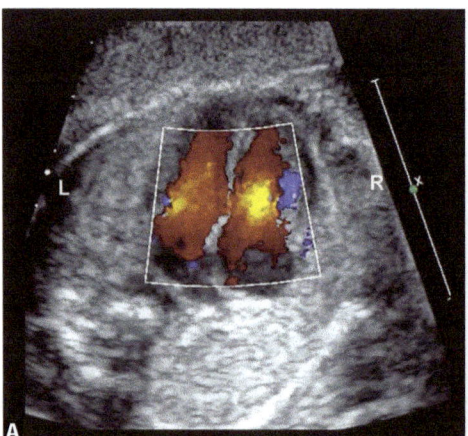 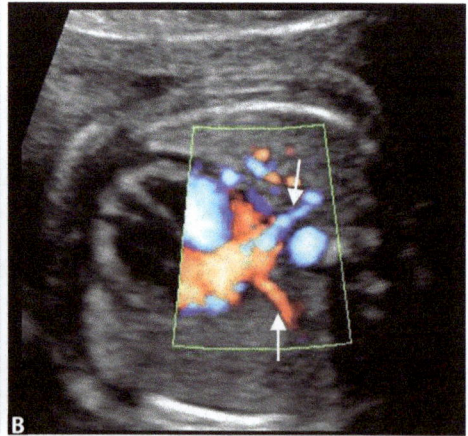

Figs 4.12A and B: Color Doppler evaluation: (A) Shows the four-chamber view color flow mapping. The atrioventricular valve flow is unidirectional with no regurgitation. The ventricular septum also is mapped for any defects. (B) Shows high definition color flow mapping of the left atrium for pulmonary veins. Two pulmonary veins (arrows) are clearly seen joining the left atrium

- Aortic and pulmonary valve annulus in systole.
- Tricuspid and mitral valve annulus in diastole.
- Right and left ventricular length.
- Aortic arch and isthmus diameter.
- Main pulmonary artery and ductus arteriosus diameter.
- End-diastolic ventricular diameter just inferior to atrioventricular valve leaflets.
- Cardiothoracic ratio.

Comparison of the diameters of the great vessels (main pulmonary artery to aorta diameter) as well as the isthmus to duct diameter ratio are useful in assessing the severity of outflow obstruction in CHD like tetralogy of Fallot and coarctation of aorta respectively.

CARDIAC FUNCTION ASSESSMENT

Right and left heart function should be qualitatively assessed in all studies. If abnormal function is suspected, quantitative assessment of the heart function should be considered and can include measures like fractional shortening, ventricular strain and the myocardial performance index. The prognosis of some forms of fetal heart failure can be assessed and followed up using the cardiovascular profile (CVP) score. This score includes parameters like venous Doppler evaluation (umbilical vein and ductus venosus), heart size, cardiac function, arterial Doppler (umbilical artery) and presence of hydrops. Similarly evaluation of the pulmonary venous Doppler patterns is found to be useful is evaluating the adequacy of the fossa ovalis in situations like hypoplastic left heart syndrome. The interested reader may refer of one of the suggested readings for a further understanding of this topic.

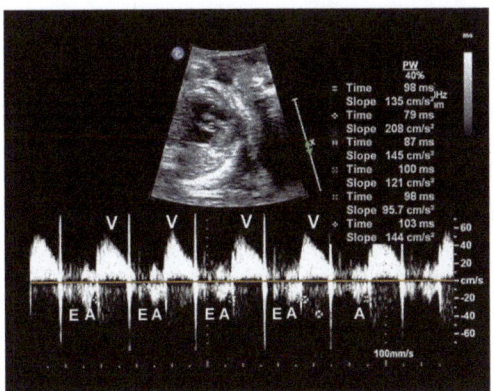

Fig. 4.13: Pulse wave Doppler for rate and rhythm: This Figure shows a typical left ventricular inflow-outflow Doppler. The atrial component shows 2 waves the E and the A wave depicting atrial filling in early and late diastole. In the fetus, typically the A wave is more dominant than the E wave suggesting the altered diastolic compliance patterns. The V wave demonstrates the outflow signal in the aorta. Note the 1:1 relation between the atrial and ventricular wave signals. The A-V interval can be measured and it indicates the mechanical PR interval in the fetus

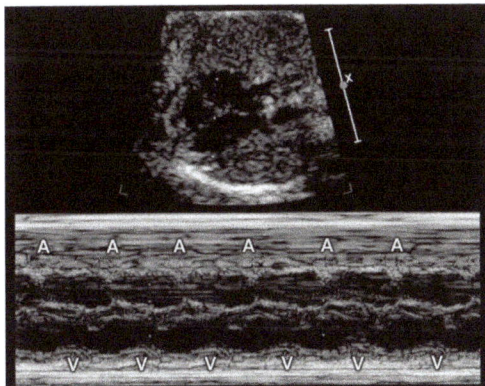

Fig. 4.14: M-mode evaluation: The M-mode cursor is used to get simultaneous sections of the atria and ventricles. The M-mode recording shows both the atrial (A) and the ventricular (V) waves showing a 1:1 relationship between them. Note that the ventricular waves follow the atrial waves depicting the normal atrioventricular conduction

COMPLEMENTARY IMAGING STRATEGIES

Newer imaging modalities like 3-and 4-dimensional sonography and spatio-temporal image correlation (STIC) have been used to evaluate anatomic defects like conotruncal malformations, aortic arch anomalies and abnormal pulmonary vein return. These modalities are also used for quantifying fetal hemodyanamic parameters like cardiac output. Tissue Doppler and strain rate imaging may help in evaluation of the fetal ventricular function.

REPORTING AND DOCUMENTATION

Reporting and documentation should be in accordance with the recognized practice guidelines for documentation and communication of diagnostic ultrasound findings. Both motion video clips as well as still images should be used to store the data. Digital video clips should include at least the following in both gray scale as well as color Doppler techniques: the 4-chamber view, left and right ventricular outflow tracts, 3-vessel and trachea view and sagittal aortic and ductal arches. Variations from normal size should be accompanied by measurements. An official interpretation (final report) of the diagnostic findings should be included in the patient's medical record.

SUGGESTED READING

1. Abuhamad A, Chaoui R. A practical guide to fetal echocardiography. Normal and Abnormal Hearts. 2010;2.
2. American Institute of Ultrasound in Medicine. AIUM practice guideline for the performance of fetal echocardiography. J Ultrasound Med. 2013;32:1067-82. Doi:10.7863/ultra.32.6.1067.
3. Carvalho JS, Allan LD, Chaoui R, Copel JA, DeVore GR, Hecher K, et al. ISUOG practice guidelines (updated): Sonographic examination of the fetal heart. Ultrasound Obstet Gynecol. 2013;41:348-59.
4. Donofrio MT, Moon-Grady AJ, Hornberger LK, Copel JA, Sklansky MS, Abuhamad A, et al. Diagnosis and treatment of fetal cardiac disease. A scientific statement from the American Heart Association. Circulation. 2014; 129:2183-242.
5. Lee W, Allan L, Carvalho JS, Chaoui R, Copel J, DeVoe G, et al. ISUOG Consensus statement: what constitutes a fetal echocardiogram? Ultrasound Obstet Gynecol. 2008;32: 239-42.

CHAPTER 5

Fetal Cardiac Defects

BS Ramamurthy

ABSTRACT

Congenital cardiac anomalies are one of the leading causes of neonatal morbidity and mortality. They are also one of the most commonly missed anomalies on antenatal scans. Most fetal cardiac defects are seen in the general low-risk pregnancy population, hence it is important to thoroughly screen all pregnancies for cardiac anomalies in the basic antenatal ultrasound examination. The etiology of cardiac defects is in most cases multifactorial. Small proportion of cases may be due to chromosomal or single gene disorders. Proper equipment settings are very important both for grey scale and color Doppler imaging. The fetal cardia should be examined as a whole organ (situs, size, axis and position) first and then the cardiac connections (sequential segmental analysis) are to be studied.

In the four-chamber view the following could be the first abnormality to be recognized leading on to the complete diagnosis: Inability to visualize the normal crux [septum primum atrial septal defect (ASD), inlet ventricular septal defect (VSD), artrioventricular septal defects (AVSD) and single ventricle pathologies], chamber disproportion (hypoplastic left heart syndrome, coarctation of aorta, critical aortic stenosis, pulmonary atresia with intact septum, Ebstein anomaly, tricuspid dysplasia and critical pulmonary stenosis), chamber attributes (congenital corrected transposition of great arteries) and area behind the heart (total anomalous pulmonary venous connection, heterotaxies).

When there is a malalignment VSD with an overriding aorta the final diagnosis could be a tetralogy of Fallot, pulmonary atresia with VSD, absent pulmonary valve syndrome or common arterial trunk. Parallel great arteries could lead to a diagnosis of congenital transposition of great arteries or double outlet right ventricle.

The three vessel trachea view in addition to aiding the diagnosis of outflow tract anomalies contributes to the diagnosis of arch anomalies (right aortic arch, interrupted aortic arch and double aortic arch).

Thus, we see that a systematic examination using the standard planes of section is necessary for the recognition of findings. Integrating these findings together yields the final diagnosis. Complementation by recognition of extracardiac anomalies, karyotype and FISH results in a total fetal diagnosis. The pediatric cardiologist is thus equipped with the whole information which is vital for counseling and for further management.

INTRODUCTION

Congenital cardiac anomalies are one of the leading causes of neonatal morbidity and mortality. They are also one of the most commonly missed anomalies on antenatal scans.

The incidence of moderate to severe forms of CHD is about 6/1000 live births. If bicuspid aortic valves, small muscular ventricular septal defects (VSD) and other trivial defects are included the incidence is as great as 75/1000 live births. The incidence of congenital cardiac anomalies is even greater prenatally considering pregnancy terminations and fetuses with severe cardiac malformations that may be still-born. This makes cardiac anomalies amongst the most common fetal defects.

Of these only 10 to 20% are found in high-risk pregnancies with known risk factors for heart defects. The remaining 80 to 90% of cases are incidentally found in low-risk pregnancies on routine antenatal screening. Hence, it is important to thoroughly screen all pregnancies for cardiac anomalies in the basic antenatal ultrasound examination.

Multiple factors have been implicated in the pathogenesis of cardiac anomalies. They include chromosomal (trisomies 13, 18 and 21, Turner syndrome and 22q deletion), genetic (Holt Oram, Apert, Noonan and Ellis-van Creveld syndromes), teratogens (rubella, mumps, lithium, alcohol, phenytoin, and diabetes). Most cases have a multifactorial etiology. The recurrence of cardiac anomalies in future pregnancies increases if the cause is multifactorial. Recurrence rates quoted are 2–5% after one affected child, 5–10% after two affected children and 1–10% if one of the parents is affected.

There are two time windows for the assessment of the fetal heart. The first is the early echocardiography done between 11 and 14 weeks. Increased NT, tricuspid regurgitation and ductus venosus late diastolic reversals are not only markers of aneuploidy but also of fetal cardiac defects. The other window is the mid-trimester anomaly scan period between 18 and 23 weeks. One can attempt to perform first trimester echocardiography only if one is well-versed with mid-trimester echocardiography.

Image optimization is by using the highest transducer frequency possible, tissue harmonics, narrow imaging field, low persistence, high contrast, optimum zoom and a single focus. Color Doppler settings would include high velocity scale, high wall filter, just big enough color box and appropriate color gain and power settings.

The scheme adopted in this Chapter is to highlight the abnormality that may be recognized by an examiner and how to proceed thereafter to arrive at a complete diagnosis. The following is the layout of this Chapter:

A. Examine the heart as a whole organ: 1. Situs, 2. Size, 3. Axis, 4. Position.
B. Examine the heart as a set of chambers, vessels and their connections: 5. Four-chamber view, 6. Left ventricular outflow tract, 7. Right ventricular outflow tract, and 8. The three vessel view.

The heart should be first examined as a whole organ in terms of situs, size, axis, position and squeeze. One should then study the cardiac structure in terms of the chambers and vessels and their connections. Sequential segmental analysis is the term used to systematically examine the cardiac connections (venoatrial, atrioventricular and ventriculoarterial).

The sign of abnormality may be encountered at any of the following stages of examination:

1. *Situs abnormality:* An abnormal situs is associated with a higher incidence of congenital heart defects. Describing below the types of situs abnormalities and the association of congenital heart defects in each

one of them. Determination of situs is the first step in fetal echocardiography. An abnormal situs could be the first clue to a cardiac defect (which may range from a simple VSD to a complex cardiac defect)(Fig. 5.1). The upper abdominal transverse section is an integral view in assessment of situs and abnormalities thereof. Liver to right, stomach to the left, descending aorta to the left and inferior vena cava (IVC) to the right and anterior to the aorta is the normal spatial arrangement. Some of the abnormalities seen in this section are:

a. Mirror image arrangement seen in situs inversus totalis.
b. Stomach to the right (heart and stomach on opposite sides), close to spine, midline large liver and absent spleen in heterotaxy. Occasionally, the stomach is in the midline in heterotaxy.
c. Juxtaposed IVC (IVC anterior and on the same side of the aorta) is seen in right atrial isomerism.
d. Absent or interrupted IVC is seen in left atrial isomerism. This is accompanied by azygos prominence (*refer* to section behind the heart).
e. The absence of ductus venosus may be recognized in this upper abdominal plane. This is a rare anomaly. In subgroup I, the umbilical venous return bypasses the liver and directly drains into the IVC, iliac vein, renal vein, right atrium or the coronary sinus. There is cardiomegaly due to cardiac volume overload (Figs 5.1 to 5.3). In subgroup II, the umbilical vein connects normally with the portal sinus, but the ductus venosus is absent. Associated cardiac/extracardiac anomalies, syndromes (Noonan, VACTERL, Smith-Lemli Opitz, etc.) and aneuploidy should be looked for.

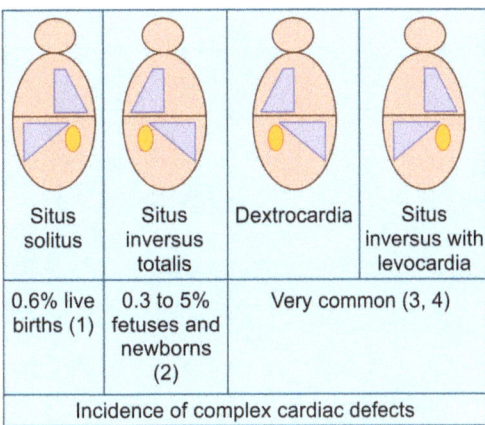

Situs solitus	Situs inversus totalis	Dextrocardia	Situs inversus with levocardia
0.6% live births (1)	0.3 to 5% fetuses and newborns (2)	Very common (3, 4)	

Incidence of complex cardiac defects

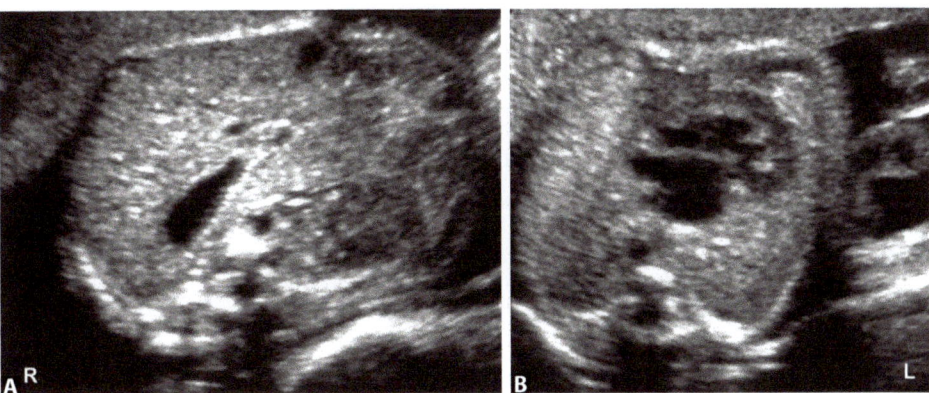

Figs 5.1A and B: Situs inversus with levocardia (stomach to the right and apex of cardia to the left). Note single inlet single ventricle (with malposed great arteries and pulmonary stenosis)

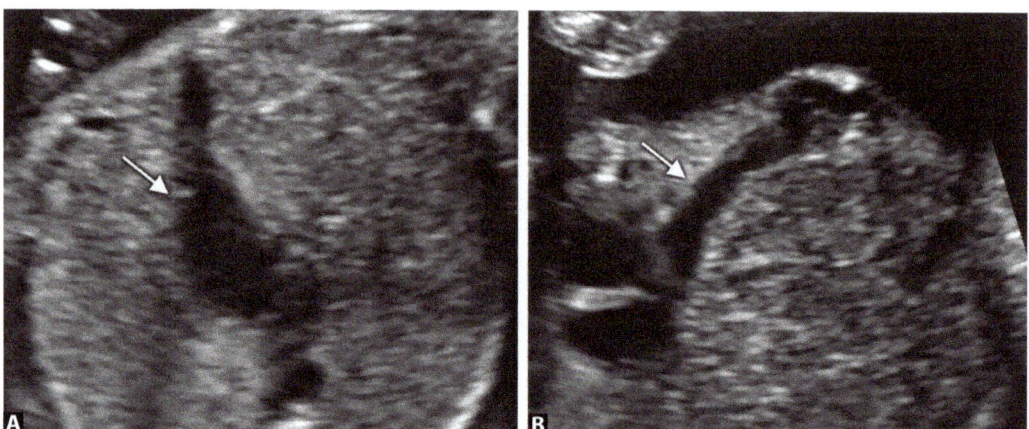

Figs 5.2A and B: Absent ductus venosus with liver bypass (A and B) Umbilical vein directly confluencing with the right atrium. Note the typical course of the umbilical vein anterior and superior to the liver

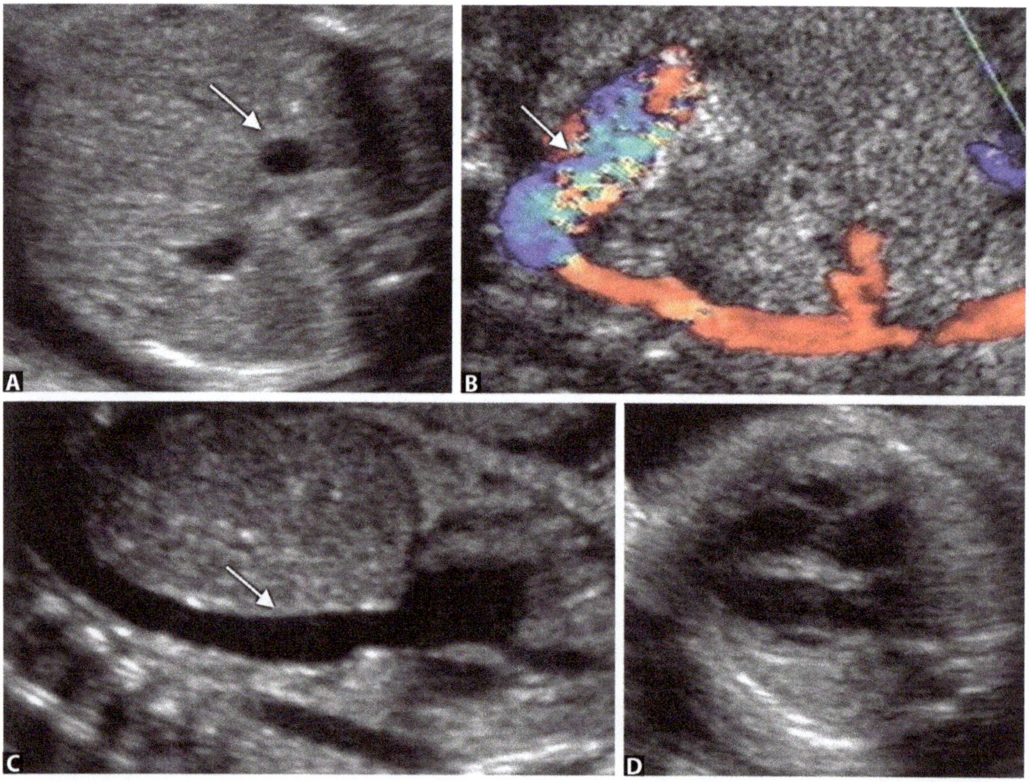

Figs 5.3A to D: Absent ductus venosus (DV) with liver bypass (A) DV not seen, IVC is dilated (arrow); (B) The umbilical vein (arrow) is draining into the right iliac vein consequently IVC is dilated (solid arrow); (C) Dilated IVC in hammock view; (D) Cardiomegaly

2. *Cardiac size:* Cardiac size is most often assessed subjectively. Objective assessment may be done by the cardiothoracic (CT) ratio. Area CT ratio and perimeter CT ratio of more than 35% and 50% respectively indicate cardiomegaly. Cardiomegaly could occur in valvular regurgitation (e.g. Ebstein anomaly), dilated cardiomyopathy, cardiac failure due to fetal acidemia, anemia or arrhythmia (Fig. 5.4).

3. *Cardiac axis:* Left axis rotation is associated with outflow tract anomalies (tetralogy of Fallot), as also in Ebstein anomaly and coarctation of aorta (Fig. 5.5). In a series of 34 cases of left axis rotation (defined as more than 75° rotation) 61.7% association with cardiac anomalies was reported.

4. *Cardiac position:* Any space occupying lesion or pathology in one hemithorax shifts the mediastinum (cardia) to the opposite side. Typical examples include congenital diaphragmatic hernia, congenital pulmonary airway malformation, pleural effusion and large bronchogenic cysts (Fig. 5.6A). Unilateral pulmonary aplasia or hypoplasia causes ipsilateral mediastinal shift (Fig. 5.6B). Cardiac shift to the right or left is referred to as dextroposition or levoposition respectively.

5. *Four-chamber view:*
   a. **Loss of AV offset/failure to identify the crux:** The crux of the cardia is not seen in septum primum atrial septal defect (ASD), inlet ventricular septal defect (VSD), and complete atrioventricular septal defect (AVSD). There is loss of offset between the mitral and tricuspid valves (linear insertion) in all these instances. The crux is also not seen in single ventricle pathology and in cases of gross chamber disproportion.

   Septum primum ASD: There is a gap in the septum primum in the region of its attachment to the crux (Fig. 5.7). In some instances, there may be a total absence of the septum primum. The mitral and tricuspid valve annuli are distinct. This lesion is also termed as partial AVSD. A dilated coronary sinus due to persistent left superior vena cava is often misinterpreted as a septum primum ASD. Associated cardiac malformations include complete AVSD,

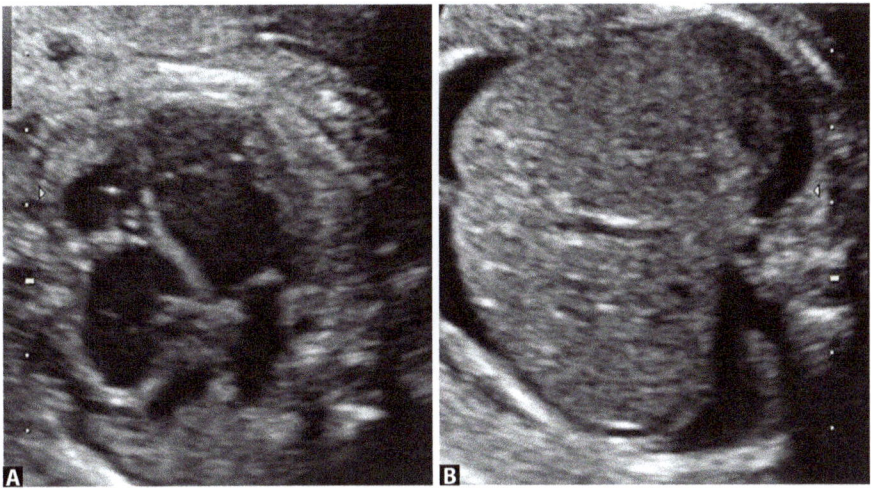

Figs 5.4A and B: Obvious cardiomegaly in a case of dilated cardiomyopathy. The myocardial contractility was poor. Note the presence of early ascites and right pleural effusion indicating cardiac failure

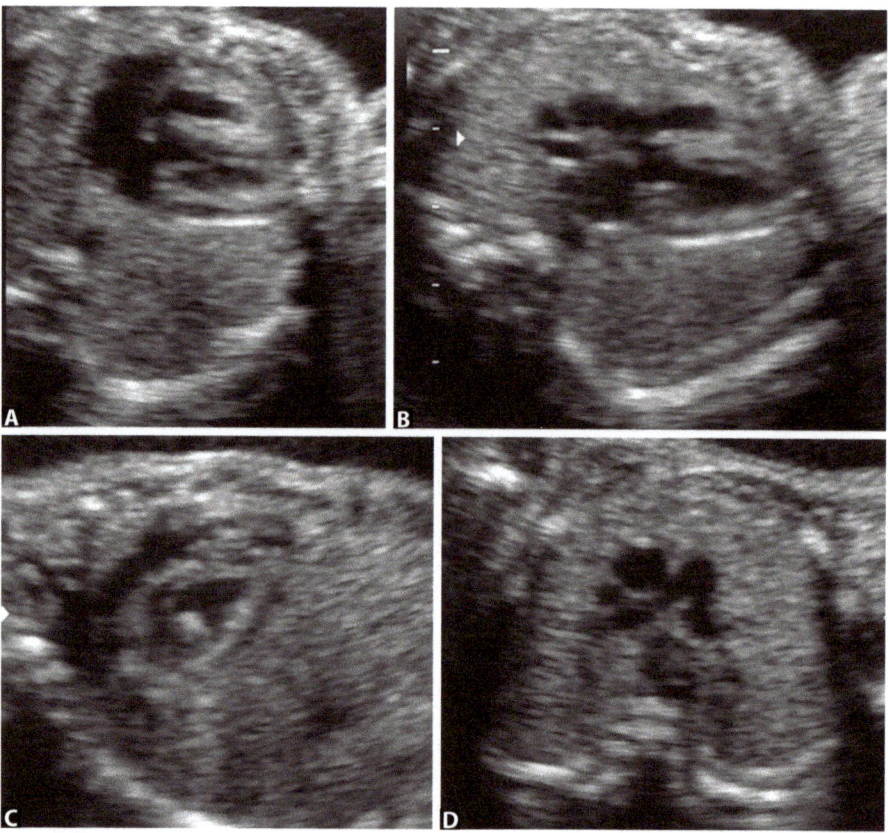

Figs 5.5A to D: Left axis deviation (A), Malalignment ventricular septal defect and overriding aortic root (B), narrow right ventricular outflow tract (C) and narrow pulmonary artery, anterior placed aorta in three vessel view (D) in tetralogy of Fallot

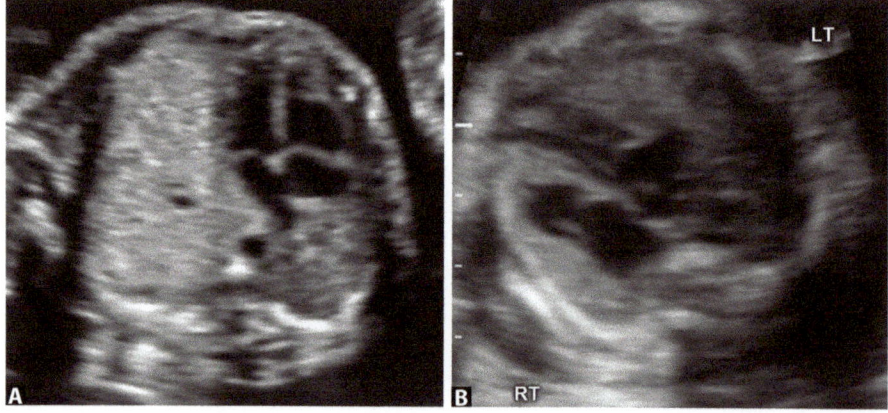

Figs 5.6A and B: (A) Cardiac shift to the right due to left lung congenital pulmonary airway malformation; (B) Cardiac shift to the right due to right lung hypoplasia

Fetal Cardiac Defects

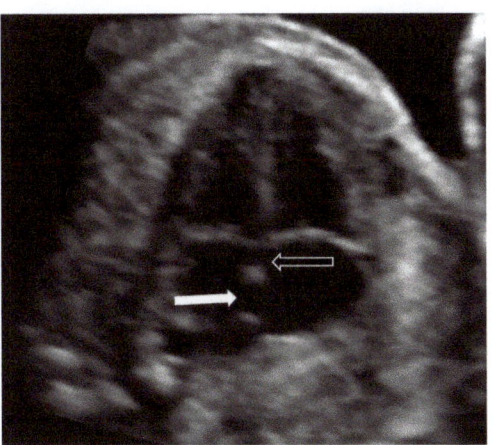

Fig. 5.7: Gap in the septum primum (open arrow) in a fetus with septum primum ASD. Note the linear insertion of the mitral and tricuspid valve leaflets. The foramen ovale is marked by the solid arrow

single ventricle, anomalous pulmonary venous drainage, Ebstein anomaly, and pulmonary atresia with intact ventricular septum. Fetal karyotyping is indicated as septum primum ASD is a marker for Down syndrome.

Fossa ovalis ASDs though commonest cannot be reliably predicted prenatally. Sinus venosus ASD has not been diagnosed in utero.

Inlet VSD: Gap in the inlet ventricular septum at the crux seen in the four-chamber view between the atrioventricular valves is diagnostic of a inlet VSD (Fig. 5.8). These defects can sometimes be very subtle. Linear insertion of the atrioventricular valves may arouse suspicion of the lesion. The mitral and tricuspid valve annuli are distinct. This lesion is also classified as a partial AVSD. The ventricular septal drop out artifact is a major pitfall. This may be resolved by a transverse or lateral four-chamber view where the ventricular septum is seen to reach up to the crux in the case of drop out artifact. Over writing by color Doppler signals (bleeding artifact)

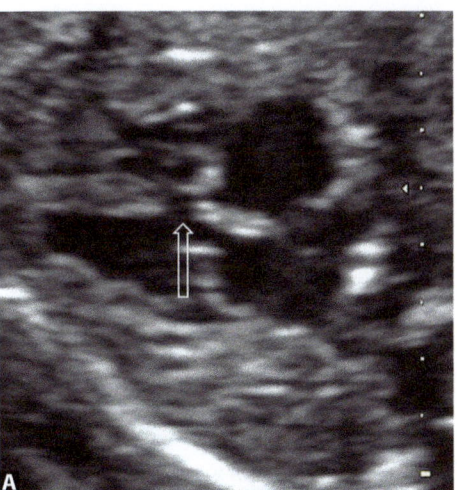

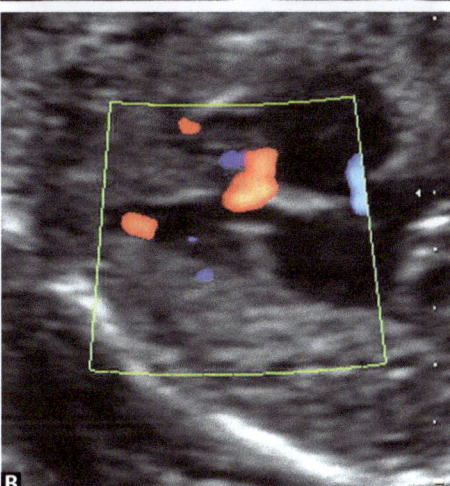

Figs 5.8A and B: (A) Gap in the inlet ventricular septum (open arrow) in a fetus with inlet VSD. Since the defect is seen in the transverse four-chamber view, the possibility of drop out artifact is ruled out; (B) Color Doppler flow across the defect

may sometimes mimic the presence of a VSD. Proper equipment settings will correct the artifact. Inlet VSDs account for only a minority of all VSDs (5 to 8%). Bidirectional flow in systole and diastole may be demonstrated by color Doppler in the lateral four-chamber view. Fetal karyotyping is indicated mainly to rule out Down syndrome.

Atrioventricular septal defect: Septum primum ASD, inlet VSD and an abnormal common (single) atrioventricular annulus are the components of the complete form of AVSD. The single atrioventricular inflow may stream selectively into one of the ventricles resulting in ventricular disproportion resulting in unbalanced complete AVSD (cf balanced complete AVSD where the ventricles are equal in size). In systole, there is loss of offset between the septal tricuspid leaflet and the anterior mitral leaflet. This results in a cycle bar or boomerang appearance of the valve leaflets. In diastole, there is a gap in the region of the crux due to absence of the septal structures (Fig. 5.9). The atrioventricular length (AVL) ratio is increased to more than 0.6 in 83% of cases.

Subtle AVSDs may be missed on the lateral four-chamber view but may be evident on apical four-chamber view. Bradycardia should prompt the presence of an atrioventricular block and appropriate evaluation with M mode and spectral Doppler. AVSD may be recognized in the first trimester around 12 to 13 weeks. Association with a thick nuchal translucency may be extant. Single atrioventricular stream dividing over the crest of the ventricular septal defect can be demonstrated on color Doppler (Fig. 5.10A). Selective streaming into the dominant ventricle may be demonstrated in the unbalanced forms. Atrioventricular regurgitation if present may be demon-strated arising from the center of the atrioventricular valve (Fig. 5.10B). Differen-tial diagnosis is single ventricle pathology.

Associated cardiac findings may include outflow abnormalities as double outlet right ventricle, conotruncal anomalies, right aortic arch, pulmonary and systemic vein anomalies. Unbalanced forms of AVSD may be associated with heterotaxy. Features which should suggest the presence of heterotaxy are situs abnormality (midline liver, asplenia), juxtaposed IVC,

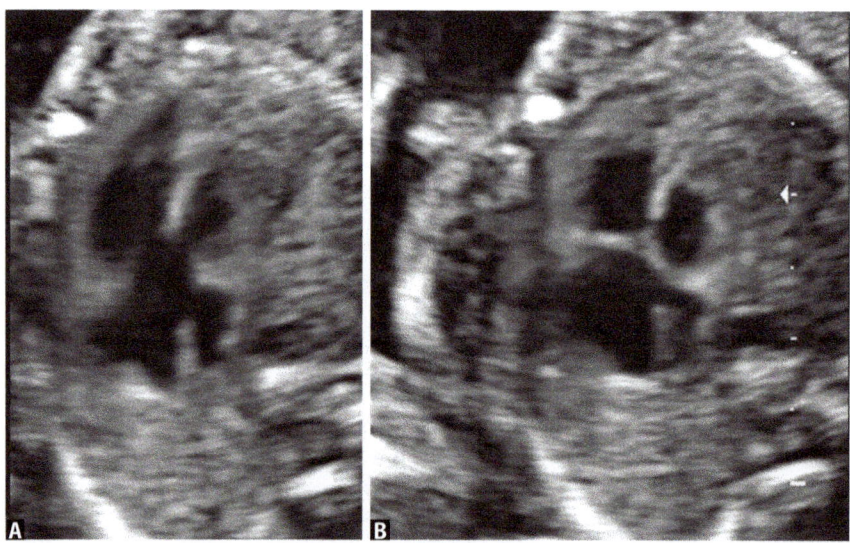

Figs 5.9A and B: Complete-balanced atrioventricular defect: (A) In diastole, the single atrioventricular tract and absent crux are notable; (B) In systole, the bar or boomerang linear form of the atrioventricular valve is well seen. The increased atrial length is evident

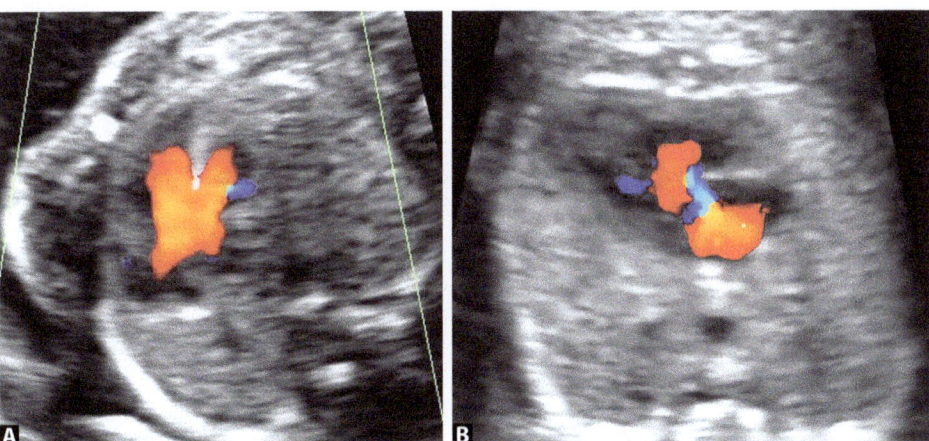

Figs 5.10A and B: Complete-balanced atrioventricular defect. (A) In diastole, the single atrioventricular flow forking over the ventricular septal defect noted; (B) In systole, the regurgitant stream is seen in blue with aliasing indicating high velocity

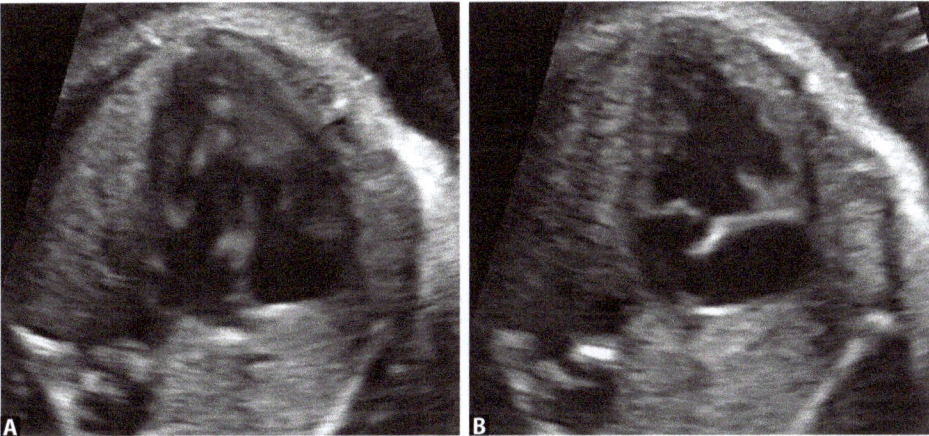

Figs 5.11A and B: Double inlet single ventricle. (A) In diastole, the two atrioventricular valves are open; (B) In systole, the two atrioventricular valves are closed

anomalous pulmonary venous connection and malposed great arteries.

Univentricular atrioventricular connection: Single functioning ventricle is the hallmark of this group of disorders. There could be two atria or one atrium connecting with the single ventricle through two or one patent atrioventricular valves resulting in either double inlet single ventricle or single inlet single ventricle (Figs 5.11 and 5.12). Very rarely there could be two atria connecting with a single ventricle through a single atrioventricular valve. The single ventricle is commonly of left ventricular morphology (smooth interior) with a rudimentary right ventricle. Double inlet left ventricle (DILV) contributes to 80% of this group of disorders. A small outlet right ventricle is seen supporting one of the great arteries. The outlet chamber

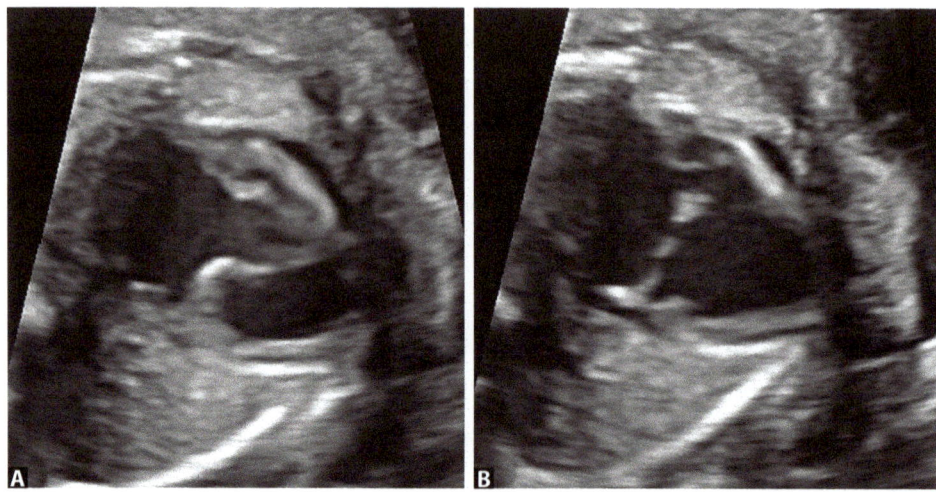

Figs 5.12A and B: Single inlet single ventricle. (A) In diastole, the single atrioventricular valve is open; (B) In systole, the single atrioventricular valve is closed

communicates with the single ventricle through a bulboventricular foramen. The outlet chamber may not be seen in the typical 'four-chamber view', but in a more cranial plane commonly to the left of the single ventricle. The great arteries are in D or L malposition. One or both great arteries may arise from the outlet chamber. Narrow caliber of one of the great arteries could be due to pulmonary stenosis or aortic coarctation. Heterotaxy should be ruled out. Chromosomal abnormality is unusual. Differential diagnosis for single ventricular pathology include pulmonary atresia with intact ventricular septum, hypoplastic left heart syndrome, unbalanced atrioventricular septal defect, tricuspid atresia with VSD and mitral atresia with VSD.

b. **Chamber disproportion:** Chamber disproportion could be due to enlargement or reduction in size of a cardiac chamber. A fetal cardiac chamber fails to grow normally if the quantity of blood flowing through it is less or absent. This typically happens in valvular stenosis or atresia. Valvular regurgitation on the other hand causes dilatation of the upstream chamber primarily and the downstream chamber secondarily. The end result in valvular lesions is chamber disproportion. Atretic lesions of the mitral or aortic valves results in hypoplastic left heart syndrome.

Critical aortic stenosis also presents as reduced left sided chamber size. The only non-valvular lesion to cause diminution of the left-sided chambers is coarctation of aorta.

Tricuspid atresia with VSD, pulmonary atresia with intact ventricular septum and critical pulmonary stenosis result in reduced right-sided chamber size. Ebstein anomaly and tricuspid dysplasia result in tricuspid regurgitation and enlargement of the right-sided chambers.

Hypoplastic left heart syndrome: In the classical form, there is atresia of the mitral and aortic valves with a very small or nearly absent left ventricle. In the other less common form, the aortic valve is atretic but the mitral valve is patent and dysplastic often with mitral regurgitation. The left ventricle is akinetic and globular with hyperechoic (endomyocardial fibroelastosis) walls. In the four-chamber

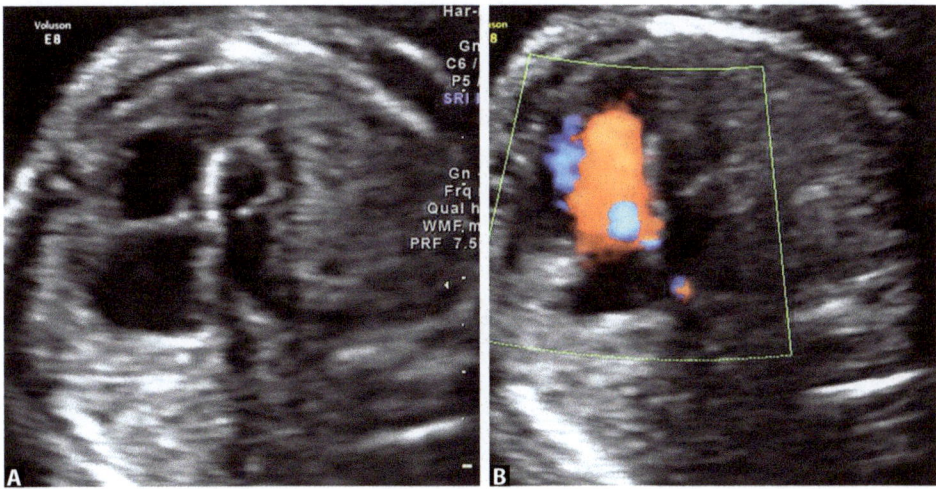

Figs 5.13A and B: Four-chamber view. (A) Smaller left atrium and left ventricle, hyperechoic interventricular septum and apex of the cardia by the right ventricle; (B) Absent transmitral and normal transtricuspid flow on color Doppler in diastole

view, the apex is taken over by the right ventricle, (Fig. 5.13). The foraminal flap bulges into the right atrium. The left atrium is generally smaller compared to the right atrium. In the presence of mitral regurgitation, the left atrium is dilated. In the five chamber and left ventricular outflow tract views, the aorta is either not identified or is very small in caliber (compared to the main pulmonary artery) (Fig. 5.14). The right ventricular outflow tract is normal. In the three vessel and three vessel trachea views, the aorta is either not visualized or small in caliber (Fig. 5.15A). Color Doppler findings include absent transmitral flow, left to right transforaminal flow, and ductus dependent reversed fill of the aortic arch in the three vessel trachea view (Fig. 5.15B). Color Doppler may be the only way to identify the presence of aorta in the three vessel trachea view. In the forms were the mitral valve is dysplastic mitral regurgitation may be documented by color Doppler. Due to the presence of dramatic findings on the four-chamber

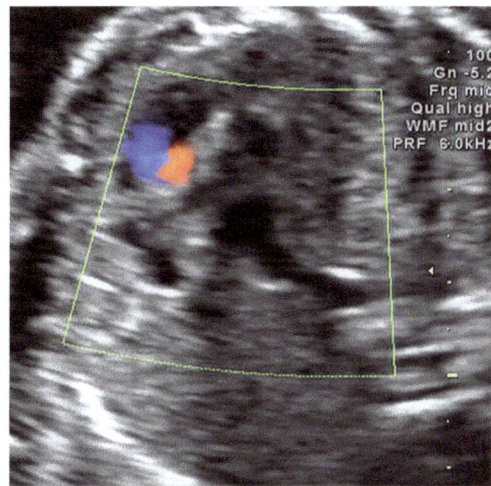

Fig. 5.14: Left ventricular outflow tract—Narrow aorta with no forward flow on color Doppler

view hypoplastic left heart syndrome can be diagnosed in the first trimester (11 to 14 weeks) ultrasonography. Chromosomal abnormality should be ruled out. Associated conditions include trisomy 13 or 18, Turner syndrome, Noonan syndrome or Holt-Oram syndrome.

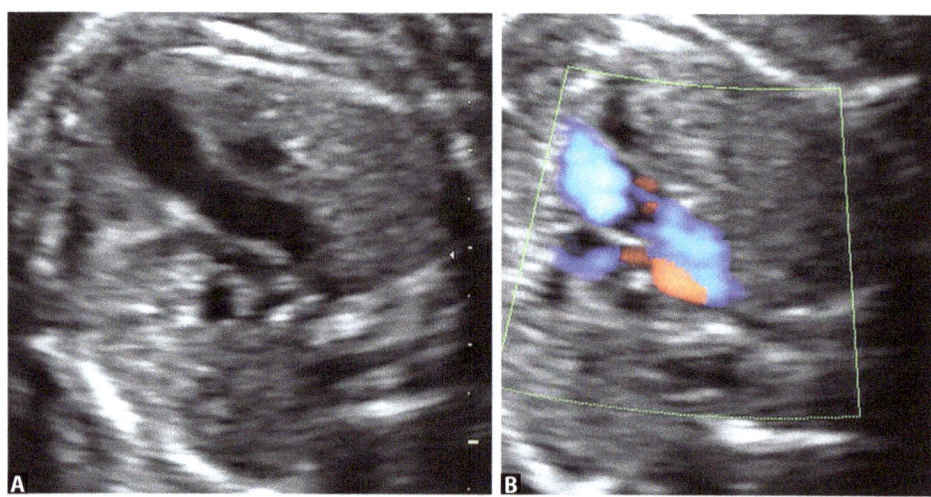

Figs 5.15A and B: Three vessel trachea view. (A) Narrow aorta compared to the pulmonary artery; (B) Ductus dependant reverse fill of the aorta in red compared to forward flow in the pulmonary artery

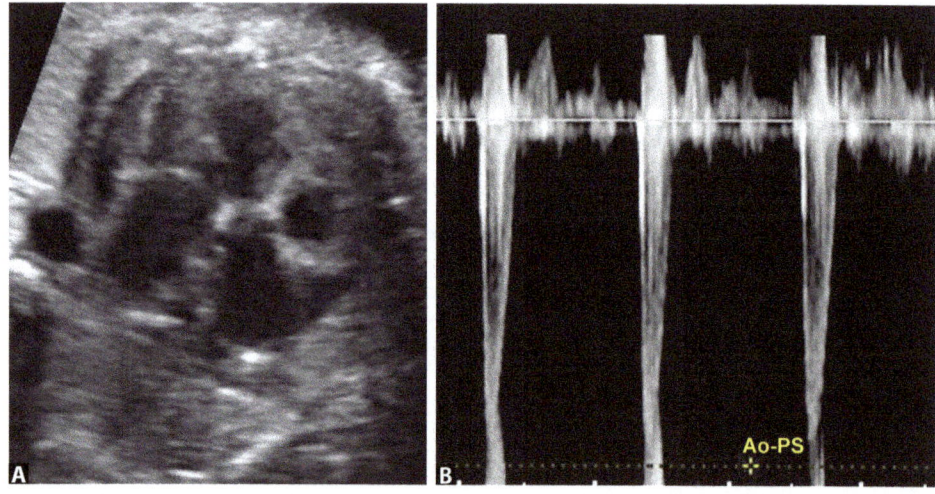

Figs 5.16A and B: Severe aortic stenosis. (A) Left ventricular outflow tract showing thick aortic valve cusps, narrow aortic annulus and post-stenotic dilatation; (B) Peak aortic systolic velocity of 194 cm/sec

Critical aortic stenosis: Aortic stenosis in the fetus is usually valvular. The milder form does not produce any changes on the four-chamber view and may be diagnosed by the presence of thickened aortic valve cusps, post-stenotic dilatation and systolic jetting (peak systolic velocity of 200 cm/sec or more)(Fig. 5.16). Critical form of aortic stenosis results in dilated left ventricle with reduced contractility and endomyocardial fibroelastosis. Forward transmitral flow is preserved. Presence of mitral regurgitation results in a dilated left atrium. In severe aortic stenosis, the aortic velocities may be attenuated due to left ventricular failure. Left to right foraminal flow and reverse flow through the ductus especially in diastole may be demonstrated on color Doppler. Follow-up scans may demonstrate evolution into a full blown hypoplastic left heart syndrome.

Coarctation of aorta: Implies discrete narrowing of the aortic isthmus (segment distal to the origin of the left subclavian artery- and proximal to the ductus arteriosus. The severest form is tubular hypoplasia of the aortic arch. Presentation may be neonatal especially after the closure of the ductus. In a proportion of cases, the presentation may be later in childhood or in adolescence. Chamber disproportion with predominance of the right-sided chambers or rather the diminution of the left-sided chambers is the first clue (Fig. 5.17). The aortic caliber is smaller compared to the main pulmonary artery (Fig. 5.18).

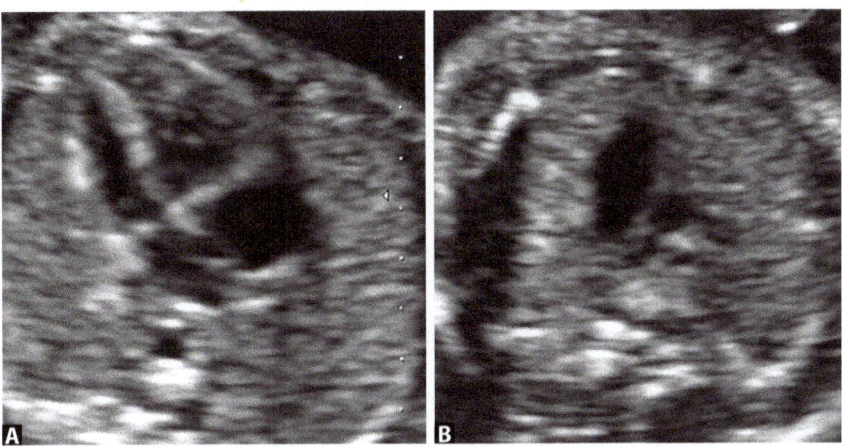

Figs 5.17A and B: Coarctation of aorta. (A) Four-chamber view with diminutive left-sided chambers; (B) Three vessel trachea view with a narrow aortic arch compared to the ductus arch

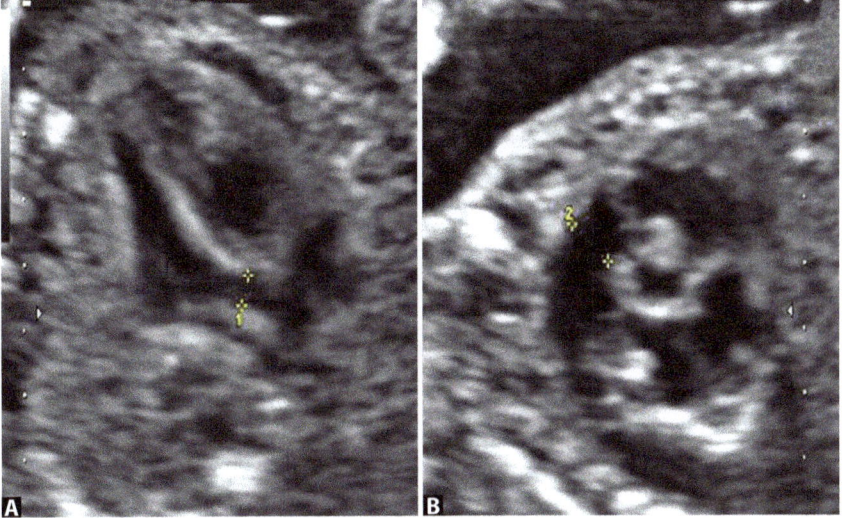

Figs 5.18A and B: Coarctation of aorta. (A) Left ventricular outflow tract with narrow aorta; (B) Right ventricular outflow tract with normal pulmonary artery

The PA/Ao ratio has been described to be of value. The aortic arch is small in caliber especially towards the isthmus in the three vessel trachea view. Color Doppler demonstrates forward flow across the mitral and aortic valves. In severe coarctation, there could be a diastolic ductus dependent reverse fill. Direct evidence of coarctation is by the demonstration of the contraductal shelf in the isthmus region in the aortic arch view (Fig. 5.19). Left superior vena cava is associated with coarctation of aorta. Diagnosis is beset by high rates of false negatives and false positives. Differential diagnosis would include hypoplastic left heart syndrome, interrupted aortic arch and total anomalous pulmonary venous drainage (will be considered in the section of the area behind the heart). Chromosomal abnormality should be ruled out. Associated anomalies are common and should be looked for.

Tricuspid atresia with VSD: Understandably, the right ventricle is small. The tricuspid valve is atretic and thick membrane like with no leaflet excursions. The small right ventricle fills through an inlet VSD (Fig. 5.20A). The bigger the VSD larger is the size of the diminutive right ventricle. Right ventricular myocardial contractility is normal. The entire right atrial volume now has to egress out through the foramen ovale into the left atrium. Consequently, the foramen is wide, the septum bulges into the left atrium with exaggerated flap excursions into the left atrium. This results in a malalignment of the interatrial and interventricular septa. In type I, the great arterial orientation is normal (common). D-transposition and L-transposition are seen in types II and III respectively (rare). The great arterial arrangement may be assessed by the outflow tract views and the three vessel trachea view. In the commonest type with normal great arterial orientation, the pulmonary artery arises from the right ventricle and its size depends on the size of the VSD and the right ventricle. The great arterial size discrepancy may be well demonstrated in the three vessel trachea view. Color Doppler shows absent transtricuspid flow with the right ventricle filling through the VSD (Fig. 5.20B). The

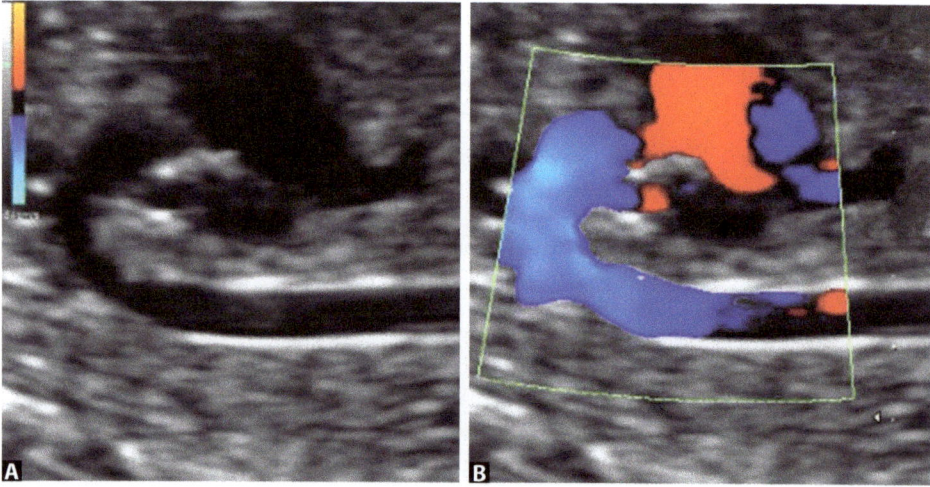

Figs 5.19A and B: Coarctation of aorta. (A) Aortic arch with isthmial narrowing; (B) Color Doppler may overwrite the isthmus narrowing

Fetal Cardiac Defects

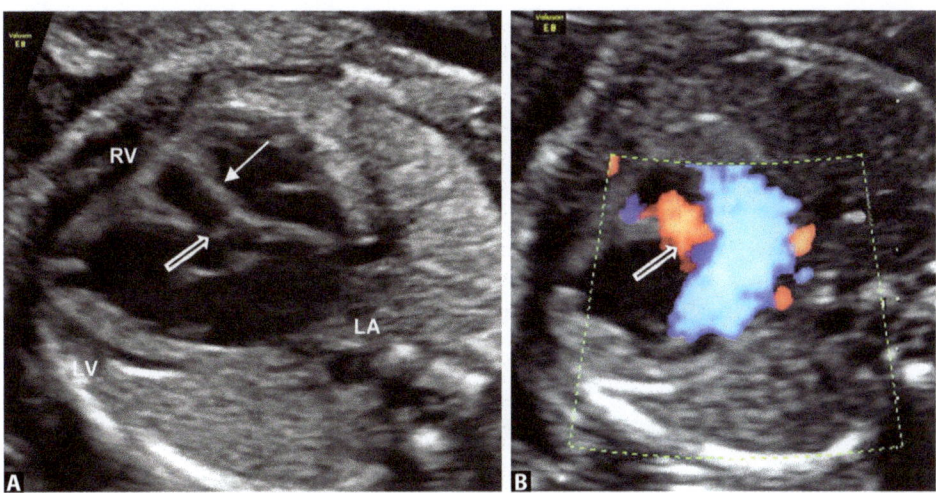

Figs 5.20A and B: Tricuspid atresia with VSD. (A) Atretic tricuspid valve (solid arrow) small right ventricle and VSD (open arrow); (B) Color Doppler left to right flow through the VSD (open arrow) and exaggerated right to left flow across the foramen ovale in blue

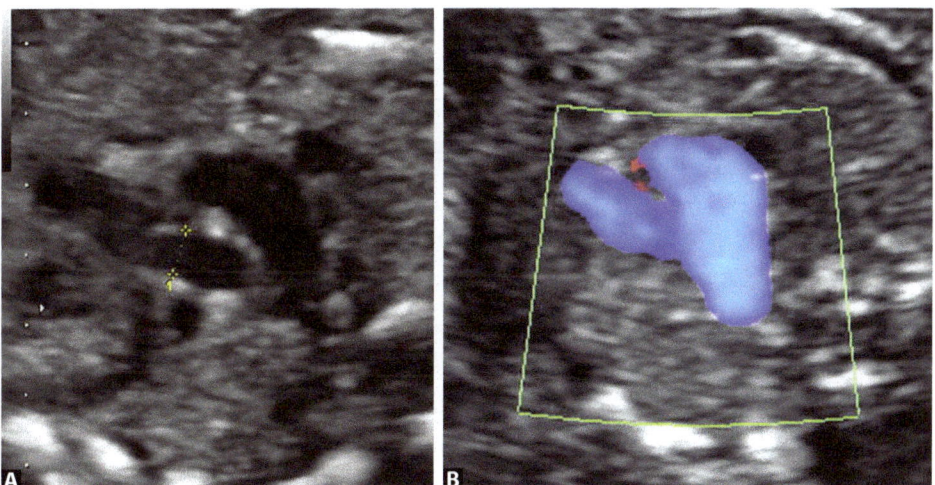

Figs 5.21A and B: Three vessel view in tricuspid atresia with VSD showing smaller pulmonary artery compared to aorta in gray scale and in color. Forward flow in pulmonary artery seen

VSD therefore shows a left to right flow direction. Since, the transforaminal flow and hence the transmitral flow is increased there is aliasing seen across the mitral valve. Normal forward ductus flow is noted (Fig. 5.21). Severe pulmonary stenosis or atresia would cause a ductus dependent pulmonary circulation with reverse filling of the pulmonary artery.

Karyotyping and FISH for 22q11 del may be offered.

Pulmonary atresia with intact interventricular septum: Majority of these cases present as a small right ventricle or even thick-walled right ventricle with no lumen (Fig. 5.22A). The tricuspid valve is without function. Less common is the form which presents as tricuspid regurgitation where the right ventricle is intact and dilated but hypokinetic. The narrow pulmonary artery is seen in the right ventricular outflow tract and the three vessel trachea views. On occasion, it may not be possible to visualize the pulmonary artery on gray scale. It presence may only be confirmed by color Doppler which demonstrates the narrow caliber and also a ductus dependant reverse filling in the three vessel trachea view.

Occasionally, the smaller pulmonary artery may demonstrate ductus dependant to and fro fill (Figs 5.23 and 5.24). Absent filling of the right ventricle may be seen in the four-chamber view (Fig. 5.22B).

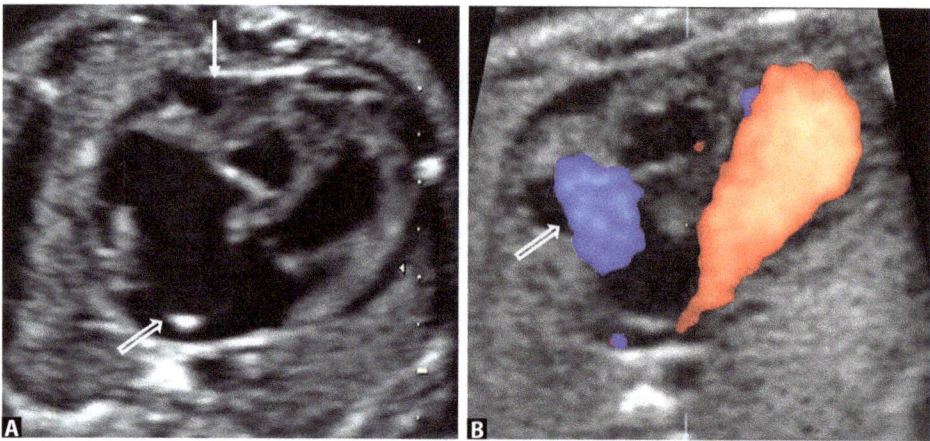

Figs 5.22A and B: Four-chamber view in pulmonary atresia with intact ventricular septum (A) Small thick-walled right ventricle (solid arrow) with a foraminal flap reaching far into the left atrium (open arrow); (B) Absent transtricuspid flow with exaggerated transforaminal right to left flow (open arrow)

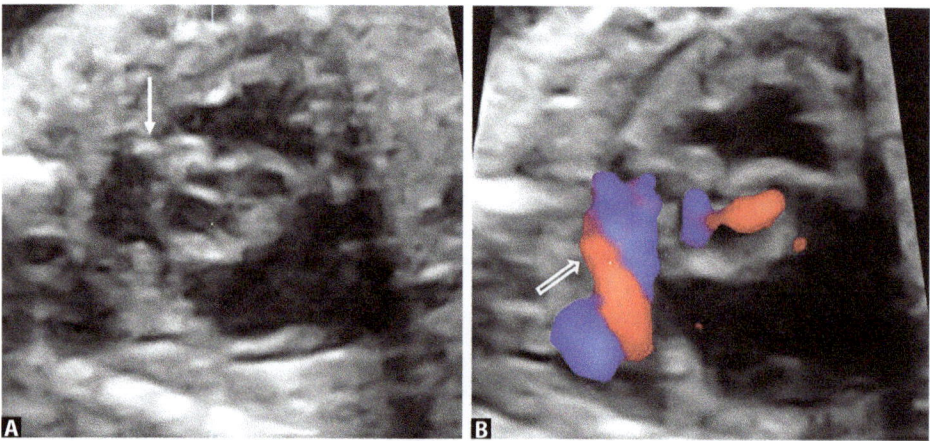

Figs 5.23A and B: Right ventricular outflow tract in pulmonary atresia with intact ventricular septum. (A) Thick atretic pulmonary valve (solid arrow); (B) Ductus dependant to and fro flow in the main pulmonary artery (open arrow)

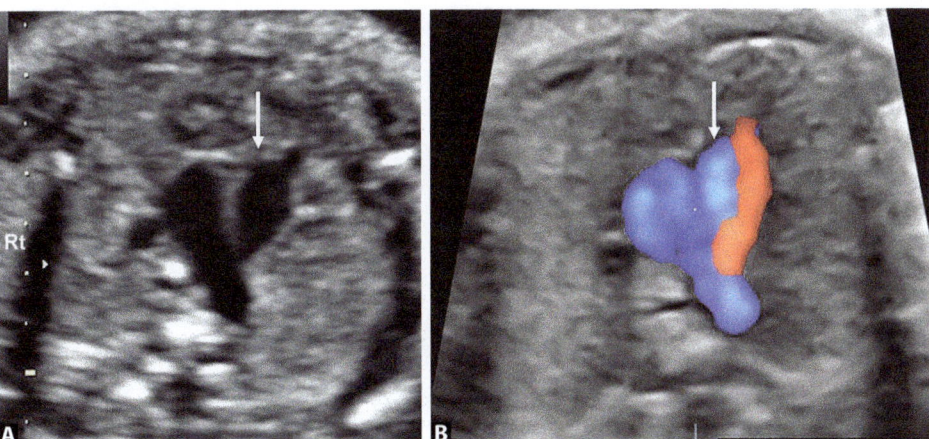

Figs 5.24A and B: Three vessel view in pulmonary atresia with intact ventricular septum. (A) Smaller pulmonary artery (arrow) compared to aorta; (B) Ductus dependent to and fro flow in pulmonary artery (arrow)

In the forms where there is a dilated right ventricle forward transtricuspid flow and holosystolic regurgitation are present. In those instances with a reasonably sized right ventricle and transtricuspid forward diastolic flow without tricuspid regurgitation the presence of ventriculocoronary shunt/s should be sought for on color Doppler. Major aortopulmonary collaterals are not a feature of pulmonary atresia with intact ventricular septum. Chromosomal abnormalities and associated anomalies are rare.

Pulmonary stenosis: Pulmonary stenosis in the fetus is valvular. In the four-chamber view, the only finding may be one of right ventricular myocardial thickening with ventricular septal bulging into the left ventricle (third trimester). Right ventricular contractility and tricuspid excursions are normal. Direct visualization of the pulmonary valve in the right ventricular outflow view reveals thickening and doming of the cusps during systole (Fig. 5.25). Normally, the valve cusps are seen only in diastole and not in systole. Post-stenotic dilatation and turbulent high velocity flow across the pulmonary valve are noted in the right ventricular outflow tract as well as in the three vessel trachea view (Fig. 5.26). Peak systolic velocity exceeds 200 cm/sec. Forward ductus flow noted. Evolution to pulmonary atresia is indicated by reversed ductus flow and the appearance of tricuspid regurgitation. Pulmonary regurgitation due to valve dysplasia may be seen and Noonan syndrome should be suspected in these cases.

Ebstein anomaly: Abnormal apical attachment of the septal and posterior tricuspid leaflets results atrialization of a part of the right ventricle (Fig. 5.27A). This may vary from a subtle to severe displacement. Cardiomegaly is mainly due to the right atrial dilatation especially in the third trimester. This could be subtle in the second trimester. Pulmonary hypoplasia may occur due to the cardiomegaly. The apically displaced attachment of the tricuspid valve leaflets may be demonstrated in the four-chamber view. This helps in differentiating from tricuspid dysplasia. The pulmonary artery is small compared to aorta and is

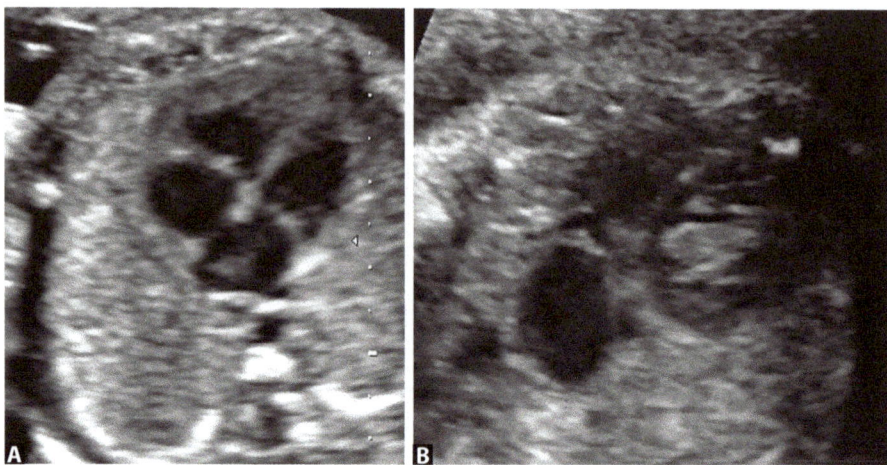

Figs 5.25A and B: Subcritical pulmonary stenosis. (A) Four-chamber view is unremarkable; (B) Right ventricular outflow tract with narrow annulus and thick pulmonary valve leaflets (arrow) and postvalvular dilatation

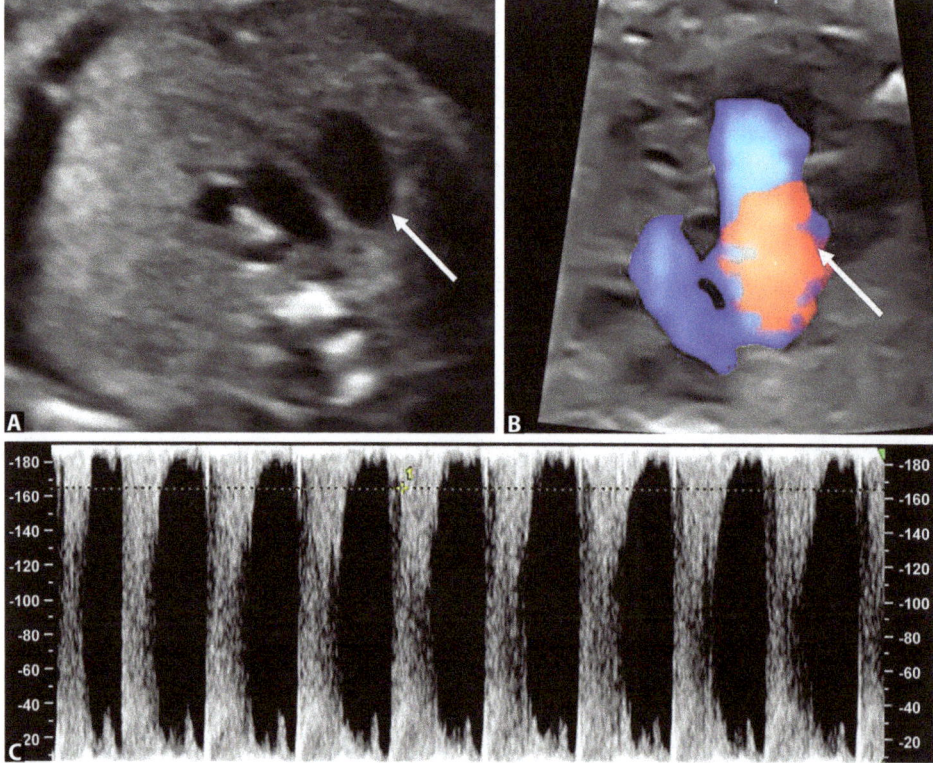

Figs 5.26A to C: Subcritical pulmonary stenosis. (A) Three vessel view shows pulmonary artery dilatation (arrow); (B) Aliasing in the pulmonary artery (arrow); (C) Pulmonary artery peak systolic velocity of close to 200 cm/sec with turbulence

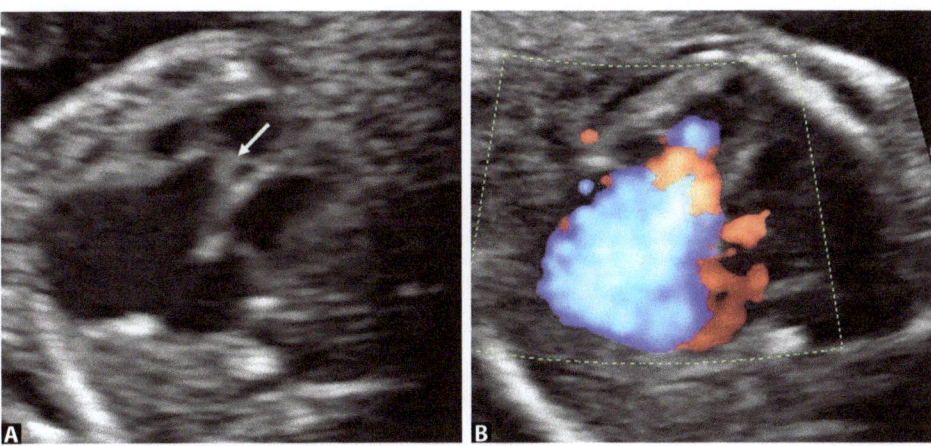

Figs 5.27A and B: Ebstein anomaly. (A) Right atrial dilatation with apical insertion of the septal leaflet of tricuspid valve (arrow); (B) Tricuspid regurgitation

most often due to functional atresia. The holosystolic tricuspid regurgitation (200 cm/sec) may be demonstrated even before atrial dilatation is manifest (Fig. 5.27B). Forward flow through a narrow pulmonary artery or ductus dependant reversed fill may be demonstrated (Fig. 5.28). The latter represents functional atresia of the pulmonary valve.

Tricuspid valve dysplasia: Thickened but normally inserted tricuspid valve leaflets constitute this anomaly. Typically, the thickened tricuspid leaflets do not close properly in systole. The right atrium is enlarged in the four-chamber view due to tricuspid regurgitation which can be demonstrated on color Doppler study (Fig. 5.29). The pulmonary artery is narrow with forward flow or ductus dependant reverse flow indicating functional atresia. Chromosomal abnormality and associated congenital anomalies are unlikely.

Chamber disproportion could also be seen due to non-valvular causes. In total anomalous pulmonary venous drainage, the pulmonary venous return is channelized into the right atrium and hence there is a right-sided chamber dominance.

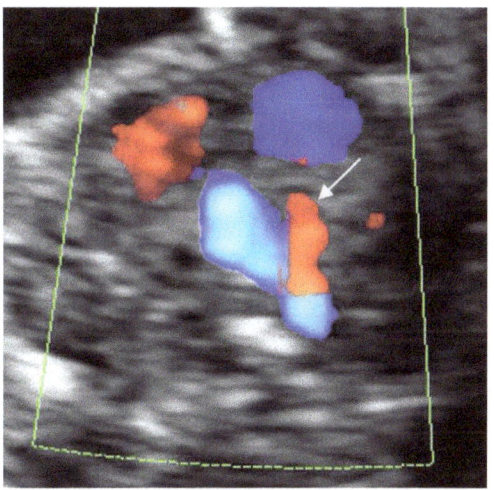

Fig 5.28: Ebstein anomaly—Three vessel view with ductus dependent reverse pulmonary artery fill indicating functional atresia. Also note the narrower pulmonary caliber compared to the aorta

This condition will be considered in the section dealing with the area behind the heart. Increased venous return to the heart (increased preload) as in chorioangioma, vein of Galen aneurysm, fetal tumor or fetal anemia result in right-sided chamber enlargement. Raised fetoplacental

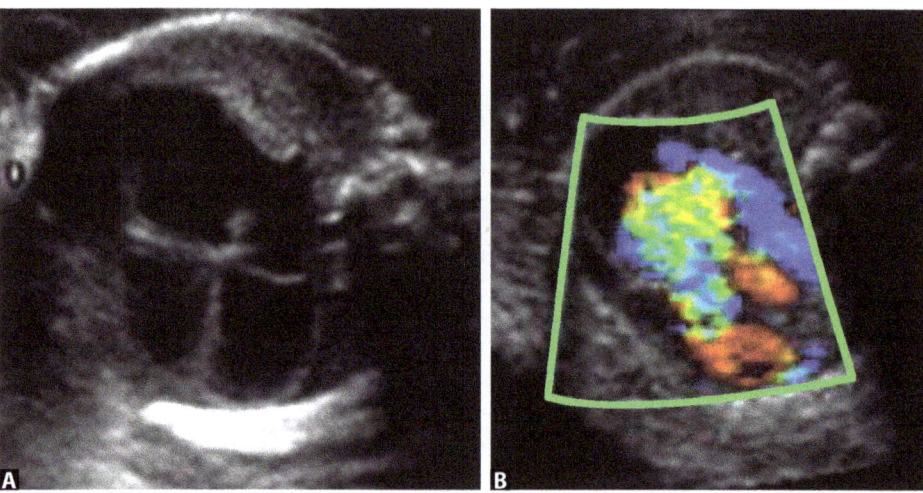

Figs 5.29A and B: Tricuspid dysplasia. (A) Four-chamber view with right atrial enlargement and thickened but normally attached tricuspid valve leaflet; (B) Tricuspid regurgitation

resistance and premature constriction of the ductus result in increased afterload which also causes right sided chamber enlargement.

c. **Chamber attributes:** The presence of atrioventricular discordance may be detected in the four chamber view as the moderator band and the normal apically inserted tricuspid septal leaflet are now seen in the left-sided ventricle. This happens in the congenitally corrected transposition of the great arteries and will be dealt later.

d. **Area behind the heart:** The area behind the heart refers to the region between the posterior wall of the left atrium and the spine. The descending aorta is the only structure seen in this region. The left atrium almost touches the descending aorta. The fluid filled esophagus may be transiently seen between the left atrium and the descending aorta. The vertical vein in total anomalous pulmonary venous drainage and the enlarged azygos vein in IVC interruption are the two pathological situations related to the cardia that may be potentially recognized in the area behind the heart. The presence of any of these vessels is termed the 'Double vessel sign'. The azygos vein is the right and subtly posterior to the descending aorta. The vertical vein in total anomalous pulmonary venous drainage (TAPVD) is seen anterior to the descending aorta. The presence of right-sided aortic arch in levocardia or left sided aortic arch in dextrocardia may be easily suspected by noting the position of the descending aorta in relation to the spine. Non-cardiac lesions like an esophageal duplication cyst or a neurenteric cyst may be occasionally be seen.

TAPVD: All four pulmonary veins drain directly or indirectly into the right atrium. The area behind the heart does not show the normal pulmonary venous connection with the left atrium (Fig. 5.30A). The left atrial posterior wall is rounded in contour. The distance between the descending aorta and the left atrium (post-LA space) is increased (Fig. 5.30A). The four pulmonary veins converge to form a vertical vein in the area behind the heart (Fig. 5.30B).

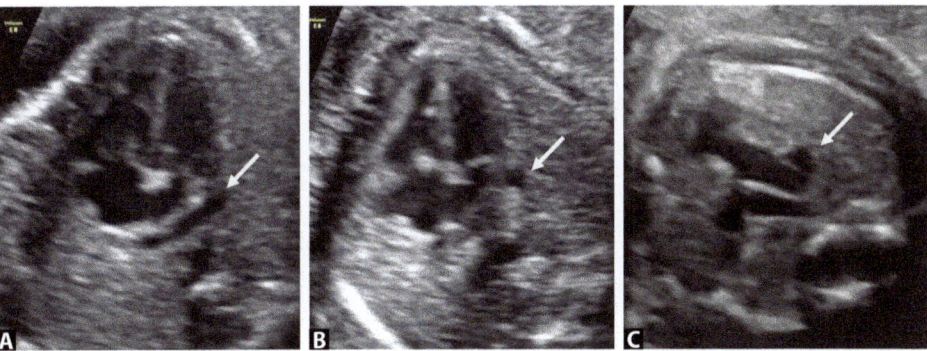

Figs 5.30A to C: Supracardiac total anomalous pulmonary venous drainage. (A) Four-chamber view with increased post-LA space and pulmonary veins not confluencing with left atrium (arrow); (B) Vertical vein axial section at four chamber level (arrow); (C) Vertical vein at the level of three vessel view (arrow). The superior vena cava is prominent

In the supracardiac type of TAPVD, this vertical vein courses superiorly to drain into the left innominate vein. In the three vessel trachea view, the vertical vein is seen as the fourth vessel to the left of the pulmonary artery (Fig. 5.30C). The superior vena cava is larger in caliber. Color Doppler cardiofugal direction of flow will help in differentiating from left superior vena cava which has cardiopetal flow. In the infracardiac type, the vertical vein courses inferiorly along the esophagus, through the diaphragm, to drain into the portal venous system. Obstruction to the vertical vein is common in the infracardiac type. The Doppler waveforms from the vertical vein is abnormal and lacks the normal pulsatility. The pulmonary veins drain into the coronary sinus in the cardiac type resulting in a dilated coronary sinus. Dilated coronary sinus in the absence of a persistent left superior vena cava should raise the suspicion for cardiac type of total anomalous pulmonary venous connection (TAPVC). The pulmonary veins may directly connect with the posterior wall of the right atrium. Right-sided chamber dominance is noted as the pulmonary venous return is directly or indirectly into the right atrium. TAPVC is commonly seen in cases of right atrial isomerism.

6. *When one rotates the transducer from the four chamber view to obtain the left ventricular tract one of the following may be encountered:*

a. **Overriding aorta:** A malalignment ventricular septal defect is diagnosed when there is an aortoseptal discontinuity with the aortic root overriding the septal defect. The aorta now receives output from both ventricles. This is a finding and not the final diagnosis. The status of the pulmonary artery yields the final diagnosis. The pulmonary artery could be (i) narrow, or (ii) atretic, or (iii) the branch arteries are dilated or (iv) it (pulmonary artery) arises from a common trunk.

   – The pulmonary artery is narrow: *Tetralogy of Fallot*: Four chamber view is basically normal. There could however be a left axis rotation (Fig. 5.31A). However in the five chamber or left ventricular outflow tract view, the malalignment VSD and aortic root overriding the VSD are visualized (Fig. 5.31B). The long axis of the ascending aorta is collinear with the interventricular septum. In the right ventricular outflow tract view and in the three vessel view, the pulmonary

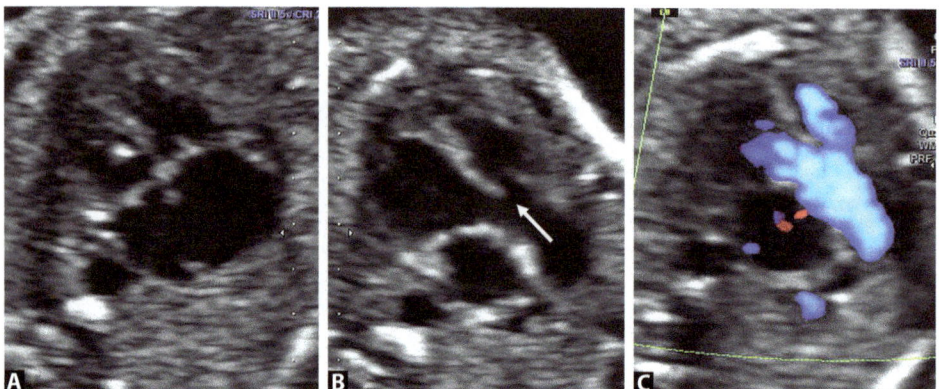

Figs 5.31A to C: Tetralogy of Fallot. (A) Four-chamber view with left axis rotation; (B) Left ventricular tract view with malalignment VSD and overriding aortic root (arrow); (C) Color Doppler of left ventricular outflow tract—aorta committed to both ventricles

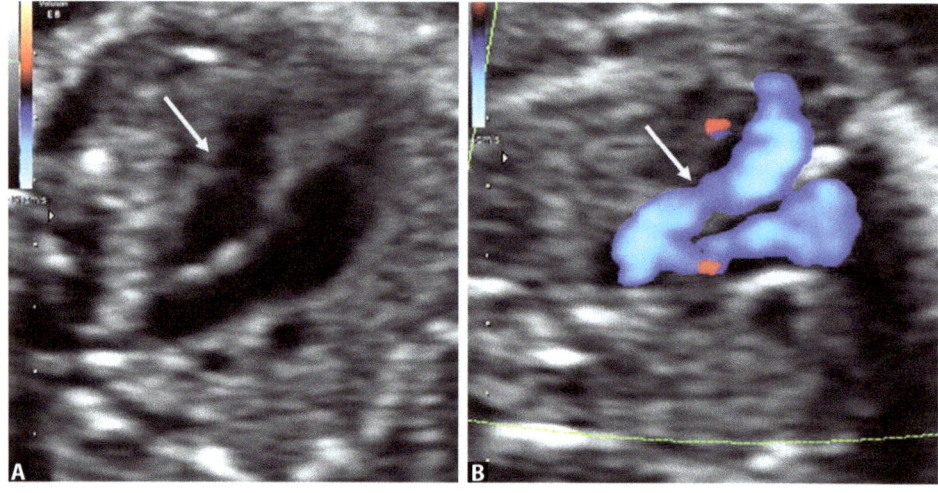

Figs 5.32A and B: Tetralogy of Fallot—Three vessel trachea view. (A) Gray scale—Pulmonary artery (arrow) is narrower than aorta; (B) Color Doppler—Forward flow in pulmonary artery (arrow)

artery is narrow in caliber (compared to the aorta)(Fig. 5.32A). This difference in caliber increases with advancing gestational age. Demonstration of the pulmonary artery bifurcation is necessary prognostication. In addition to the great arterial size discrepancy, the anteriorly placed aorta is seen in the three vessel view. The three vessel trachea view should also be used to rule out or confirm a right aortic arch. Aortic comitance to both ventricles can be demonstrated by color Doppler in the apical five chamber view (Fig. 5.31C). Forward flow through the narrow pulmonary artery must be demonstrated to rule out pulmonary atresia (Fig. 5.32B). Reversed ductus dependant filling of the pulmonary artery could also occur in severe pulmonary stenosis.

Chromosomal abnormalities and FISH for 22q11 deletion should be done. Thymic hypoplasia may be quantified by the thymic thoracic ratio. Associated extracardiac congenital anomalies must be looked for. Follow-up scans every four weeks is necessary to monitor the pulmonary caliber and flow direction. Increasing aortopulmonary discrepancy is of poor prognosis.

- The pulmonary artery is not seen—*Pulmonary atresia with VSD*: The pulmonary artery is not visualized. Blood supply to the lungs is through the ductus or directly from the descending aorta (major aortopulmonary collaterals—MAPCA's). The four-chamber view is unremarkable (Fig. 5.32A). The five chamber and the left ventricular outflow tract view show a large artery (aorta) overriding a malalignment VSD (Fig. 5.33B). The aorta is larger than in tetralogy of Fallot as the entire output of both ventricles pass through it given that the pulmonary artery is atretic. The only vessels to be seen in the three vessel view are the aorta and SVC (Fig. 5.34A). Right aortic arch and thymic hypoplasia should be looked for. On color Doppler, the aorta is committed to both ventricles. The right ventricular tract is not demonstrable. A thin pulmonary artery with retrograde fill from the ductus may be identified in the three vessel view (Fig. 5.34B). Occasionally, the pulmonary valve is atretic, but distal to the valve, the pulmonary artery is well seen and is of reasonable caliber. In these cases, there is a to and fro movement of blood in the main pulmonary artery (ductus dependant). The descending aorta should be carefully studied with color Doppler in the transverse and coronal planes to look for major aortopulmonary collaterals especially in those cases where there is no ductus dependant pulmonary artery fill. Karyotyping and FISH for 22q11 deletion may be planned.
- The branch pulmonary arteries are markedly dilated—*Absent pulmonary valve syndrome*: The pulmonary valve cusps are rudimentary or absent. Consequently, there is a free unhindered to and fro movement of blood across

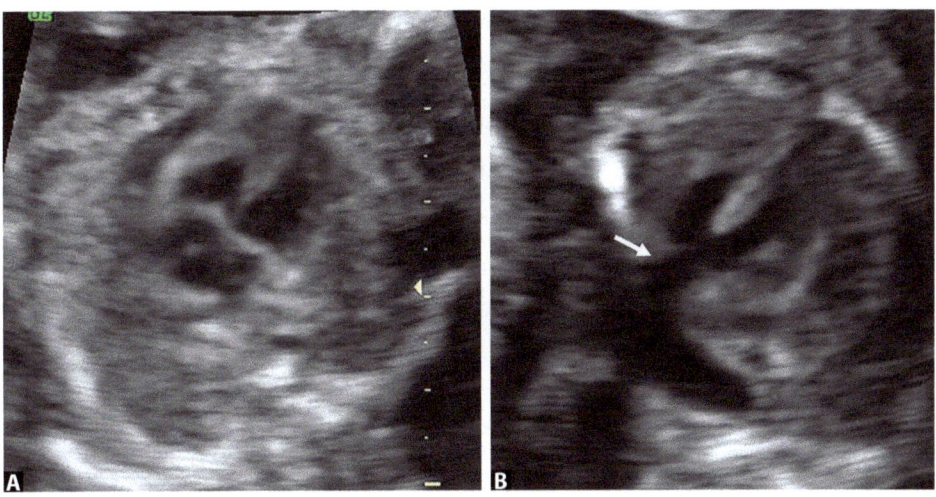

Figs 5.33A and B: Pulmonary atresia with VSD. (A) Normal four-chamber view; (B) Overriding large aorta on a malalignment VSD (arrow)

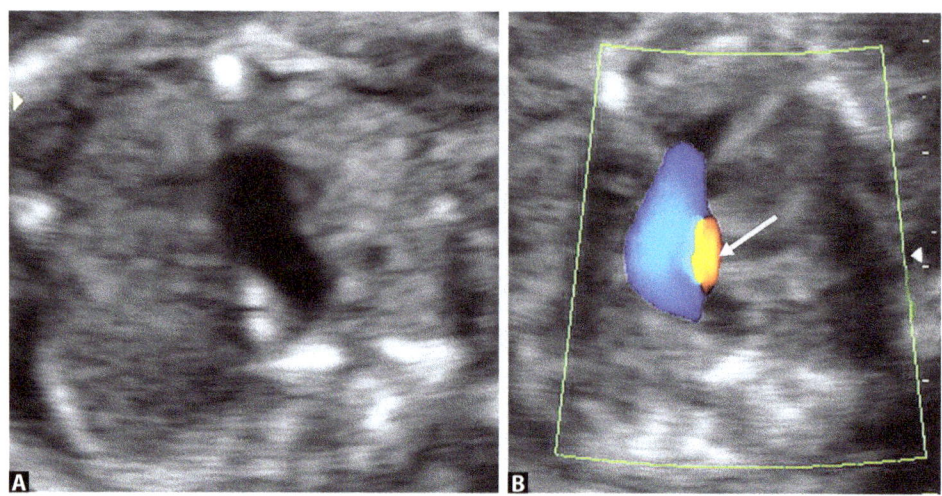

Figs 5.34A and B: Pulmonary atresia with VSD. (A) Only aorta and SVC are seen in the three vessel view; (B) Small pulmonary artery with reverse ductus dependant fill in red (arrow) on color Doppler

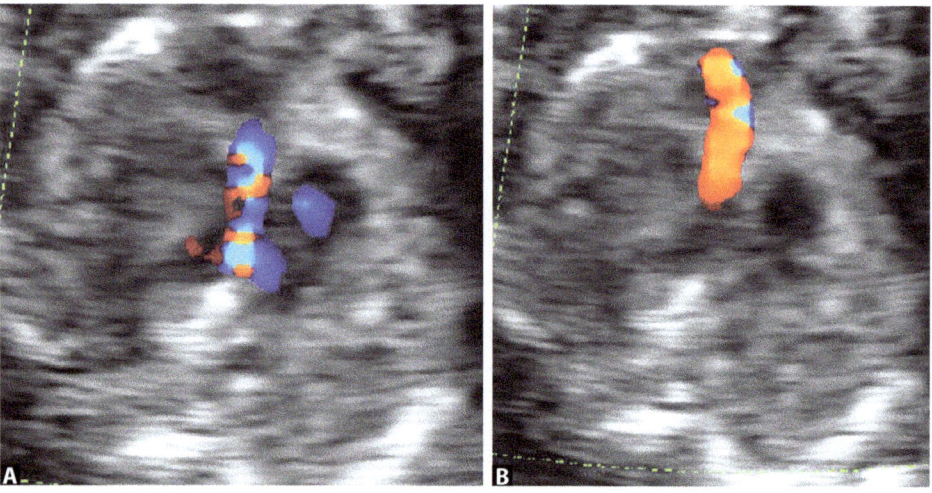

Figs 5.35A and B: Absent pulmonary valve syndrome. (A) Forward flow in pulmonary artery in systole with Doppler aliasing indicating stenosis at the valve; (B) Reverse flow in diastole indicating pulmonary regurgitation. The ductus arteriosus is absent

the pulmonary annulus (Figs 5.35A and B). The main, right and left pulmonary arteries are severely dilated (Figs 5.36A and B). The ductus arteriosus may be absent (Figs 5.36A and B). The pulmonary annulus itself may be narrow (Fig. 5.36A). The aorta root is overriding a malalignment VSD. The dilated pulmonary arteries may cause airway compression. This condition is a subtype of Fallot's tetralogy. The four chamber view shows a right ventricular dominance due to the pulmonary regurgitation. The three vessel and short axis view shows dramatically dilated (three, to four-fold) aneurysmal

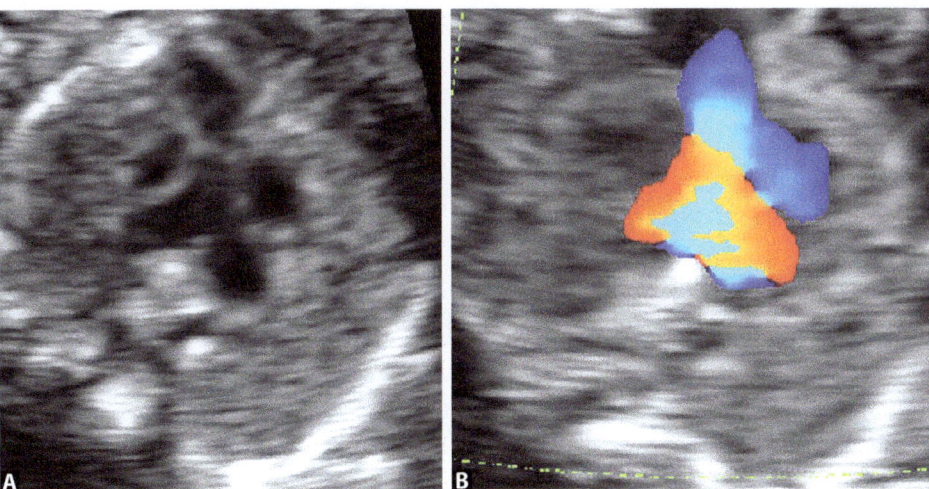

Figs 5.36A and B: Absent pulmonary valve syndrome. (A) Short axis right ventricular outflow tract with relatively narrow pulmonary annulus and dilated branch pulmonary arteries; (B) Color Doppler fill of the dilated branch pulmonary arteries. The ductus arteriosus is absent

branch pulmonary arteries. Right aortic arch and thymic hypoplasia should be sought for. Spectral Doppler peak systolic velocity across the pulmonary annulus could be as high as 200-250 cm/sec. Karyotyping and FISH for 22q11 deletion must be offered.

- The pulmonary artery and the aorta arise from a common trunk—*Common arterial trunk*: The common arterial trunk overrides a malalignment VSD and hence the trunk is committed to both ventricles. Occasionally the common trunk arises solely from the right ventricle. Depending on the anatomic origin of the pulmonary artery/ies from the trunk three types are described. Type I is when there is a pulmonary trunk arising from the common arterial trunk. The pulmonary trunk bifurcates into the right and left pulmonary arteries. In types II and III, the right and left pulmonary arteries arise independently from the common trunk either close to each other (type II) or at a distance from each other (type III). The previously categorized type IV (pulmonary artery arising from the isthmial segment of the common truncal arch) is now considered as pulmonary atresia with VSD. The four-chamber view appears normal. On moving to the five chamber and left ventricular outflow tract views, the malalignment VSD and an overriding large artery are detected (Fig. 5.37A). Demonstration of the pulmonary artery/ies arising from the large outflow tract just beyond the annulus confirms it to be the common arterial trunk (rules out pulmonary atresia with VSD)(Fig. 5.37B). The truncal valves are often thickened and may be tricuspid or tetracuspid. Only two vessels are seen in the three vessel view. Right aortic arch and thymic hypoplasia should be sought for. The ductus is absent in most cases. Color Doppler confirms the common trunk committed to both ventricles and may help in tracing the pulmonary arteries (Fig. 5.37C).

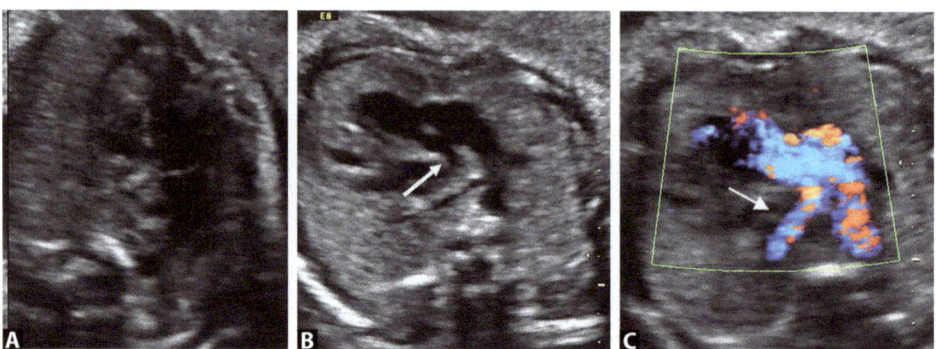

Figs 5.37A to C: Common arterial trunk. (A) Large single outflow tract overriding the malalignment VSD, truncal valve closed, (B) pulmonary artery arising from trunk just distal to the truncal valve closed (arrow); (C) Pulmonary artery arising from the trunk (arrow) on color Doppler

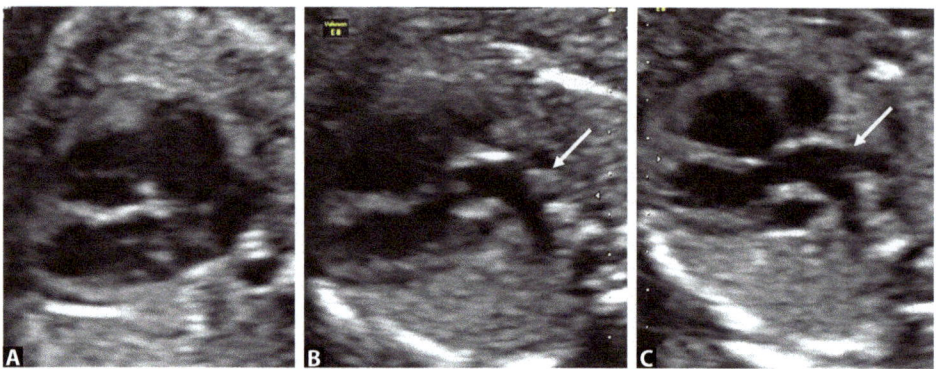

Figs 5.38A to C: Complete transposition of great arteries. (A) Normal four-chamber view; (B) Left ventricular outflow tract showing the artery to abruptly turn and point to the spine (arrow); (C) Left ventricular outflow tract is bifurcating in the axial plane (arrow) indicating that it is the pulmonary artery

Truncal regurgitation if present may be detected. Non-specific extracardiac anomalies should be ruled out and a karyotype and FISH for 22q11 del must be planned.

b. **Parallel great arteries:** The great arteries run parallel to each other. This can happen in two groups of conditions (i) Ventriculoarterial discordance—Transposition of great arteries (complete or congenitally corrected) and (ii) Both arteries majorly arise from the right ventricle—Double outlet right ventricle.

Complete transposition of great arteries: Venoatrial and atrioventricular connections are normal. The ventriculoarterial connections are discordant, i.e. the aorta and pulmonary artery arise from the right and left ventricles respectively. The great arteries course parallel to each other the aorta being anterior and to the right of the pulmonary artery. VSD and pulmonary stenosis are the associated cardiac anomalies. The four chamber view is typically normal (Fig. 5.38A). The pulmonary artery is seen to arise from the left ventricle in the five chamber and left ventricular outflow tract views. It bifurcates shortly after its origin (Figs 5.38B and C). The aorta arises from the right ventricle and courses anterior and parallel to the pulmonary artery (seen in an oblique plane)

(Figs 5.39A and B). The three vessel trachea view shows a single large artery, i.e. the aorta with the superior vena cava. The pulmonary artery is not seen in this plane as it is inferior to the aorta. The aortic arch is broad and its origin is anteriorly placed. Color Doppler displays the parallel relation of the great arteries. It also helps to assess ventricular defect and pulmonary stenosis. The 4D (STIC) coronal view of the atrioventricular and semilunar orifices may be used to assess the exact relation between the origins of the great arteries. A side-to-side relation has a high association with coronary artery abnormalities. Associated extracardiac anomalies are rare. Karyotyping is not indicated. FISH for 22q11 del may be offered.

Congenitally corrected transposition of great arteries: Venoatrial connections are normal. The atrioventricular and ventriculoarterial connections are discordant. This results in the systemic venous blood reaching the pulmonary circulation and the pulmonary venous blood reaching the systemic circulation. Dextrocardia or mesocardia are a common association (Fig. 5.40A). The morphologic left atrium (pulmonary venous drainage) connects with the morphologic right ventricle (moderator band, apically attached atrioventricular valve, and septal chorda tendinae). The morphologic right atrium (systemic venous drainage) connects with the morphologic left ventricle (apex forming, absent moderator band and absent septal chorda tendinae)(Fig. 5.40B). The morphological left ventricle supports an axially branching pulmonary artery (Fig. 5.41A). The arching aorta arises from the morphological right ventricle (Fig. 5.41B). The great arteries are parallel to each other with the aorta anterior and to the left of the pulmonary artery (Figs 5.42A and B). On the five-chamber view, the first outflow tract to be seen is from the morphological left ventricle (right sided) pointing to the left of the spine. This artery branches and is hence the pulmonary artery. The aorta arises from the morphological right ventricle (left-sided) and courses parallel and to the left of the pulmonary artery. Sequential segmental approach thus helps in reaching the correct diagnosis. Color Doppler aids

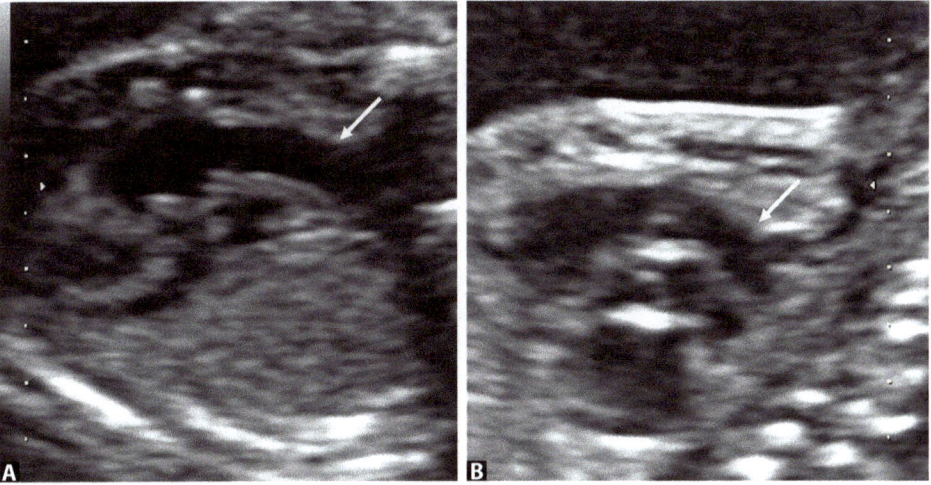

Figs 5.39A and B: Complete transposition of great arteries. (A) The arching outflow tract (aorta) arising from the substernal right ventricle (arrow); (B) Parallel course of the great arteries on the oblique view

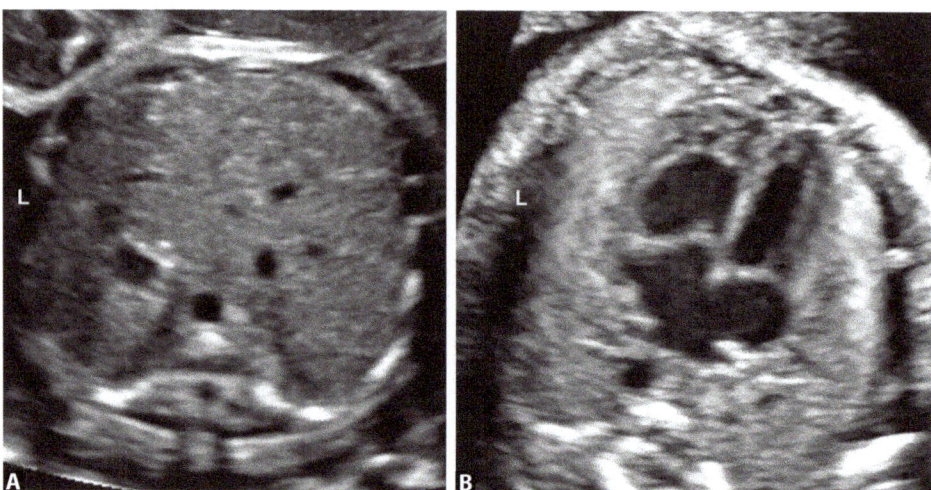

Figs 5.40A and B: Congenitally corrected transposition of great arteries. (A) Upper abdominal plane with stomach to the left side; (B) Mesocardia with apex substernal, the left-sided atrium is the left atrium marked by the pulmonary venous connection, the left-sided ventricle is the morphological right ventricle marked by the apical insertion of the tricuspid valve and the moderator band, this clearly demonstrates atrioventricular discordance

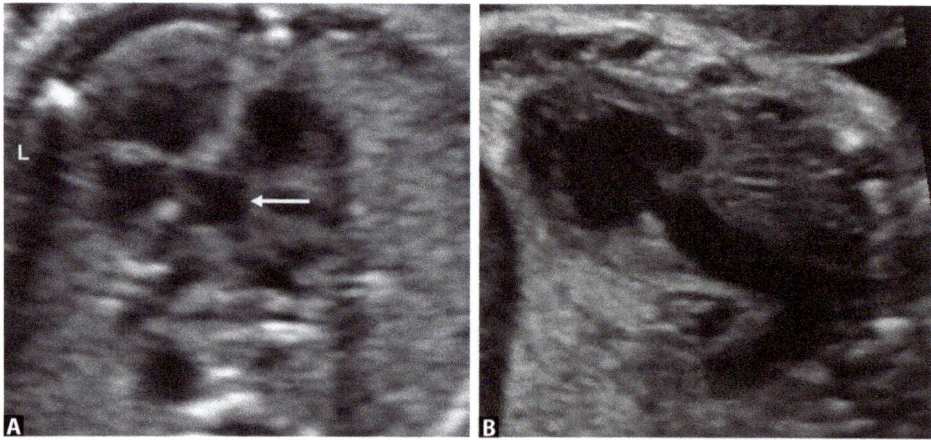

Figs 5.41A and B: Congenitally corrected transposition of great arteries. (A) Cephalad angulation from four-chamber view shows the dividing pulmonary artery (arrow) to arise from the right-sided morphological left ventricle; (B) The morphological right ventricle is seen to support the aorta, indicating ventriculoarterial discordance

in the diagnosis of ventricular septal defect, tricuspid regurgitation and pulmonary stenosis which may coexist. It is also useful in demonstrating the parallel course of the great arteries. Extracardiac abnormalities are rare. Karyotype is normal as a rule. FISH for 22q11 del is recommended particularly if there are associated anomalies.

Double outlet right ventricle (DORV): This term encompasses a group of anomalies

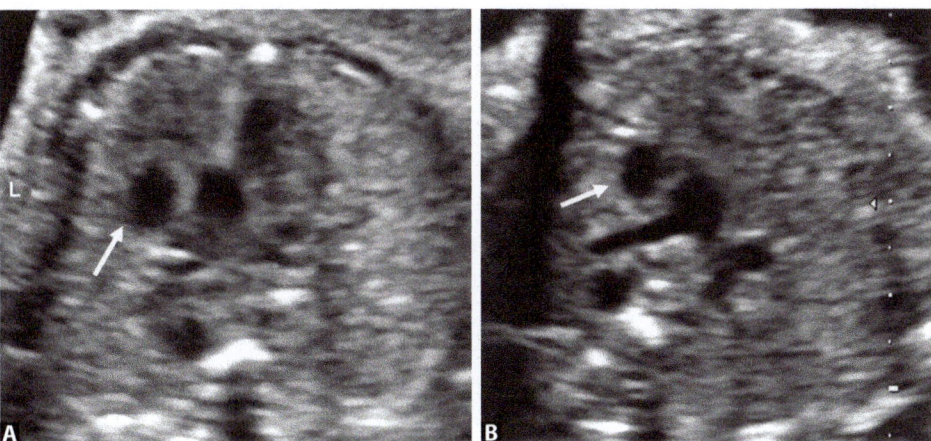

Figs 5.42A and B: Congenitally corrected transposition of great arteries. (A) The short axis of both great arteries seen side-to-side with the aorta (arrow) being to the left of the pulmonary artery; (B) The aorta (arrow) seen to the left of the pulmonary artery (dividing) in the three vessel view

where both the aorta and the pulmonary artery arise wholly or predominantly from the morphological right ventricle. A ventricular septal defect is almost always present. There may be associated aortic or pulmonary stenosis. The great arterial origins may bear any of the following relationships: (A) Aortic valve to the right of the pulmonary valve (side-to-side type), (B) Aortic valve is anterior and to the right of the pulmonary valve (D-transposition type), (C) Aortic valve is posterior and to the right of the pulmonary valve (Tetralogy of Fallot type), and (D) Aortic valve is anterior and to the left of the pulmonary valve (L-transposition type). The VSD may be subaortic, subpulmonary, remote or doubly committed. Exact position of the VSD is sometimes difficult to assign. The four-chamber view of the heart may be unremarkable. There may be ventricular disproportion due to left-sided smallness and right-sided dominance. DORV may be associated with atrioventricular septal defect, mitral atresia or double inlet ventricle. In these instances, the four chamber view will obviously be abnormal. Aorto-septal discontinuity (VSD) is seen

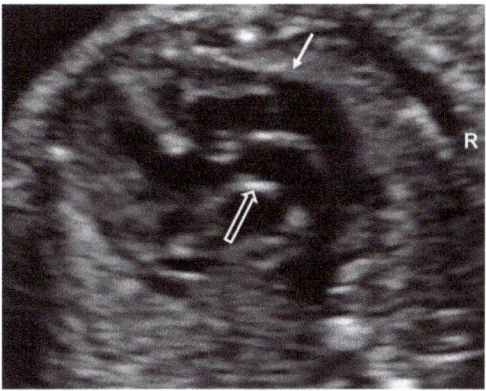

Fig. 5.43: Double outlet right ventricle—Both great arteries are arising from the right ventricle and are parallel to each other (malposed) the aortic origin (arrow) being to the right and anterior to the pulmonary artery origin (open arrow) (D TGA type), the VSD is subpulmonic

on the five-chamber view/left ventricular outflow view. Both the great arteries arising from the right ventricle (substernal chamber) is also seen in the same views. Parallelism of the great arteries can be demonstrated by angling the probe cephalad towards the three vessel view (Fig. 5.43). The arterial calibers should be recorded to detect stenosis. A right-sided aortic arch which may be associated with DORV can be picked up on the three vessel trachea view. Due to the malposition of the arteries, only one artery (commonly the aortic arch) may be seen on the three vessel trachea view (with the pulmonary artery coursing at an inferior plane). Color Doppler helps in demonstrating: (i) left to right flow across the VSD, (ii) blood flow into both great arteries from the right ventricle, (iii) presence of great arterial stenosis (turbulence), (iv) reversed flow in either great artery in the case of atresia.

7. *In the plane of the three vessel view or three vessel trachea view one may encounter any one of the following findings:*

a. **Size abnormality of any of the vessels:** Normally, the aorta is slightly smaller in caliber compared to the pulmonary artery. The aorta is significantly small in caliber in aortic coarctation (Fig. 5.44) and hypoplastic left heart syndrome. The pulmonary artery is small in caliber in tricuspid atresia, pulmonary atresia with intact ventricular septum, tetralogy of Fallot and pulmonary atresia with ventricular septal defect. These entities have already been dealt with.

b. **Abnormal flow direction in any of the vessels:** The aorta and the pulmonary artery display the same flow direction on color Doppler examination in the three vessel trachea view (normal). In hypoplastic left heart syndrome, the aorta is small in caliber and displays retrograde (ductus dependent) flow direction (Fig. 5.15). In pulmonary atresia, the pulmonary artery is small in caliber and displays retrograde (ductus dependent) flow direction (Fig. 5.35B). In absent pulmonary valve syndrome, there is to and fro movement of blood in systole and diastole respectively indicating free pulmonary regurgitation.

c. **Abnormal spatial arrangement of the vessels:**
   - Spatial arrangement abnormality amongst the vessels: Typically seen in tetralogy of Fallot or in double outlet right ventricle (tetralogy of Fallot type) where the aorta is anteriorly placed in relation to the superior vena cava and pulmonary artery (Fig. 5.45).
   - Spatial arrangement abnormality in relation to the trachea: The 'V' configuration of the great arteries in the three vessel trachea view has its apex

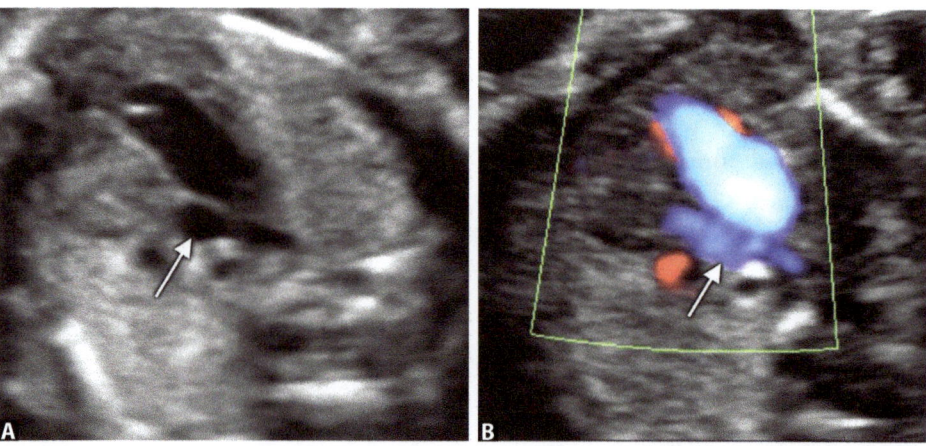

Figs 5.44A and B: Coarctation of aorta. (A) The aorta (arrow) is much smaller compared to the pulmonary artery; (B) Forward flow noted in the aorta in the three vessel trachea view

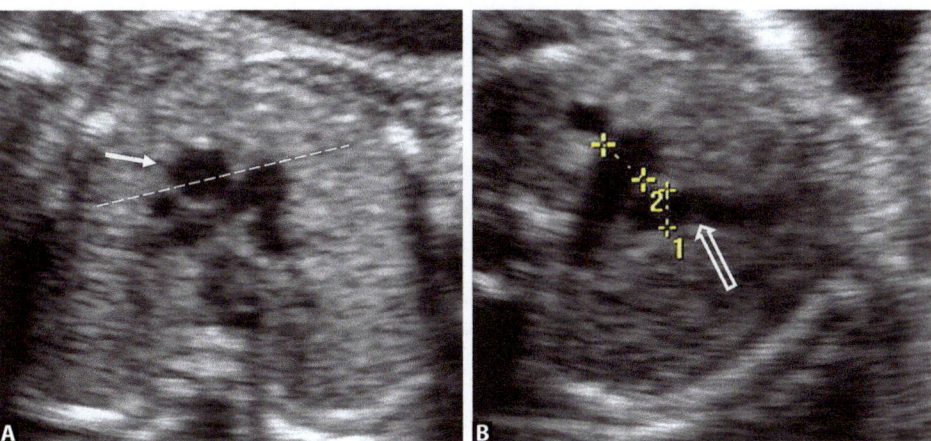

Figs 5.45A and B: Tetralogy of Fallot. (A) The aorta (solid arrow) is anteriorly placed in relation to the pulmonary and superior vena cava in the three vessel view; (B) The pulmonary artery (open arrow) is smaller in caliber

to the left of the trachea and points to the left of the spine indicating a normal left-sided aortic and ductus arch. In right aortic arch with right ductus arch, the apex of the 'V' is to the right of the trachea and points to right of the spine (Fig. 5.46A). In right aortic arch with left ductus arch, the great arteries are in a 'U' configuration forming a loose sling around the trachea and the esophagus (Fig. 5.46B). In double aortic arch, a tight vascular ring is formed around the trachea and esophagus with the left aortic arch passing anteriorly and right aortic arch passing posteriorly to converge posterior to trachea and esophagus. Situs abnormalities (including heterotaxy) and 22q11 del are associated with aortic arch anomalies. Left aortic arch with aberrant right subclavian artery (ARSA) is a common variant where the right subclavian artery is the last artery to arise from the aortic arch (normally the right subclavian artery is a branch of the brachiocephalic trunk which is the first branch of the aortic arch). It then courses posterior to the trachea and esophagus from the apex of the 'V' in the three vessel trachea towards the right shoulder (Fig. 5.46C). ARSA is best sought for in the three vessel trachea view with a lower PRF and higher gain setting. Presence of ARSA with other markers of aneuploidy necessitates fetal karyotyping. ARSA with a conotruncal anomaly increases the risk for 22q11 del.

- Spatial arrangement abnormality in relation to the sternum: When the thymus is hypoplastic or absent the vessels in the three vessel trachea view are too close to the sternum (Fig. 5.47). This should prompt the presence of possible 22q11 del.

d. **Abnormality in the number of vessels:** There may be only two vessels seen in the three vessel trachea view. This happens in common arterial trunk where there is only one great arterial trunk arising from the ventricles (Fig. 5.48A). In complete transposition of great arteries, the pulmonary artery and the ductus arch are inferior to the aortic arch and hence in the three vessel trachea view only the aorta

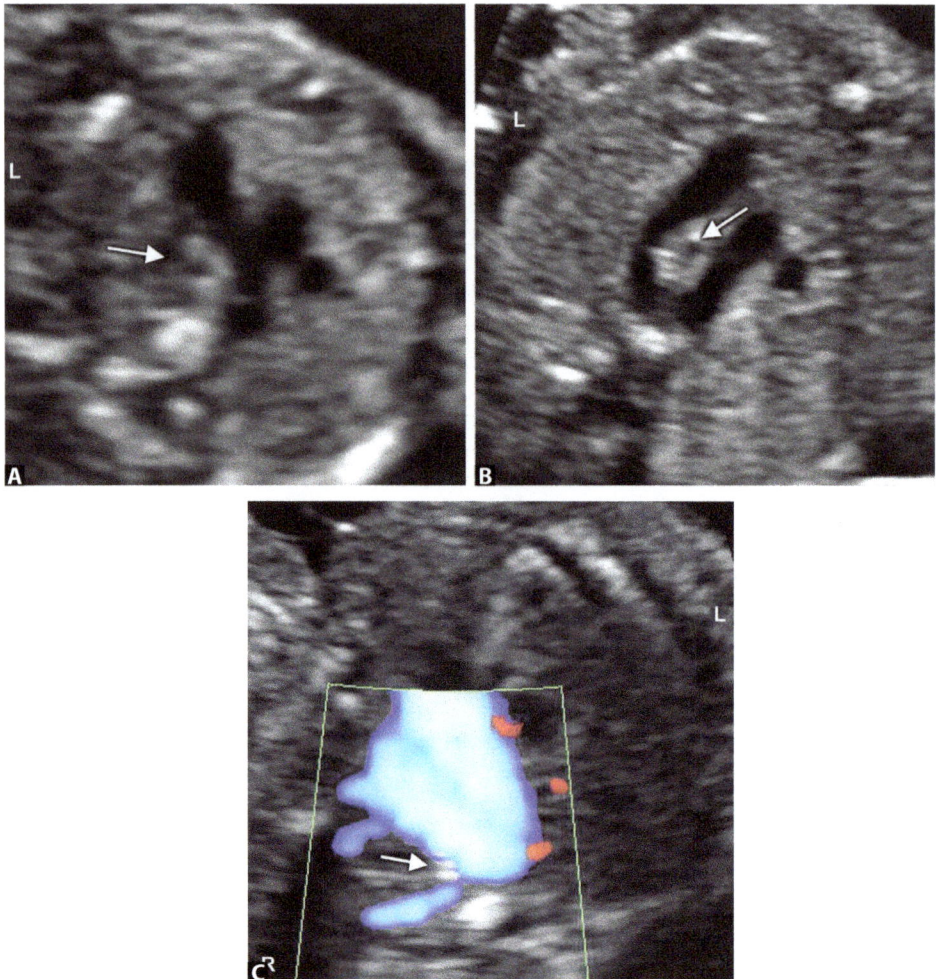

Figs 5.46A to C: (A) Right aortic arch with right ductus arch, V to the right sign (arrow indicates the trachea); (B) Right aortic arch with left ductus arch - U sign forming a sling around the trachea (arrow) and esophagus, (C) Left aortic arch with aberrant right subclavian artery. Three vessel trachea view with ARSA seen arising from the apex of the 'V' and coursing to the right side. The trachea is marked by arrow

is seen. The aorta and pulmonary artery in hypoplastic left heart syndrome and pulmonary atresia with intact ventricular septum respectively may be so small in caliber that they may not be identified by gray scale ultrasound thus causing only two vessels to be seen in the three vessel trachea view. Color Doppler helps in identifying the vessel.

There may be four vessels seen in the three vessel trachea view. This happens in persistent left superior vena cava (SVC).

Persistent left SVC: This is the most common venous variant in the thorax. Coexisting cardiac malformation (heterotaxy, conotruncal abnormalities and left ventricular outflow tract obstruction) is seen in about 5% of cases. The right superior

Fetal Cardiac Defects

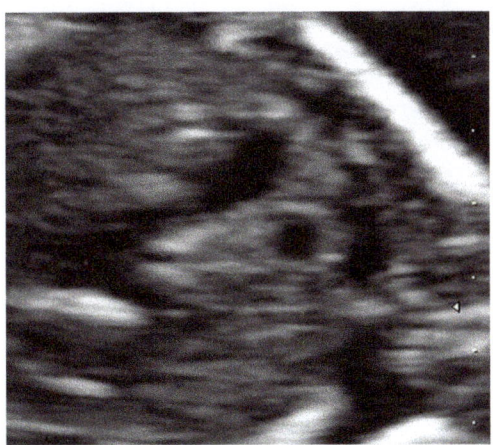

Fig. 5.47: The great vessels in the three vessel view are placed too close to the anterior chest wall in this case of double outlet right ventricle. The thymus is either absent or grossly hypoplastic

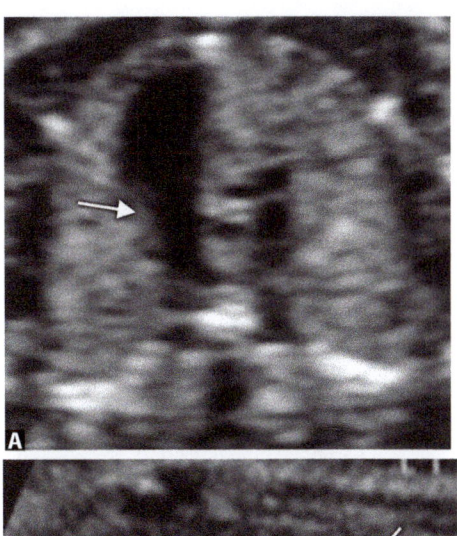

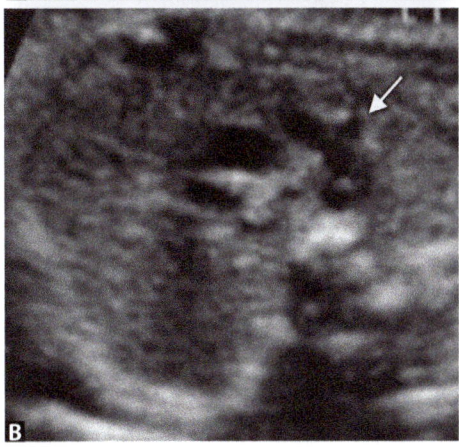

Figs 5.48A and B: (A) Single artery (aorta— arrow) seen in the three vessel view in a case of common arterial trunk; (B) Persistent left superior vena cava (arrow) in the three vessel view is the fourth vessel

vena cava may or may not be present. The left superior vena cava is identified as an extra vessel to the left of the pulmonary artery in the three vessel view (Fig. 5.48B). It may also be identified in the left atrioventricular groove in the four chamber view. The coronary sinus (into which it drains) is prominent (3 to 7 mm) and can be recognized when the probe is angled caudally from the four-chamber view. Differential diagnosis is the vertical vein in supracardiac total anomalous venous drainage. Color Doppler will demonstrate caudocranial flow direction in a vertical vein (in contrast to craniocaudal flow direction in the left superior vena cava).

e. **Miscellaneous:** Tracheal dilatation may be recognized in the three vessel view in congenital high airway obstruction sequence (CHAOS). An esophageal duplication cyst or a neurenteric cyst may be picked up in the three vessel view.

Thus, we see that a systematic examination using the standard planes of section is necessary for the recognition of findings. Integrating these findings together yields the final diagnosis. Complementation by recognition of extracardiac anomalies, karyotype and FISH results in a total fetal diagnosis. The pediatric cardiologist is thus equipped with the whole information which is vital for counseling and for further management.

SUGGESTED READING

1. Berg C, Georgiadis M, Geipel A, Gembruch U. The area behind the heart in the four-chamber view and the quest for congenital heart defects. Ultrasound Obstet Gynecol. 2007;30:721-7.
2. Chaoui R, Bollmann R, Goldner B, et al. Fetal cardiomegaly: echogardiographic findings and outcome in 19 cases. Fetal Diagn Ther. 1994;9:92-104.
3. Chaoui R, Heling KS, Kalache KD. Caliber of the coronary sinus in fetuses with cardiac defects with and without left persistent superior vena cava and in growth restricted fetuses with heart sparing effect. Prenat Diagn. 2003;23:552-7.
4. Chaoui R, Heling KS, Sarut Lopez A, Thiel G, Karl K. The thymic-thoracic ratio in fetal heart defects: A simple way to identify fetuses at high risk for microdeletion 22q11. Ultrasound Obstet Gynecol. 2011;37:397-403.
5. De Vore GR, et al. Prenatal diagnosis of cardiovascular malformations in the fetus with situs inversus viscerum during the second trimester of pregnancy. J Clin Ultrasound. 1986;14:454-7.
6. Fuglestad S, Puga G, Danielson G. Surgical pathology of the truncal valve: A study of twelve cases. Am J Cardiovasc Pathol. 1988;2:39-47.
7. Gindes L, Hegest J, Barkai G, Jacobson JM, Achiron A. Isolated levocardia—Prenatal diagnosis, clinical importance, and literature review. J Ultrasound Med. 2007;26:361-5.
8. Hoffman JIE, Kaplan S. The incidence of congenital heart disease. J Am Coll Cardiol. 2002;39(12):1890-900.
9. Hornberger LK, Sanders SP, Rein AJ, Spevak PJ, Parness IA, Colan SD. Left heart obstructive lesions and left ventricular growth in the mid trimester fetus. A Longitudinal study. Circulation. 1995;92(6):1533-8.
10. Kawazu Y, Inamura N, Shiono N, Kanagawa N, Narita J, Hamamichi Y, et al. 'Post-LA space index' as a potential novel marker for the prenatal diagnosis of isolated total anomalous pulmonary venous connection. Ultrasound Obstet Gynecol. 2014;44:682-7.
11. Kirklin JW, Barratt-Boyes BG. Complete transposition of great arteries. In: Kirklin JW, Barrat-Boyes BG (Eds). Cardiac surgery. New York: Churchill Livingstone. 1993:1383-467.
12. Lincoln C, Jamieson S, Joseph M, Shinebourne E, Anderson RH. Transatrial repair of ventricular septal defects with reference to their anatomic classification. J Thoracic Cardiovasc Surg. 1977;74:183-90.
13. Losekoot TG, Becker AE. Discordant atrioventricular connection and congenitally corrected transposition. In: Anderson RH, Macartney FJ, Shinebourne EA, et al. (Eds). Pediatric Cardiology. Edinburgh: Churchill Livingstone. 1987:867-88.
14. Machlitt A, Heling KS, Chaoui R. Increased atrioventricular length ratio in fetal four chamber view: A new marker for atrioventricular septal defect. Ultrasound Obstet Gynecol. 2004;24(6):618-22.
15. Smith RS, Comstock CH, Kirk JS, Lee W. Ultrasonographic left cardiac axis deviation—a marker of fetal anomalies. Obstet Gynecol. 1995;85(2):187-91.
16. Sridaromont S, Reldt RH, Ritter DG, Davis GD, Edwards JE. Double-outlet right ventricle: Hemodynamic and anatomic correlations. Am J Cardiol. 1976;38:85.
17. Tandon R, Edwards JE. Tricuspid atresia: A re-evaluation and classification. J Thorac Cardiavasc Surg. 1974;67:530-42.
18. Todros T, Paladini D, Chiappa E, Russo MG, Gaglioti P, Pacileo G, et al. Pulmonary stenosis and atresia with intact ventricular septum during prenatal life. Ultrasound Obstet Gynecol. 2003;21(3):228-33.
19. Van Praagh R, Van Praagh S, Vlad P, Keith JD. Diagnosis of the anatomic types of single or common ventricle. Am J Cardiol. 1965;15:345-66.
20. Vijaykumar V, Brandt T. Prolonged survival with isolated levocardia and situs inversus. Cleveclin J Med. 1991;58(3):243-7.
21. Wong SF, Ward C, Lee-Tannock A, Le S, Chan FY. Pulmonary artery/aorta ratio in simple screening for fetal outflow tract abnormalities during the second trimester. Ultrasound Obstet Gynecol. 2007;30:275-80.

CHAPTER 6

Pitfalls in Fetal Echocardiography

Reeth Sahana, Prathima Radhakrishnan

INTRODUCTION

With an estimated incidence of around six infant morbidity/mortality per 1000 live births, the congenital heart disease (CHD) is considered to be one of the major birth defect worldwide. In India, abundant data is available on the incidence of CHD at birth. The incidence of CHD varies from as low as 2.25–5.2/1000 live births to as high as 8–10/1000 live births in different studies. Going by the crude birth rate of 27.2/1000 (2001 Indian Census data), the total live births are estimated to be nearly 28 million per year. With an average incidence rate of 6–8/1000 live births; nearly 180,000 children are believed to be born with heart defects each year in India. Of these, nearly 60,000–90,000 suffer from critical cardiac lesions requiring early intervention. Approximately 10% of present infant mortality in India may be accounted for CHDs alone.

Although, the incidence of congenital heart defects is high, the detection is still very low in India. The accurate prenatal diagnosis would help to improve the outcome for these affected babies, especially in those cases that are likely to require prostaglandin infusion to maintain patency of the ductus arteriosus. This helps both the obstetrician and the parents to decide the place for delivery as this requires tertiary-level care in neonatal and cardiac intensive care units. The parents must be better informed prior, to prepare themselves for emotional and financial implications owing to the high costs of these services.

Fetal echocardiography is defined as a detailed sonographic evaluation that is used to identify and characterize fetal heart anomalies before the delivery. Echocardiography should be performed with the lowest possible ultrasonic exposure settings to gain the necessary diagnostic information. Although, it is impossible to detect all the fetal abnormalities, adherence to appropriate guidelines will maximize the probability of detecting most cases of clinically significant CHD. Fetal echocardiography is generally performed between 18 and 24 weeks' gestational age. Optimal views of the heart are usually obtained when the cardiac apex is directed towards the anterior maternal wall.

EQUIPMENT TO PERFORM FETAL ECHOCARDIOGRAPHY

The equipment used for performing a fetal echocardiography needs to have an excellent B-mode, with a good cine-loop facility, so that one can scroll back frame-by-frame and capture the frame of interest. The spatial and temporal resolution needs to be very good. The system should have color Doppler, pulsed Doppler and continuous wave Doppler. In addition to these, STIC, tissue Doppler and multiplanar imaging are added advantages.

A special preset for fetal heart evaluation needs to be created with a high frame rate, decreased persistence and increased compression. The system should have the ability to zoom the image without causing deterioration in the image quality. A higher pulse repetition frequency (PRF) setting is required for color Doppler in the fetus as compared to the routine obstetric color Doppler.

TIMING OF FETAL ECHOCARDIOGRAPHY

Ideally all fetuses that have an anomaly scan at 18-24 weeks must have the 'basic cardiac exam', which is a 'screening scan' that involves the gray scale visualization of the four chambers and the outflow tracts. The highest incidence of cardiac defects is found in the 'extended cardiac scan', which is done if there is any suspicious image found during the 'basic cardiac scan'. In addition, maternal pre-gestational diabetes, anti-depressants like lithium intake, presence of anti-Ro/SSA and anti-La/SSB antigen-antibodies, family history of cardiac defects, presence of other fetal anomalies, etc. should prompt a more detailed cardiac scan. The International Society of Ultrasound in Obstetrics and Gynecology (ISUOG) has issued standard guidelines for basic and extended cardiac screening.

In spite of the many advances in technology and skills, there are certain limiting factors in performing a fetal echocardiogram and diagnosing certain fetal cardiac defects. These can be considered as 'pitfalls'.

PITFALLS IN FETAL ECHOCARDIOGRAPHY

Pitfalls may be due to fetal, maternal or operator limitations. The most common fetal limitations are the fetal position, gestational age or reduction in the amniotic fluid. Maternal habitus is a common limitation. Other limitations are as follows:
- Commonly missed/incorrect diagnosis
- Conditions which may progress in utero
- Conditions not evident in utero.

TECHNICAL LIMITATIONS

Most common reason for technical limitation is poor image quality which could be due to various reasons which may be either maternal or fetal, e.g. maternal obesity, prone fetal position and late or very early gestation. Technical limitations make a detailed heart evaluation very difficult due to acoustic shadowing, especially during the third trimester. It is necessary to examine the patient at different time points if the heart is poorly visualized. The examiner can optimize sonograms by appropriate adjustment of technical settings, such as acoustic focus, frequency selection, signal gain, image magnification, temporal resolution, harmonic imaging and Doppler-related parameters (e.g. velocity scale, frequency wall filter and frame rate). As the heart is a dynamic structure, a complete evaluation can only be made if a real-time imaging with acquisition of analog recordings or digital video clips is used as a standard part of every fetal echocardiogram.

FIRST TRIMESTER CARDIAC SCAN

Early fetal echocardiography, which involves assessment of the heart biometry and visualization of cardiac structures done between 10 and 15 weeks of gestation, is

Table 6.1: Rate of successful visualization of all cardiac structures by TVS and TAS

	Full cardiac examination								
	TVS				TAS				TVS and TAS
	B-Mode		Color Doppler		B-Mode		Color Doppler		
GA, week	n	%	n	%	n	%	n	%	n	%
10	0/9	0	0/9	0	0/9	0	0/9	0	0/9	0
11	1/22	5	10/22	45	0/22	0	2/22	9	10/22	45
12	0/41	0	36/41	88	0/41	0	15/41	37	37/41	90
13	1/24	4	19/24	79	0/24	0	16/24	67	21/24	88
14	1/12	8	9/12	75	3/12	25	10/12	83	11/12	92
15					4/15	27	15/15	100	15/15	100

Successful visualization of fetal heart by transvaginal (TVS) and transabdominal (TAS) scan in the first trimester of pregnancy
Source: J Ultrasound Med. 2006;25:173-82.

technically difficult. The rate of successful visualization of cardiac structures by transvaginal sonography (TVS) and transabdominal sonography (TAS) was studied by Smrcek et al. between the gestational age of 11 and 14 weeks, and they found to be as low as 0% with M-Mode to 9% with color Doppler and improved up to 45% with combined TAS and TVS mode. At 14 weeks with the combined approach, the fetal cardia can be satisfactorily assessed to about 90%. However, the study concluded that the ideal time would be 12 weeks and an adequate assessment was about 90% when a combined TAS and TVS approach was used with study of heart in both M-mode and color Doppler (Table 6.1).

THIRD TRIMESTER CARDIAC SCAN

Late fetal echocardiography performed during the third trimester is technically difficult due to shadowing by the overlying ribcage. Due to persistent unfavorable fetal position which is not uncommon especially in the third trimester, as it takes fetuses longer time to turn from prone to supine position.

FETAL POSITION

The fetal echocardiography is best performed in the apical view, but ideally needs to be assessed on lateral views where in outflow tracts and interventricular septum is well-visualized. In addition, the transverse view helps to study the systemic veins, aortic and ductal arches much clearer. However, all these are very much dependent on the optimal fetal position during scanning.

AMNIOTIC FLUID

For the satisfactory assessment of fetal study, adequate amount of amniotic fluid is very much necessary. In case of reduced amniotic fluid, the fetal cardiac study could be suboptimal due to reduced acoustic window and takes long time for the fetus to come to a favorable position. In case of polyhydramnios, the fetal echocardiography could take a much longer time due to increased fetal movements.

MATERNAL HABITUS

Maternal obesity is known to be associated with a variety of maternal and fetal complications which increases the risk for fetal structural abnormalities, especially cardiac defects independent of other maternal risks such as diabetes. High body mass index (BMI) adversely affects the ability to visualize fetal structures, especially cardiac and spinal anatomy owing to the thick maternal abdominal wall which causes poor penetration of ultrasound beams, due to which the cardiac assessment will take a longer time and could be suboptimal. Maternal adipose tissue thickness is one of the main reason for suboptimal ultrasonographic visualization (SUV) of the fetal heart. A direct relationship is observed between the rate of SUV of the cardiac structures and maternal BMI.

Advanced ultrasound equipment, skilled technician, increased duration and repetition of examination cannot completely eliminate the deleterious effect of obesity on visualization which may lead to decreased anomaly detection rates. In order to overcome these limitations, it is necessary to understand the different techniques of transducer movements that takes for an assessment of the heart and different approach can be used which include use of three-dimensional ultrasonography harmonic imaging and transumbilical placement of the probe. Adequate training and technical skills are an absolute necessity to provide a quality service in ultrasonographic examination of fetal cardiovascular system. The mother has to be informed that to get a clear image, she has to wait for the fetus to come to a favorable position.

In early gestational period if the fetal heart appears normal then the mother is advised for anomaly scan between 18 and 20 weeks. However, in case of suspicion of major heart defect, mother will be advised for an early fetal well-being scan at 16–17 weeks followed by another review scan at 20–22 weeks, if the early scan is found to be normal.

Due to any limitations if the transabdominal ultrasonography is not satisfactory or any anomaly is suspected, then the fetal MRI is advised especially to study the fetal cardia. However, the availability of fetal MRI for cardiac studies is limited to very few centers across the world.

COMMONLY MISSED OR INCORRECT DIAGNOSIS

Right to Left Disproportion

Most of the time, the referrals to a fetal medicine unit especially in the third trimester is with the diagnosis of right chambers of the heart appearing larger than the left chambers or the left-sided chambers appearing smaller than the right, i.e. suspicion of hypoplastic left heart syndrome. This may be due to:
- Large outlet ventricular septal defects (VSD)
- Small aortic valve
- Diffuse transverse arch hypoplasia
- Small apex forming left ventricle
- Small mitral valve
- Patent foramen ovale shunting left to right.

However, the cardiac scan done by specialist antenatally or on postnatal fetal echocardiography performed by pediatric cardiologists are often found to be normal (Fig. 6.1).

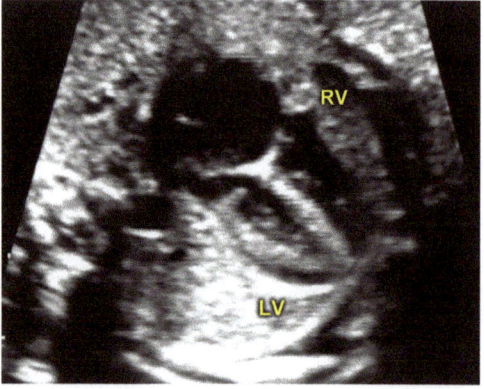

Fig. 6.1: Right ventricular dominance in a normal third trimester fetus

Perimembranous VSD

The mistaken diagnosis of a perimembranous VSD or an apical VSD is because of echocardiogram dropout zone in membranous septum or apex. This usually depends on the transducer placement. These findings could also be associated with right–left disproportion but is of no functional significance (Figs 6.2 to 6.4).

FETAL ARRHYTHMIA

Fetal echocardiography is the most important diagnostic tool for arrhythmia diagnosis in the fetal period. On using M-mode many times, it is very difficult to obtain signal. Hence pulsed Doppler is preferred. Transient bradycardia, which is falsely reported sometimes, causes unnecessary anxiety to the parents. This is due to excessive pressure on the maternal

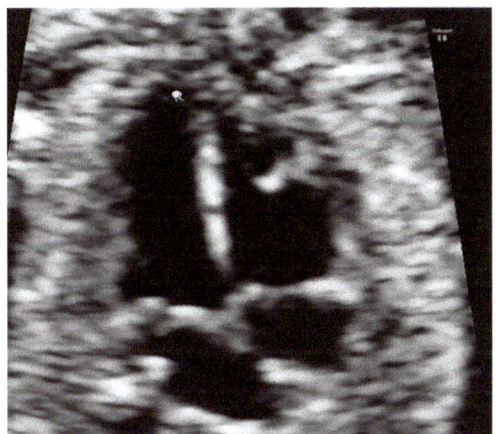

Fig. 6.2: Four-chamber view of heart, the arrow pointing at apical dropout zone which appears like an apical VSD

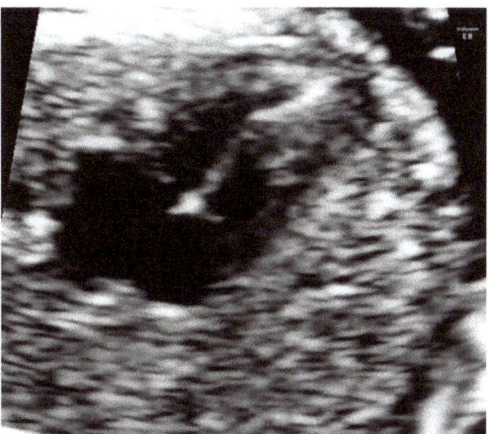

Fig. 6.3: Four-chamber view. Slight change in the position of the transducer, the complete septum without any discontinuity is noted

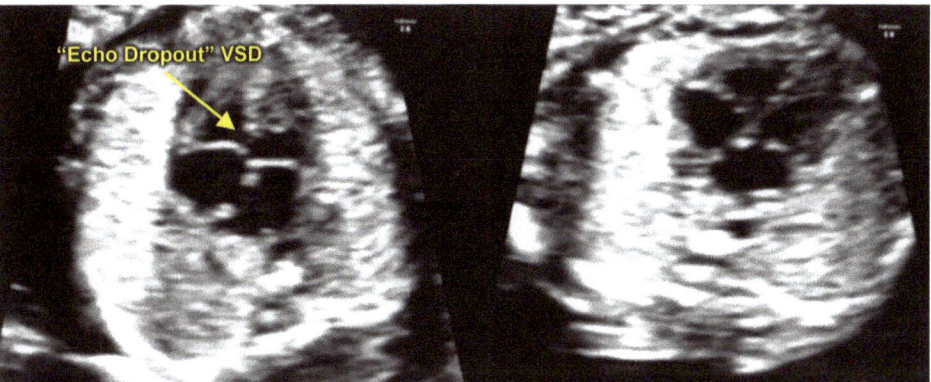

Fig. 6.4: "Echo Dropout VSD" in apical four-chamber view and same fetus in slightly lateral view shows an intact ventricular septum

abdomen and hence fetal cardia that initiates vagal stimulation and transient bradycardia. However, normal fetal rhythm is usually established once the pressure is released.

OVER-DIAGNOSIS OF TETRALOGY OF FALLOT

Incorrect orientation of transducer may demonstrate apparent septoaortic discontinuity in a normal fetus. The mechanism of this artifact is probably related to the angle of incidence of sound beam. Careful visualization of the left ventricular outflow tract with different insonation angles as well as use of color Doppler and the absence of other elements of tetralogy should virtually eliminate this problem (Fig. 6.5).

SACROCOCCYGEAL TERATOMA

The fetal cardiac scan can sometimes show features of hyperdynamic circulation in an otherwise anatomically normal appearing heart. Although, the fetal heart looks structurally normal, still we need to look out for any non-cardiac anomalies like sacrococcygeal teratoma that causes the functional abnormality in the heart at later stages. It is always recommended for follow-up assessment if any anomalies are found as it may result in heart failure due to size of the mass.

CONDITIONS THAT ARE DETECTED LATE IN PREGNANCY

Some of the cardiac anomalies through their natural course develop ultrasonographic manifestations and become amenable to diagnosis only later in the course of pregnancy or even after birth. Although comprehensive fetal cardiac anatomy can be assessed by the end of the first trimester, alterations in chamber size, small VSDs, and differences in size between the great vessels may not become apparent until later in fetal or neonatal life. The natural histories of the hypoplastic heart syndrome, coarctation of the aorta, endocardial fibroelastosis secondary to aortic or pulmonary stenosis, tetralogy of Fallot, and cardiac tumors are all examples of evolving cardiac lesions.

DELAYED OR MISSED DIAGNOSIS DUE TO LIMITED RESOLUTION

Although VSDs can be readily diagnosed in utero, they are probably the most commonly missed lesions during prenatal echocardiographic examinations. The small size of most of these lesions is apparently beyond the resolution of most currently available gray-scale ultrasound scanners. Therefore, the prenatal diagnosis of VSD is often very difficult if not impossible. Moreover, in many cases, VSDs can undergo spontaneous closure during pregnancy or shortly after birth, which makes the rate of undiagnosed lesions even higher. However, new higher-frequency transducers (5 to 7 MHz) and color Doppler may enhance the diagnosis of some cases with VSD.

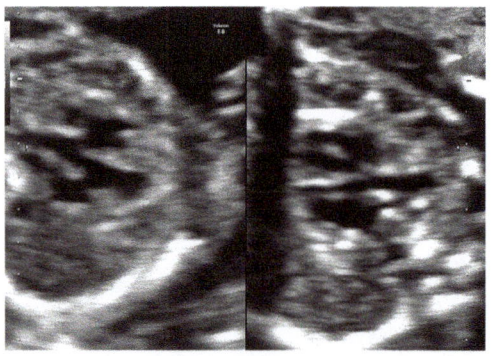

Fig. 6.5: Septoaortic discontinuity in lateral view of the heart and same fetus with slight transducer adjustment showing normal continuity

PROGRESSION OF LESIONS IN UTERO, LEADING TO LATE ONSET CARDIAC MALFORMATIONS

Examples for lesions which progress in utero include major vessel stenosis and ventricular outflow tract obstruction. These forms of obstructive outflow tract lesions may not be obvious in the first half of pregnancy, mainly because the process of arrest of growth in narrowing the vessel is not significant enough to be detected by bidimensional ultrasound scanning. For example, aortic stenosis tends to be a progressive disease. Mild pulmonary stenosis diagnosed early in the second trimester may progress to critical pulmonary stenosis and hypoplasia of the right ventricle, or alternatively in cases in which the pulmonic valve and right ventricle appeared normal on early fetal echocardiography, serious pulmonary stenosis developed by the end of pregnancy. Hypoplasia of the aortic arch and pulmonary arteries can develop with coarctation of aorta and tetralogy of Fallot respectively. The late development of left and right ventricular outflow tract lesions may render this group of congenital heart defects discernible only in the second or even third trimester.

The delayed diagnosis of tetralogy of heart may be caused by a combination of limited ultrasonographic resolution early in the course of pregnancy with in utero progression of the typical lesions.

Some lesions tend to acquire a typical late-onset appearance. Endocardial fibroelastosis, fetal cardiac rhabdomyoma, hypertrophic cardiomyopathy, and ventricular aneurysm are all examples of late-onset appearance of fetal cardiac pathology. Endocardial fibroelastosis is an excellent example of cardiac lesion that may develop and present at any time in utero. A debate is currently under way as to whether endocardial fibroelastosis is a primary or secondary disease, and Coxsackie virus or mumps virus infections have been suggested. Therefore, the appearance of fetal endocardial fibroelastosis, following normal fetal cardiac evaluation, supports the hypothesis that this peculiar cardiac lesion may be secondary and that its appearance depends on the time of possible inutero infection. Alternatively, its initial manifestations may be subtle; therefore, they might escape early diagnosis. Fetal cardiac rhabdomyoma is another example of congenital cardiac disease that evolves in utero. Rhabdomyomas have been detected during the third trimester after a normal ultrasound examination during the first half of pregnancy, clearly indicating that rhabdomyoma may develop during late gestation, infancy, and childhood. No data exist on the natural history of this anomaly during fetal life. However, Sonesson, et al. described one case where they showed that rhabdomyomas were not evident on first examination at 23 weeks but became evident only at the second examination 12 weeks later, at 35 weeks.

Premature closure of the foramen ovale is another abnormality that may develop later in gestation and may even escape accurate in utero diagnosis. Although most cases with premature closure of the foramen ovale will present as hypoplastic left heart some may show normal- or nearly normal-sized left heart. The only possible hint of this abnormality that could be detected was that instead of having a normal flapping motion, the foramen ovale showed ballooning into the left atrium, where a clear color filling the aneurysmal flap that reached the surface of the mitral valve was noted.

ERRONEOUS DIAGNOSIS

The main reason for late diagnosis of fetal cardiac malformation during pregnancy should be attributed to erroneous diagnosis. The ability to obtain a correct diagnosis on the initial scan can be compromised if pulsed and color Doppler studies are not included.

One should understand that major cardiac defect like transposition of the great vessels, AV canal defects, heterotaxy syndrome, double outlet of the right ventricle, total anomalous pulmonary venous connection, truncus arteriosus, and Ebstein anomaly are cardiac malformations that do not evolve from a normal-looking heart during pregnancy.

Third-trimester 'routine' ultrasound examination for fetal growth and well-being usually does not include detailed fetal echocardiography. However, a brief glance at the fetal heart by experienced operators is enough to raise suspicion of an abnormality. This is followed by a comprehensive cardiac evaluation. Whether routine third-trimester fetal echocardiography would further reduce the rate of undiagnosed cases with cardiac malformations is a matter of speculation.

CONDITIONS THAT ARE EVIDENT ONLY AFTER BIRTH

Some congenital heart anomalies may present soon after birth. The fetal structures such as foramen ovale, ductus venosus and ductus arteriosus, which are vital for fetal circulation is no longer needed for survival following birth and begin to close. Non-closure of these structures lead to congenital heart defects like atrial septal defects and patent ductus arteriosus.

Infants with life-threatening heart defects may not initially have symptoms or the clinical signs may be obscure, serious condition may not be recognized on the routine physical examination in majority of cases. Therefore, diagnosis of such conditions require high degree of suspicion by the neonatologist and appropriate investigation and timely management.

SUMMARY

- Fetal echocardiography is a useful tool for the diagnosis of CHD with a sensitivity and specificity rate of 98% and 99%, respectively.
- Fetal echocardiography is performed when there is a specific maternal or fetal indications detected or suspected on basis or targeted ultrasound examination.
- Pitfalls of fetal echocardiography may be either due to technical limitations or related to interpretation.
- Technical limitations may be due to poor image quality, fetal position, maternal habitus, multiple gestations, presence of oligohydramnios and poor windows.
- Advanced ultrasound equipment, skilled technician, increased duration and repetition of examination can help in overcoming technical limitations and increasing the detection rates of CHD.
- Pitfalls due to interpretation may be due to incorrect/missed diagnosis like minor VSDs or due to conditions that progress in utero such as bicuspid aortic valve or due to anomalies which are evident only later on in the neonate.

CONCLUSION

Congenital heart disease is the most common congenital anomaly found in the fetus and with the increase in the detection rates of CHD, the demand for fetal echocardiography has also proportionally increased. Fetal echocardiography is a very useful tool for the prenatal diagnosis of CHD despite the pitfalls associated with it. Several studies have focused on the effectiveness of fetal echocardiography in detecting CHD since its introduction in the 1980's. The studies have provided convincing evidence about the reliability and high scan quality of fetal echocardiography. The accurate prenatal diagnosis of CHD via fetal echocardiography has many benefits. In addition to helping in management of the pregnancy, it also improves the perinatal outcome of the neonate with significant CHD avoiding the onset of hemodynamic compromise. The prenatal diagnosis of CHD via fetal echocardiography also allows for appropriate parental counseling which allows the families to make informed decisions regarding the outcome of pregnancy. Improved operator skill, a low threshold for echocardiography referrals and convenient access to fetal cardia specialists are important factors that can improve the effectiveness of screening programs. Hence, it is imperative to develop screening programs that will help to improve prenatal detection of cardiac anomalies during routine ultrasound scan and thus decrease the mortality and morbidity rate associated with CHD.

SUGGESTED READING

1. Achiron R, Weissman A, Rotstein Z, Lipitz S, Mashiach S, Hegesh J. Transvaginal echocardiographic examination of the fetal heart between 13 and 15 weeks' gestation in a low-risk population. J Ultrasound Med. 1994; 13:783-9.
2. Allan LD, Crawford DC, Henderson RH, Tynan MJ. Spectrum of congenital heart disease detected echocardiographically in perinatal life. Br Heart J. 1985;54:523-6.
3. Allan LD. Diagnosis of fetal cardiac abnormalities. Arch Dis Child. 1989;64:964-8.
4. American Institute of Ultrasound in M. AIUM practice guideline for the performance of fetal echocardiography. Journal of ultrasound in medicine: Official journal of the American Institute of Ultrasound in Medicine. 2013;32(6):1067.
5. Carvalho JS, Allan LD, Chaoui R, Copel JA, DeVore GR, Hecher K, et al. ISUOG Practice Guidelines (updated): Sonographic screening examination of the fetal heart. Ultrasound Obstet Gynecol. 2013;41(3):348-59.
6. Chang RK, Gurvitz M, Rodriguez S. Missed diagnosis of critical congenital heart disease. Arch Pediatr Adolesc Med. 2008;162: 969-74.
7. Hendler I, Blackwell SC, Bujold E, Treadwell MC, Mittal P, Sokol RJ, et al. Suboptimal second-trimester ultrasonographic visualization of the fetal heart in obese women should we repeat the examination. J Ultrasound Med. 2005;24(9):1205-9.
8. Hiraishi S, Agata Y, Nowatari M, Oguchi K, Misawa H, Hirota H, et al. Incidence and natural course of trabecular ventricular septal defect: two-dimensional echocardiography and color Doppler flow imaging study. J Pediatr. 1992; 120:409-15.
9. Naeye RL, Blanc WA. Prenatal narrowing or closure of the foramen ovale.Circulation. 1964; 30:736-42.
10. Revel A, Ariel I, Rein AJJ, Anteby E, Lavie Y, Yagel S. Fetal endocardial fibroelastosis. J Clin Ultrasound. 1993;22:355-6.
11. Rychik J, Ayres N, Cuneo B, Gotteiner N, Hornberger L, Spevak PJ, et al. American Society of Echocardiography guidelines and standards for performance of the fetal echocardiogram. J Am Soc Echocardiogr. 2004;17(7):803-10.
12. Silverman NH, Schmidt KG. Ultrasound evaluation of the fetal heart. In: Callen BW, (Ed). Ultrasonography in Obstetrics and Gynecology, 3rd ed. Philadelphia, Pa: WB Saunders; 1994:310-32.
13. Smythe JF, Dyck JD, Smallhorn JF, Freedom RM. Natural history of cardiac rhabdomyoma in infancy and childhood. Am J Cardiol. 1990; 66:1247-9.
14. Sonesson SE, Fouron JC, Lessard M. Intrauterine diagnosis and evolution of a cardiomyopathy in a fetus with Noonan's syndrome. Acta Pediatr. 1992;81:368-70.
15. Tegnander E, Eik-Nes SH, Johansen OJ, Linker DT. Prenatal detection of heart defects at the routine fetal examination at 18 weeks in a non-selected population. Ultrasound Obstet Gynecol. 1995;5:372-80.
16. Thornburg LL, Miles K, Ho M, Pressman EK. Fetal anatomic evaluation in the overweight and obese gravida. Ultrasound Obstet Gynecol. 2009;33(6):670-5.

17. Treadwell MC, Seubert DE, Zador I, Goyert GL, Wolfe HM. Benefits associated with harmonic tissue imaging in the obstetric patient. Am J Obstet Gynecol. 2000;182(6):1620-2.
18. Wang PH, Chen GD, Lin LY. Imaging comparison of basic cardiac views between two- and three-dimensional ultrasound in normal fetuses in anterior spine positions. The International Journal of Cardiovascular Imaging. 2002;18(1):17-23.
19. Working Group on Management of Congenital Heart Diseases in I. Consensus on timing of intervention for common congenital heart disease. Indian Pediatrics. 2008;45(2):117.

CHAPTER 7

Fetal Arrhythmias: Evaluation and Management

Shardha Srinivasan

ABSTRACT

Fetal arrhythmias are common in clinical practice and are usually benign. However in some cases, they may result in hemodynamic compromise and may be associated with adverse fetal outcomes including hydrops or fetal loss. They are also one of the few fetal cardiac conditions that are amenable to successful inutero therapy. As seen in postnatal life, these may present with an irregular rhythm, tachyarrhythmia or a bradyarrhythmia; either in isolation or in the setting of associated congenital heart defects. Fetal echocardiography is the cornerstone for evaluation of fetal arrhythmias, providing insight into the mechanism of arrhythmia as well as important information with regards hemodynamic effects of the arrhythmia and an important tool for monitoring the course over the pregnancy. Newer techniques such as fetal magnetocardiogram (fMCG) and fetal electrocardiogram (fECG) are emerging as important adjuncts especially in the study of repolarization abnormalities. This Chapter provides a general overview and basic guidelines for the evaluation and management of fetal arrhythmias, with a focus on ultrasound evaluation of rhythm disorders in the fetus.

INTRODUCTION

Fetal arrhythmias are commonly seen in routine obstetric practice. Though the majority of cases have a benign course, a small percentage of cases may result in significant hemodynamic compromise in the fetus either due to a persistent course, associated congenital heart defects or as a result off the underlying etiology. In such cases, early recognition and appropriate diagnosis allows for consideration of appropriate fetal therapy. Ultrasound has remained the corner stone in the clinical assessment of the fetal rhythm and well-being and as a guide to therapy and management. Ultrasound however, is limited in its ability to evaluate repolarization changes that may lead to malignant fetal arrhythmias. Our understanding of the fetal phenotype in the setting of these channelopathies is evolving due to the application of newer techniques such as magnetocardiography and fetal electrocardiograms. Identification of the fetus at risk allows for closer monitoring using standard clinical tools, when a higher index of suspicion warrants it. This Chapter will provide an overview of the basics of diagnosis and management of the different kinds of fetal rhythm disturbances in clinical practice.

INCIDENCE AND PRESENTATION

Abnormalities of fetal rhythm may be seen in about 1-3% of pregnancies, and account for about 10-14% referrals to tertiary care obstetric centers. The majority are benign transient ectopic beats with sustained and significant arrhythmia being noted in a smaller percentage of cases.

Most cases are noted incidentally during a routine obstetric visit, presenting as an irregular, too fast or too slow a rhythm. Some may be noted as incidental pickup as part of a routine OB ultrasound. A small percentage off cases may present with diminished fetal movements and/or hydrops fetalis in setting of persistent arrhythmia, with or without associated heart defects.

Normal fetal heart rate ranges from 110-160 beats per minute (BPM) however this does vary some with gestational age. Though persistent bradycardia is defined as heart rates below 100 BPM and tachycardia as heart rates over 180 BPM, in general persistent fetal hearts in the 110-100 range as well as 160-180 BPM range with diminished variability is not normal and merits further evaluation and monitoring for both abnormalities in rhythm as well as noncardiac causes.

CLASSIFICATION

Based on clinical presentation, fetal arrhythmias are generally classified into:
- Irregular rhythms
  - Premature atrial beats
  - Premature ventricular beats
  - Second degree heart block (Mobitz type I and some types of Mobitz type II)
- Tachycardia
  - Sinus tachycardia
  - Supraventricular tachycardia.
    - Atrioventricular reentrant tachycardia (AVRT)
    - Paroxysmal junctional reciprocating tachycardia (PJRT)
    - Atrial ectopic tachycardia (AET)
  - Atrial flutter
  - Ventricular/Junctional tachycardia
- Bradycardia
  - Sinus bradycardia
  - Blocked atrial bigeminy
  - Second degree heart block
    - Mobitz type II
    - Secondary to QT prolongation
  - Complete heart block
    - Immune mediated
    - Idiopathic
    - Associated with congenital heart disease.

Differentiation is aided by evaluation of atrioventricular (AV) and ventriculoatrial (VA) relationship and time intervals (described later in text).

DIAGNOSIS AND MONITORING OF FETAL ARRHYTHMIA

- *Cardiotocography:* External fetal monitoring is widely used for monitoring the fetus over extended periods of time and provides information on sudden changes in heart rate and heart rate variability. The device is attached via two probes over the maternal abdomen, one of which records fetal heart rate via a Doppler probe and the second uterine contractions. Several limitations exist, including inability to track very rapid heart rates due to under-counting secondary to aliasing, interference from maternal heart rates, fetal movements leading to poor tracing and poor sensitivity in the setting of an irregular fetal rhythm. Fetal scalp electrode monitoring is also used for fetal heart rate analysis during labor.

Fetal Arrhythmias: Evaluation and Management

- *Ultrasound evaluation is the cornerstone for the diagnosis and monitoring of the fetus with suspected arrhythmia. Goals include:*
  - Evaluate fetal heart rate.
  - Elucidate type and mechanism of arrhythmia.
  - Evaluate persistence of arrhythmia. Incessant or intermittent.
  - Assess for associated cardiac malformations.
  - Assess for associated noncardiac conditions such as fetal goiter, anemia.
  - Evaluate fetal hemodynamics and well-being. Role for fetal CHF score in serial evaluations (Refer to Chapter 8, Table 8.1.)
  - Evaluate the impact and efficacy of fetal therapy using serial scans.

Evaluation of the type and mechanism of fetal arrhythmia using ultrasound involves using surrogate markers for atrial and ventricular contractions. Systematically analyze:

- Atrial rate and relationship between consecutive atrial beats
- Ventricular rate and relationship between consecutive ventricular beats
- Relationship between the atrial and ventricular beats and pattern of sequential activation of these chambers (AV relationships)
- Measure time intervals: AV and VA conduction times.

By using mechanical measures of contraction (as with M-mode) or alterations in Doppler flow patterns that result from chamber contraction (Doppler flow patterns) or a combination of the two, a ladder diagram for various patterns of activation can be formulated to assist with the diagnosis (Table 7.1).

Table 7.1: Algorithm for echocardiographic diagnosis of fetal arrhythmia, utilizing relationships between atrial and ventricular contractions, atrial and ventricular rates and possible underlying rhythm

Atrial rate	Ventricular rate	A-V relationship	Additional findings	Likely diagnosis
Normal 120–160	Normal 120–160	A A A A A / V V V V V	Variability + Normal AV interval	Normal sinus rhythm
Faster ~180–220	Faster ~180–220	A A A A A A / V V V V V V	Variability + VA>AV	Sinus tachycardia
Faster ~220–280	Faster ~220–280	A A A A A A A / V V V V V V V	VA<AV	SVT Likely AVRT
Faster 170–240	Faster 170–240	A A A A A A A / V V V V V V V	Sudden onset VA>AV	PJRT/AET
~170–220 or Normal	~170–220	A A A A A A A / V V V V V V V	Simultaneous V-A or AV dissociation	JET or VT
300–500	Variable block 80–250	A A A A A A A A A A / V V V V	Regular A Irregular A	AF CAT
120–160	120–160	A A A A A / V V V V V	AV prolongation	1° HB

Contd...

Contd...

Atrial rate	Ventricular rate	A-V relationship	Additional findings	Likely diagnosis
120–160	Irregular	A A A A A / V V V V	Gradual AV prolongation with non-conducted beat	Mobitz I 2nd degree AV block
120–160	Irregular or bradycardia <100	A A A A A / V V V	Variable ratio	Mobitz II 2nd degree block
120–160	<100	A A A A A / V V V	AV dissociation	CHB
110–160	170–220	A A A A A / V V V V V V V V	AV dissociation	VT

Abbreviations: AV, atrioventricular interval; VA, ventriculoatrial interval; SVT, supraventricular tachycardia; AVRT, atrioventricular re-entrant tachycardia; PJRT, paroxysmal junctional reciprocating tachycardia; AET, atrial ectopic tachycardia; JET, junctional ectopic tachycardia; AF, atrial flutter; CAT, chaotic atrial tachycardia; HB, heart block; CHB, complete heart block; VT, ventricular tachycardia.

Methods in common practice include:
M-mode techniques (Fig. 7.1):
- Simultaneous recording of M-mode through the atrium (A) and ventricle (V) by aligning the M-mode beam is used to study atrioventricular sequential contraction pattern (Fig. 7.1A).
  Advantages include:
  - Technique is available on all machines. Easy to use.

  Disadvantages:
  - Adversely affected by fetal movement and fetal position.
  - Atrial signals may be too small or weak for reliable interpretation. In these cases, aligning the M-mode with region of the crista terminalis in the right atrium or the junction of the atrium with the atrial appendage provides the most reliable and distinct atrial signals.
  - Difficult to reliably assess AV and VA intervals especially in tachycardia.
- Color M-mode tracings: Utilizes a combination of M-mode to demonstrate atrial contractions and as a surrogate for 'P' waves and color Doppler evaluation of flow through a valve or vessel (commonly the LVOT or aorta) as a surrogate for ventricular events (V). Easy to obtain by aligning M-mode through the left ventricular outflow tract and opposite atrial wall. The M-mode cursor is optimized for the best atrial signal as it is easy to capture aortic flow (Fig. 7.1B). Alternatively, the M-mode cursor can be aligned through both atria in a horizontal four-chamber view and Doppler flow captured in the aorta as is crosses anterior to the atria (Fig. 7.1C). It is beneficial to keep the Doppler color box as narrow as possible and aliasing velocity high to obtain clean signals without color bleed obscuring M-mode signals. This technique allows for optimization of atrial contraction signals and AV relations are easy to assess.
- Anatomic M-mode: It is available on the newer machines and allows for either nonstandard orientation of the M-mode beam or two simultaneous M-mode planes allowing for simultaneous assessment of atrial and ventricular contraction pattern (Fig. 7.1D).
  - Limited availability depending on the machine.
  - Some degradation of M-mode signal.

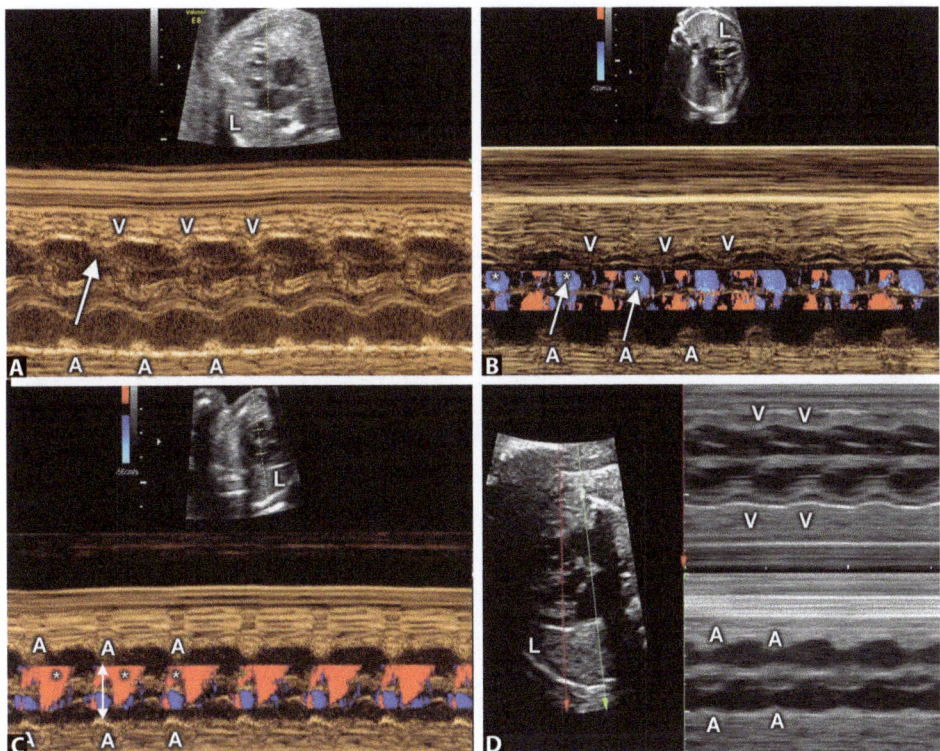

Figs 7.1A to D: Use of M-mode in the diagnosis of fetal arrhythmia. (A) The M-mode cursor is aligned through the ventricle (V) as well as atrium (A) to record contraction signals from the respective chambers. The reference 2D image is shown on top of the M-mode recording with the ventricle on top and atrium at the bottom. A-V synchrony is demonstrated (↑) in this fetus with normal sinus rhythm; (B) Color M-mode in a similar orientation with the cursor passing through the ventricle (V) on top, across the ventricular outflow tract (*) and the opposite atrium (A). In this image, ventricular ejection results in flow in the left ventricular out flow tract that is oriented away from the transducer demonstrated in blue (*). This is superimposed on M-mode signal and atrioventricular synchrony demonstrated by arrow (↑). Given proximity of the left ventricular outflow tract and aorta to the atrium, the M-mode can be optimized to provide the best atrial contraction signals; (C) color M-mode with M-mode signal going through both atria and the aorta. Atrial contractions are demonstrated on M-mode (A) while ventricular ejection is shown as color flow in the aorta demonstrated by the *. (↔) Demonstrates simultaneous atrial signals on M-mode; (D) Anatomic M-mode using two simultaneous M-mode cursors. The reference 2D image demonstrates the red line aligned through the ventricles and associated M-mode is shown on the top and the green line passing through the atria with associated M-mode on the bottom.

Abbreviations: A, atrial contraction; V, ventricular contraction; L, fetal left
* color flow in the aorta or left ventricular outflow.

Doppler Techniques (Fig. 7.2)

Doppler flow patterns are easily obtained and provide reliable surrogates for atrial and ventricular events. Crisp signals lend themselves better to measurements of time intervals and hence they provide useful information for elucidation of arrhythmia mechanisms. Interpretation of Doppler signals is aided by a good understanding of the events responsible for the signals seen

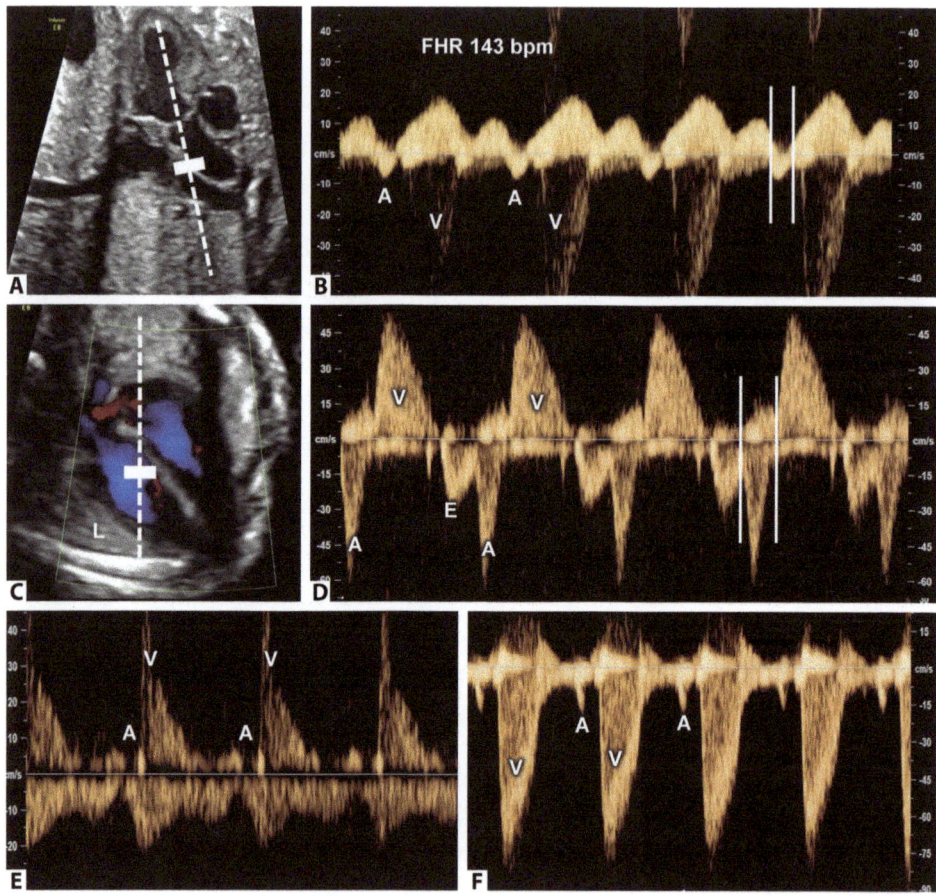

Figs 7.2A to F: Demonstration of normal sinus rhythm in the fetus using Doppler techniques. (A and B) Superior vena cava-aorta Doppler. A demonstrates optimal placement of the Doppler gate. B representative Doppler tracing demonstrating flow reversal in the superior vena cava with atrial contraction (A) followed by ejection signal in the aorta (V). Parallel lines denote the A-V interval; (C and D) Left ventricular inflow (mitral valve)- outflow (Aorta) Doppler. Atrial contraction results in augmented filling of the left ventricle (A) followed by flow in the outflow tract during ventricular contraction (V). Parallel lines denote the atrioventricular (AV) interval, also known as mechanical PR interval; (E) simultaneous Doppler of the pulmonary vein and pulmonary artery. The flow reversal in the pulmonary vein is not as marked and is better seen as cessation off forward flow with atrial contraction and ventricular contraction is noted by ejection Doppler in the artery (V); (F) Pulmonary artery Doppler. Atrial flow propagation into the pulmonary artery (A) followed by systolic flow in the pulmonary artery (V)

Abbreviation: A: atrial flow signal V ventricular ejection.

and the basic techniques noted here can be adapted for use in different vessels where in proximity of arterial venous structures allows for sequential assessment of cardiac events. Some of the common methodologies in clinical use are described here, but several variations are reported.

- *Inflow-outflow Doppler or mitral valve-aorta (Mv-Ao) Doppler:* Placing the Doppler gate in the left ventricular outflow tract in close proximity to the mitral valve provides simultaneous Doppler signals from the two structures. In normal sinus rhythm, the mitral valve inflow 'a' wave follows atrial depolarization and is a surrogate for 'P' wave on the ECG while ventricular contraction results in ventricular ejection and flow in the aorta, a surrogate for 'QRS' on the ECG (Figs 7.2C and D).

- *Simultaneous arterial–venous Doppler:* Simultaneous Doppler evaluation of an artery and vein is utilized to study physiologic consequence of atrial and ventricular contraction. Atrial contraction results in flow reversal in the veins and ventricular contraction results flow in the artery or lack of flow if ineffective. Such information can be obtained from simultaneous sampling of the superior vena cava and aorta (SVC-Ao)(Figs 7.2A and B), pulmonary artery and vein (Fig. 7.2D) as well as azygous vein and descending aorta in cases with interruption of the inferior vena cava.
- *Other methods:* Doppler flow patterns in the pulmonary artery (Fig. 7.2E) as well as venous Doppler in hepatic veins has been used for arrhythmia assessment.

Tissue Doppler analysis can also provide arrhythmia analysis but is more time consuming.

Doppler techniques are most commonly used for measurement of time intervals and evaluation of AV-VA intervals. It is important to recognize that these intervals are influenced by the electromechanical properties of the ventricle. The measurement of AV interval (used as a surrogate for the PR interval on ECG) by the MV-AO method is the most affected by this and less so from the SVC-AO technique. Reference values have been published and are specific for a given technique. Current methods of ultrasound evaluation do not provide us with information regarding repolarization abnormalities. In addition, it is important to recognize the impact of the arrhythmia on Doppler flow patterns in the veins as augmented flow reversal may be seen, and this makes assessment of fetal well-being difficult. It is important to reassess this in the absence of the arrhythmia (Fig. 7.3).

Technical factors
- Clarity of signals is influenced by the angle of evaluation
- Choose optimal gate size to obtain a crisp signal. Too big a gate will lead to inclusion of extraneous signals. Too small a gate will make it difficult to sample adjacent structures simultaneously. In our laboratory we start with a 2 mm gate and narrow it down or open it further based on signals obtained.
- Gain: Too high a gain will mask events that are buried within other events (Fig. 7.4).

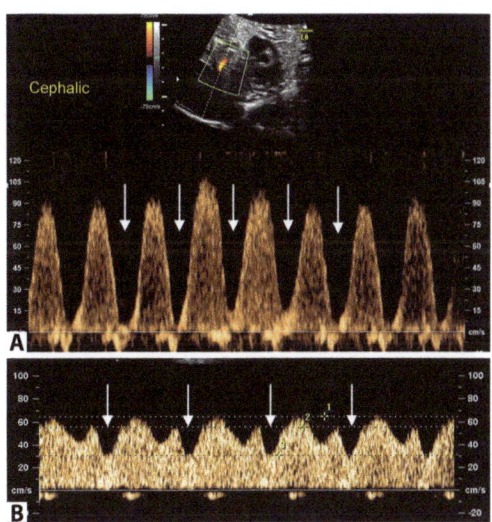

Figs 7.3A and B: (A) Doppler signal in the ductus venosus showing cessation of flow during atrial systole in a fetus with supraventricular tachycardia. FHR 260 BPM; (B) The flow pattern normalizes once normal sinus rhythm is established FHR 136 BPM. These changes may impact the ability to assess fetal well-being and the congestive heart failure score in tachycardia. ↑ denotes impact of atrial contraction on forward flow in the ductus venosus

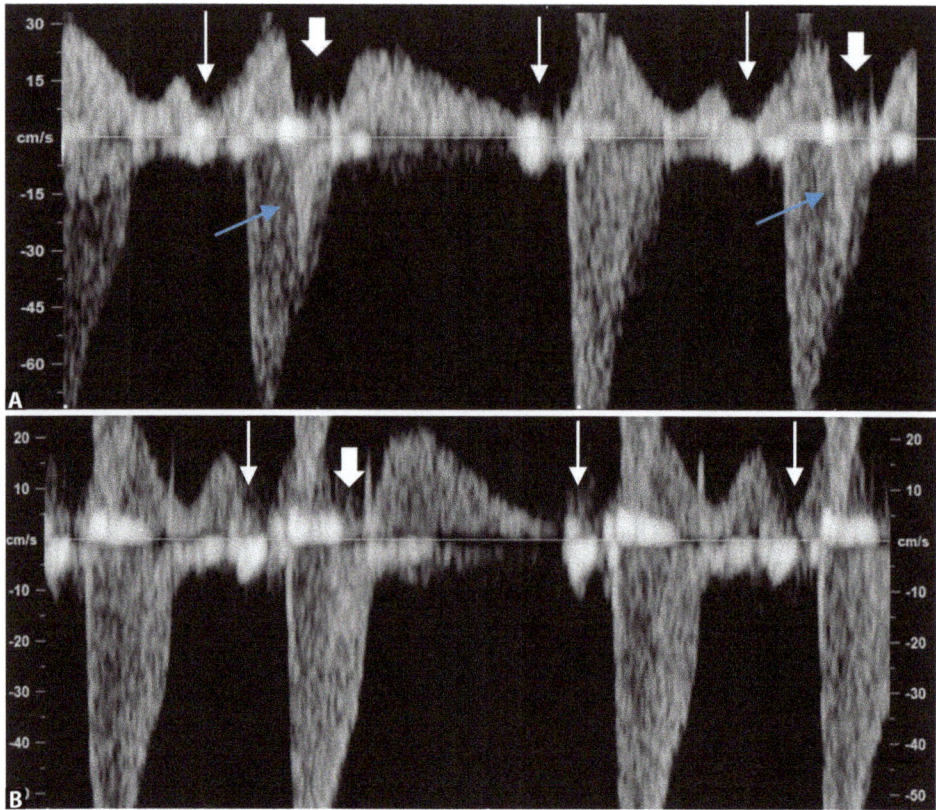

Figs 7.4A and B: Impact of gain on the ability to detect superimposed Doppler signals. SVC-AO tracing in a fetus with blocked or non-conducted premature atrial beats. White arrows denote atrial flow reversal with sinus atrial beats, bold white arrows denote the premature atrial beats. Aortic flow signal (V) follows conducted sinus atrial beats. There is prominent atrial flow reversal signal associated with the premature atrial beats (blue arrow) noted within the ventricular flow signal in A, but is masked by the high Doppler gain in B

Fetal Magnetocardiograms (fMCG) and Fetal Electrocardiograms (fECG)

Every electrical signal is associated with a magnetic signal. The fetal ECG which is a recording of fetal cardiac electrical activity is hampered by the fact that the vernix caseosa is electrically insulating in later pregnancy while the signals are small earlier. Newer machines overcome this with signal processing and amplification but the methodology remains cumbersome. Magnetocardiograms are obtained by collecting the magnetic signals associated with fetal cardiac activity with a squid magnetometer and then analyzing the signals. Good signal strength is obtained as vernix does not interfere however the technology is currently not portable and limited in availability to a few centers. However, it has contributed significantly to our understanding of fetal arrhythmias especially those associated with repolarization abnormalities.

TYPES OF ARRHYTHMIA: EVALUATION AND BASIC MANAGEMENT STRATEGY

Irregular Rhythms

- *Premature atrial contractions (PAC):* Most common cause for an irregular rhythm noted in the fetus. Most resolve spontaneously. There is 1-3% risk for tachycardia to develop in this setting. Risk factors for tachycardia in this setting include: persistent atrial bigeminy (~10% risk) and presence of atrial couplets and triplets. A fixed coupling interval between the sinus atrial beat and the ectopic atrial beat noted on ultrasound evaluation can be indicative of a re-entrant etiology. Associated congenital heart disease is rare and reported in up to 2% of cases.

  Diagnosis of premature atrial beats is established by documenting premature or earlier than expected atrial contractions on M-mode or on Doppler evaluation (Fig. 7.5). Premature atrial beats may be conducted to the ventricle resulting in an early ventricular beat presenting as an 'extra beat' on auscultation or Doppler evaluation or may be 'blocked' resulting in a 'dropped or skipped beat'.

  The main differential is from other causes for an irregular rhythm, i.e. premature ventricular complexes and second degree heart block. Arial flutter with variable conduction and high grade block will also be irregular on auscultation with variable rates. Hence ultrasound evaluation by a person familiar with the techniques of fetal rhythm assessment is indicate in setting of persistent irregular fetal rhythm.

  Blocked atrial bigeminy confers a higher risk for tachycardia. It is sometimes challenging to differentiate some types of blocked atrial bigeminy from 2:1 second degree heart block especially when the premature atrial beat is marginally premature. In such cases, evaluation of maternal anti-Ro and anti-La status is recommended to rule out antibody mediated conduction abnormalities. Many cases will resolve spontaneously, but if persistent, the possibility of underlying repolarization abnormality such as QT prolongation should be considered and close follow-up in pregnancy and neonatal EKG is recommended. Evaluation of electromechanical properties as a means to distinguish blocked atrial bigeminy from other more sinister causes has been described and is promising.

- *Premature ventricular complexes (PVCs):* Account for about <10% of cases with irregular rhythm. Diagnosis is established by documenting regular atrial contractions at a normal rate with early ventricular depolarization (Figs 7.6A to C). Doppler evaluation of the great veins will usually demonstrate a deeper A wave reversal due to atrial contraction against a closed AV valve (Fig. 7.6C).

  PVC's may be seen in the setting of cardiac tumors, fetal myocarditis and other myocardial diseases such as cardiomyopathy, congenital heart disease and channelopathies though the majority are idiopathic and resolve spontaneously in the absence of a secondary cause. A good family history is indicated.

- *Irregular rhythm due to second degree heart block:* Both Mobitz type I (Wenkebach) as well as higher degrees of Mobitz type II block such as 3:1 or 4:1 block may present as an irregular rhythm and cannot be reliably differentiated without ultrasound evaluation. Again both demonstrate a regular atrial rhythm. The gradually increasing AV interval is easier demonstrated on Doppler evaluation or color M-mode evaluation than standard M-mode assessment (Fig. 7.7). Potential causes and management are discussed under heart block.

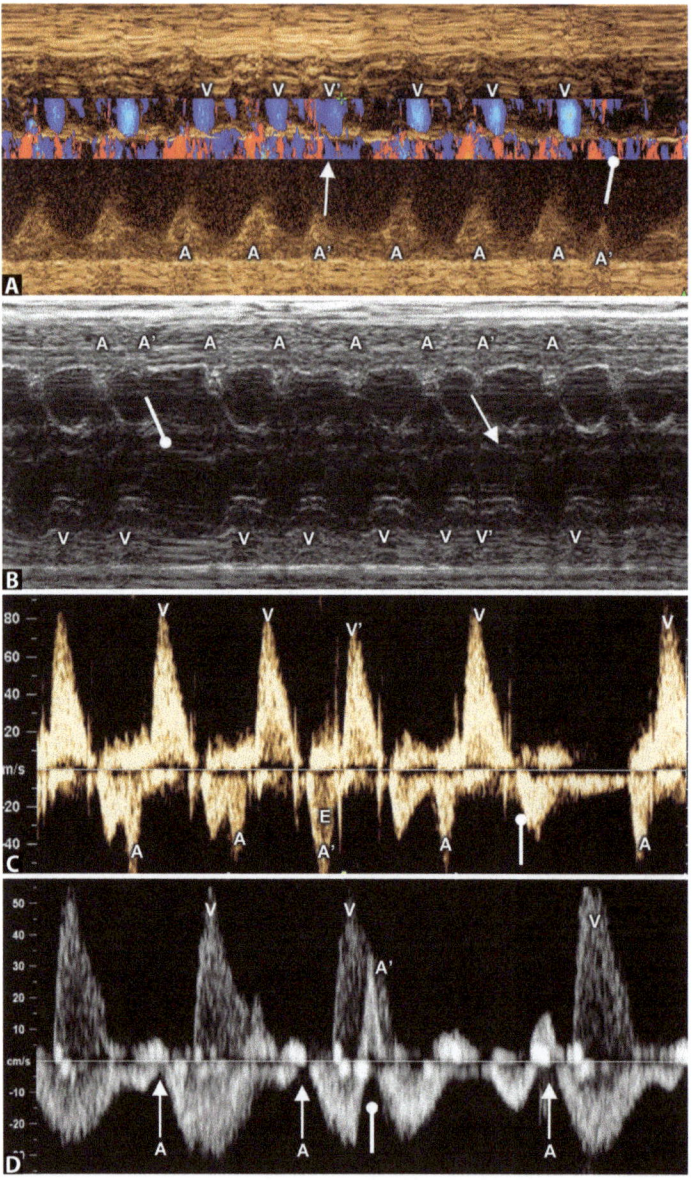

Figs 7.5A to D: Premature atrial complexes. (A) color M-mode demonstrating regular atrial contractions below (A) interspersed with premature atrial beats (A') that come early. Ventricular ejection (V) is represented as color flow in the left ventricular outflow tract moving away from the transducer. Conducted premature atrial beat (solid arrow) results in an early ventricular beat (V'). Blocked atrial beats are denoted by round tip arrow; (B) Simultaneous M-mode through the atrium (A) on top and ventricle (V) on bottom; (C) Left ventricular inflow outflow Doppler. Premature atrial beat (A') results in a fusion with preceding E wave and a taller signal. Blocked atrial beat denoted by closed end arrow results in a dropped ventricular beat; (D) SVC-Aorta tracing showing blocked atrial beat (A') superimposed on previous aortic flow (V). A: atrial, V: ventricular, A': premature atrial beat, V': premature ventricular activation, Arrow: conducted premature atrial beat, Arrow with closed end: non-conducted premature atrial beat

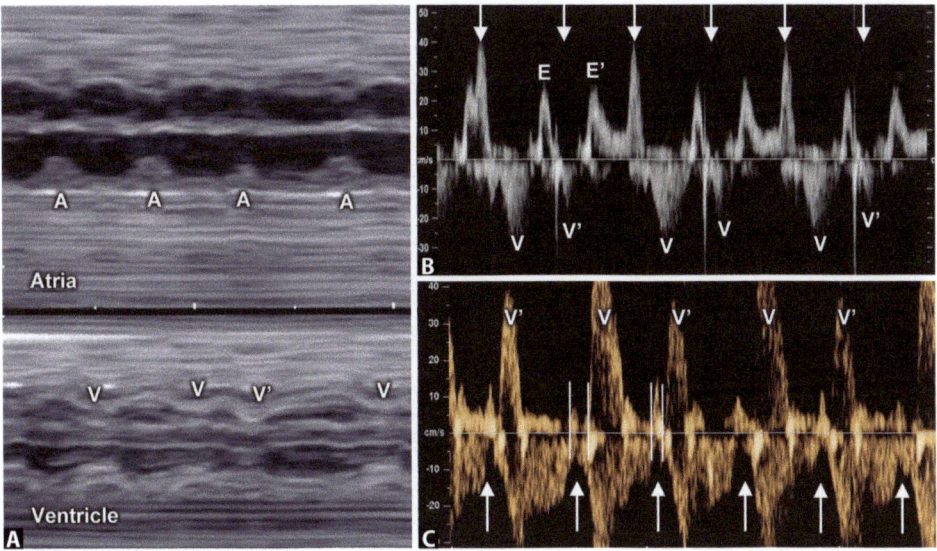

Figs 7.6A to C: Premature ventricular complexes. (A) Anatomic M-mode with atrial contractions in the top panel. Atrial contractions (A) are regular. Simultaneous ventricular contractions (V) shown in bottom demonstrates an early ventricular complex (V'); (B) Left ventricular inflow-outflow Doppler demonstrating ventricular bigeminy. Ventricular contractions result in flow in aorta (V) and this is followed by early filling wave (E) in mitral inflow. However an early ventricular contraction (V') results in non-visualization of the atrial filling wave and an early E wave (E') Arrows denote regular atrial contractions; (C) SVC-Aorta tracing demonstrating regular atrial contractions (arrows) with a variable ventricular (V) relation. Every other ventricular ejection (V) is early (V'). Parallel lines denote the atrioventricular time interval which is shorter in the setting of ventricular ectopy. Note mild prominence of atrial flow reversal signals associated with the premature ventricular beats due to atrial contraction against a closed AV valve. Arrows atrial flow signal

Management of Irregular Rhythms

Premature atrial and ventricular beats
- Evaluate and rule out secondary causes such as myocarditis especially for premature ventricular beats.
- Observation with weekly outpatient monitoring of fetal heart rate by obstetrician till arrhythmia resolves.
- Repeat ultrasound evaluation may be indicated in setting of persistent premature ventricular ectopic beats, concern for tachycardia or presence of secondary causes. Blocked atrial bigeminy confers a higher risk for recurrence.
- Neonatal EKG may be considered in those with persistent ectopy through the pregnancy especially for ventricular extrasystole and atrial ectopy with fixed coupling intervals.
- Some centers advocate kick counts as a way for monitoring fetal well-being especially in later gestation though data is minimal.

Management of irregular rhythm due to second degree heart block is similar to that of a fetus with higher grade AV-block and is discussed under bradycardia.

Guidelines for management of the fetus with different arrhythmias were outlined in a recent American Heart Association document.

Fetal Tachyarrhythmias

Fetal tachycardia is generally classified as sustained heart rates above 180 BPM though most cases of pathologic tachycardia will

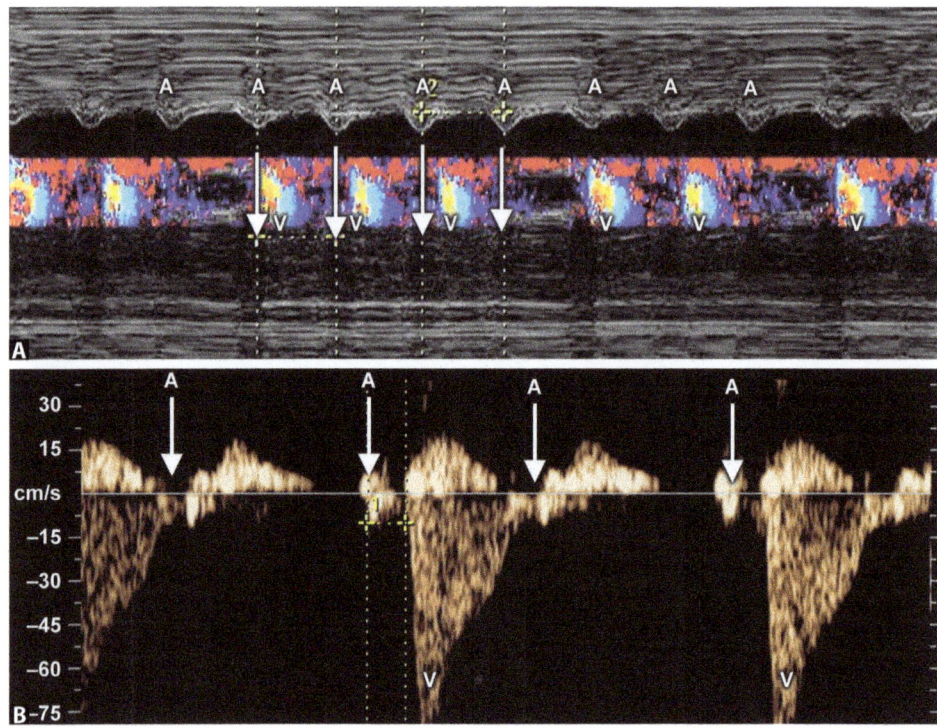

Figs 7.7A and B: (A) Color mode demonstrating Mobitz type 1 or Wenkebach rhythm. Regular atrial contractions (A) are demonstrated. Ventricular contractions results in flow signal in the aorta (V). Progressive lengthening of the atrioventricular interval as denoted by the distance between the arrow and ventricular signals finally results in a non-conducted atrial beat; (B) Mobitz type 2 block with 2:1 conduction demonstrated on SVC-Aorta Doppler. Regular atrial signals (arrows) are noted at about 150 BPM with every other atrial signal being blocked or non-conducted with a resultant slow ventricular (V) rate of about 75 BPM

present with heart rates above 200 BPM. Sustained heart rates between 160–200 BPM merit close evaluation to distinguish between sinus tachycardia and other potential abnormal rhythms. Many of the algorithms used to distinguish causes for tachycardia in postnatal life are applicable to fetal diagnosis with some modifications. The evaluation of VA and AV time intervals are integral to the analysis and differentiation of fetal tachycardias (Fig. 7.8). Further tachyarrhythmias are arbitrarily classified as intermittent, if present for less than 50% of time and incessant if present >50% of the monitoring time. Fetal tachycardia has been associated with a higher risk for hydrops, perinatal morbidity and mortality and premature delivery.

1. *Sinus tachycardia:* Sinus tachycardia may be seen in the fetus in association with maternal febrile states, stimulant use, chorioamnionitis and fetal anemia and thyrotoxicosis. Ultrasound evaluation demonstrates 1:1 AV relationship with some variability and a long VA interval.
2. *Supraventricular tachycardia:* The majority of fetal tachyarrhythmias are supraventricular in origin as distinct from primary atrial flutter or ventricular tachycardia. Based on the determination of AV and VA intervals these can be divided

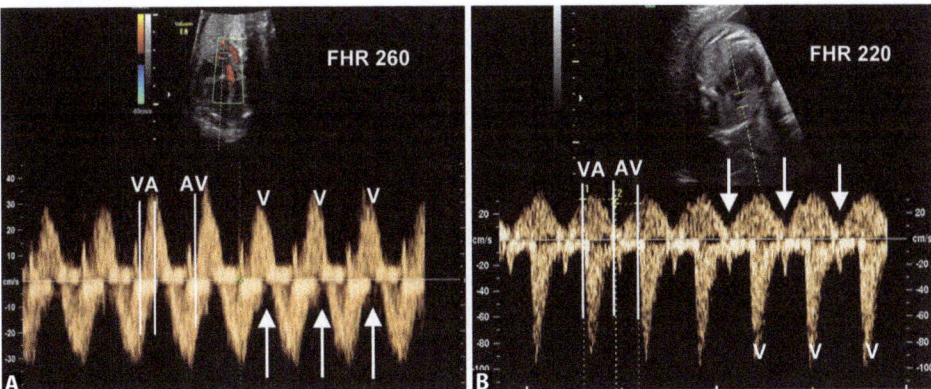

Figs 7.8A and B: Superior vena cava and aorta (SVC-AO) tracing in fetal supraventricular tachycardia demonstrating. (A) A short VA tachycardia (VA<<AV) likely atrioventricular re-entry tachycardia; (B) a long VA (VA> AV) tachycardia, diagnosed atrial ectopic tachycardia in another fetus. Note the slightly slower fetal heart rate in B versus A. Arrows show atrial flow reversal in the superior vena caval tracing

Abbreviations: V, aortic flow or ventricular ejection; AV, atrioventricular time interval; VA, ventriculoatrial time interval

into different subgroups akin to ECG stratification of arrhythmias into short and long RP tachycardia. Fetal SVT has been associated with hydrops especially with higher heart rates and incessant tachycardia. Underlying congenital heart disease may be seen in a small percentage of cases.

Short VA tachycardia: Atrioventricular re-entry tachycardia (AVRT) is the most common of these. Heart rates are typically in 220–280 BPM range with 1:1 AV relationship and the VA interval is shorter than the AV interval (Fig. 7.8A). An accessory pathway is noted in about 10% of cases after birth. Abrupt onset and termination is typical. Intermittent premature atrial beats may be noted during periods of sinus rhythm.

Long VA tachycardia: These are characterized by 1:1 AV relationship with a VA interval that is longer than the AV interval (Fig. 7.8B). Fetal heart rates range from 180–220 BPM though faster rates may be noted. Causes include paroxysmal junctional reciprocating tachycardia (PJRT), some atrial ectopic tachycardias (AET) and sinus tachycardia (ST).

3. *Junctional tachycardia:* Simultaneous VA activation.
   Near simultaneous VA activation with one-to-one AV relationship may be seen with congenital junctional ectopic tachycardia (JET). Though not classically a supraventricular tachycardia this may not be readily differentiated from AVRT without analysis of AV-VA time intervals. JET may be seen in the setting of SSA isoimmunization of the fetus and familial cases are reported. Junctional ectopic tachycardia may result in VA dissociation in some cases and will be difficult to distinguish from ventricular tachycardia in these cases. Atrioventricular nodal reentry tachycardia is rare in fetus and will also demonstrate near simultaneous AV activation.

4. *Atrial re-entry tachycardia (atrial flutter):* Accounts for about 30% of cases of fetal tachycardia. Rapid atrial rates of 300–400 BPM are associated with slower ventricular rates in the setting of variable conduction and thus a range of fetal heart rates may

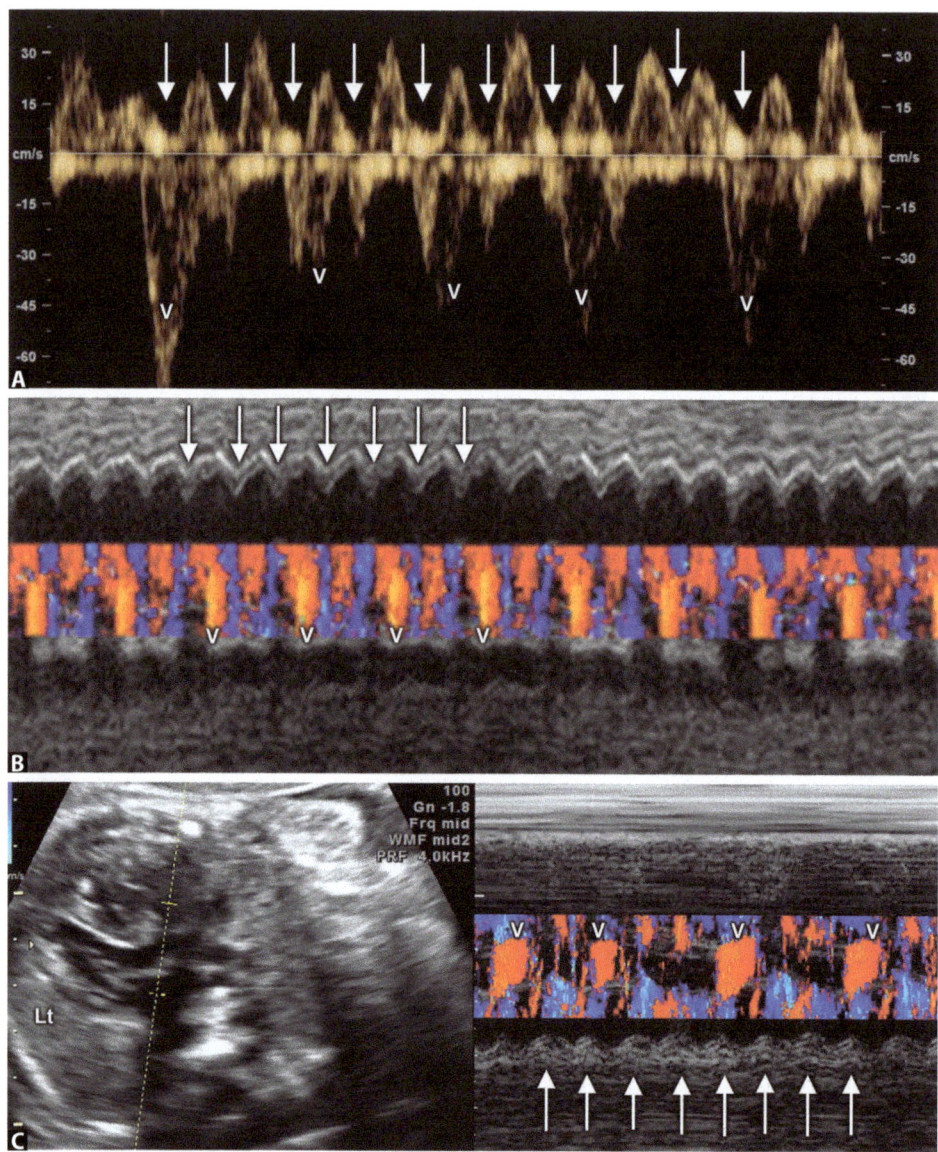

Figs 7.9A to C: Echo evaluation of fetal atrial flutter. (A) SVC-AO tracing with aortic flow being demonstrated below the baseline (V). Rapid atrial contractions at 400 BPM are denoted by the arrows with variable atrial flow reversal signal. There is 2:1 block with a ventricular rate that is approximately 200–210 BPM; (B) Color M-mode in atrial flutter. Down arrows point to the rapid atrial contractions which are noted on top. Atrial rate is 450 BPM with 2:1 conduction and ventricular rate (V) of about 225 BPM. Ventricular ejection is denoted by color flow in the aorta (V); (C) Color M-mode in another fetus demonstrating variable ventricular response. Fetal left is on the bottom (Lt). Color gate is positioned across the left ventricular outflow tract demonstrating red flow towards the transducer (V) and left atrial M-mode signal on the bottom (arrows). There is variable block between 2:1 to 4:1, with a resultant irregular ventricular rate (V)

be noted, ranging from bradycardia in the setting of high-grade block to tachycardia with 2:1 conduction (Figs 7.9A to C). Atrial flutter may co-exist with supraventricular tachycardia in about 30% of cases. Significant variations in heart rate in a fetus with SVT from bradycardia to normal to tachycardia should raise suspicion for coexisting atrial flutter. Sudden changes in heart rate while being monitored especially with initiation of medical therapy has often resulted in unnecessary emergent delivery of the fetus due to concerns for fetal distress. This can be avoided with education and close involvement of staff comfortable with bedside evaluation of the fetal rhythm. Rare cases off chaotic atrial tachycardia may mimic atrial flutter but is distinguished by fast but irregular atrial rhythm as against the regular atrial beats in atrial flutter. Atrial flutter has been reported in association with structural heart disease, heart block, myocarditis.

5. *Ventricular tachycardia:* Characterized by atrioventricular dissociation in the setting of a faster ventricular rate and normal atrial rates. It is rare in the fetus and may be seen in the setting of a sick myocardium as with myocarditis, cardiomyopathy; fetal congenital heart disease, tumors, immune mediated heart block and channelopathies. Rarely retrograde VA conduction may be seen, making it difficult to distinguish this from junctional ectopic tachycardia and rare slow forms of atrioventricular nodal re-entry tachycardia.

Management of Fetal Tachyarrhythmia

Untreated persistent fetal tachyarrhythmia has a potential for progression to fetal hydrops and rarely fetal loss. Though management strategies remain somewhat institution and practice specific some general guidelines are available. Multidisciplinary care is essential to make sure that maternal as well as fetal well-being and risk benefit ratios are considered.

Management of supraventricular tachycardia and atrial flutter is impacted by several general factors (*see* Flowchart 7.1):

- *Incessant (lasting >50% of time monitored) versus intermittent (<50% of time monitored):* Intermittent SVT in the absence of hydrops and ventricular dysfunction can be managed conservatively, as long as close observation for change in persistence and evolution of hydrops and ventricular dysfunction is feasible. Incessant SVT is more likely to benefit from antiarrhythmic therapy.
- *Gestational age:* Fetuses that are at or close to term (at or above 35 weeks) may be monitored closely in the absence of hydrops or delivery may be considered if at or over 37 weeks gestation.
- Maternal risk factors including underlying EKG abnormalities, cardiac dysfunction or other noncardiac risk factors, twin gestation may sway the risk benefit ratio as well as choice of antiarrhythmic drug.
- *Hydrops fetalis:* Hydrops signifies the presence of cardiac decompensation in the fetus and a mortality of 8–14% is reported in this setting. This will often resolve with control of the fetal rhythm. However, fetal transfer of most antiarrhythmics is impaired in the setting of hydrops, except for Flecainide and Sotalol.
- *Type of arrhythmia:* In the absence of hydrops initial transplacental therapy has been reported with Digoxin or Flecainde or Sotalol alone as primary or secondary therapy. Primary drug choices may vary slightly by underlying arrhythmia and is outlined in Flowchart 7.2, however, in clinical practice, acceptable results have been shown with all three and choices are often dictated by institutional practice and comfort. Transplacental transfer of Digoxin

is low in the setting of hydrops and it is used with either Flecainide or Sotalol as primary therapy in such cases. Amiodarone as well as direct fetal therapy with intramuscular Digoxin has been used in cases with hydrops refractory to primary therapy.

Given potential for risk to mother as well as baby a multidisciplinary approach is essential for the management of fetal arrhythmias by personnel who are experienced in the evaluation of both mother and fetus.

Ventricular tachycardia: May be seen in a diverse settings. Dexamethasone and IV immunoglobulin may be of benefit in setting of underlying immune mediated conduction defects. Underlying sinus bradycardia should raise concern for associated ion-channelopathy. Management of ventricular tachycardia with intravenous short-term magnesium in mother, lidocaine infusion, propranolol and mexilitine has been reported. QT prolonging drugs should be avoided, if

Flowchart 7.1: Evaluation and management of fetal tachycardia. This flowchart explores general guidelines for evaluation of the fetus with fetal tachycardia based on gestational age and associated risk factors.

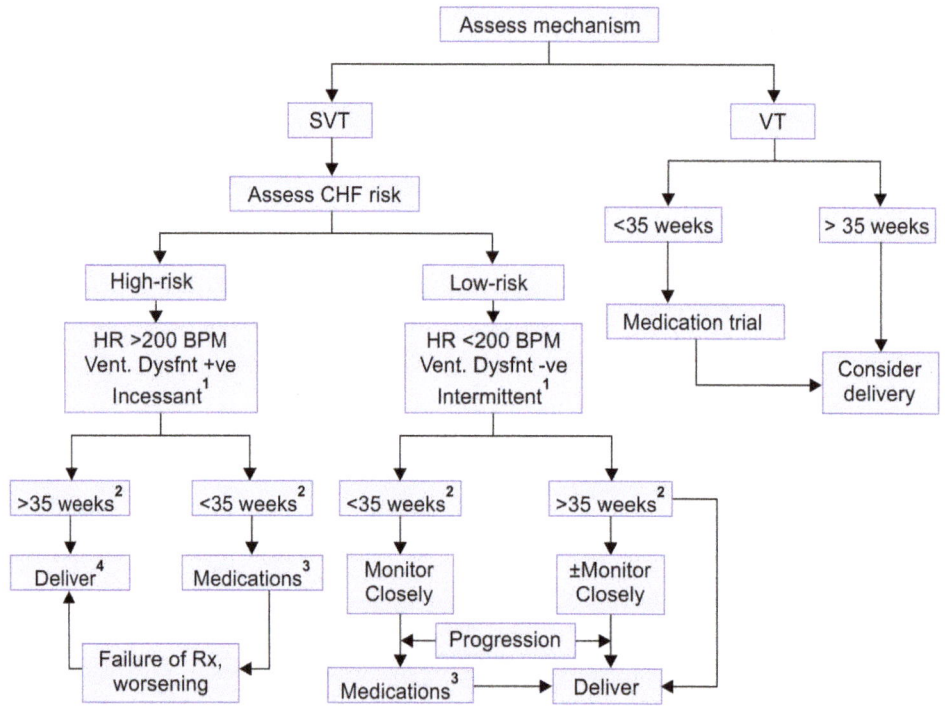

1. Incessant is defined as tachycardia lasting >50% of monitoring period, typically over a day while intermittent tachycardia is present for <50% of time. 2. Although 35 weeks is taken as a cut off here, monitoring through 37 weeks would be entertained if close surveillance is possible or a short trial of first line agent may be considered in the absence of hydrops. 3. Antiarrhythmic therapy is described in greater detail on page 112. 4. Decision to deliver a patient is complex and will take into account several factors including risk to fetus and mother and the risk of therapy versus prematurity. Ventricular tachycardia in general is more diverse in etiology and more likely to result in fetal decompensation, hence options are for a trial of medications or delivery if close to term.

Abbreviations: vent. Dysfnt., ventricular dysfunction; –ve : absent; +ve present; SVT, supraventricular tachycardia; VT, ventricular tachycardia.

Flowchart 7.2: Antiarrhythmic therapy choices for the management of fetal tachyarrhythmia. There are no universal therapy guidelines and this flowchart outlines some generally used strategies tailored to the underlying diagnosis. In general, Digoxin is not used as monotherapy for fetal supraventricular tachycardia in the setting of fetal hydrops, though it is often used as first line in the absence of hydrops.

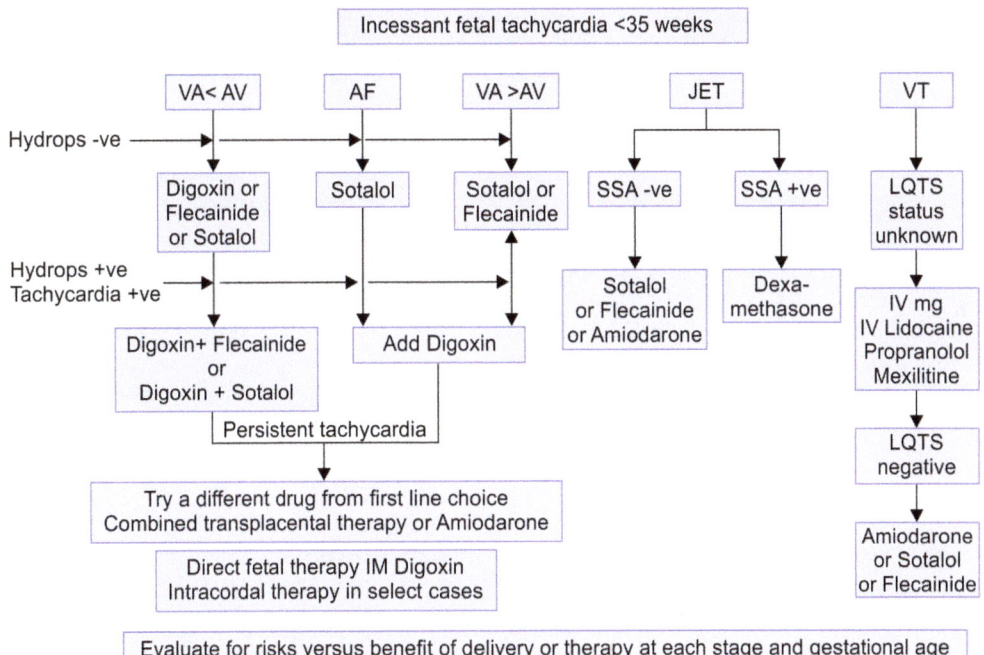

Abbreviations: VA, ventriculoatrial interval; AV, atrioventricular interval; AF, atrial flutter; JET, junctional ectopic tachycardia; VT, ventricular tachycardia; +ve, present; –ve, absent; LQTS, long QT syndrome. Please see text for doses and description. It is important to reassess the fetus and mother frequently for side effects, progression and response to therapy and management decisions are made in the context of fetomaternal well-being, prematurity risk and gestational age

possible till an underlying channelopathy has been ruled out.

The American Heart Association put out a consensus statement in 2014, with general guidelines for management which serves as a good reference.

- *Maternal-fetal monitoring:* Once there is control of the fetal rate and rhythm ongoing close monitoring of the mother as well as fetus for drug effects and toxicity, recurrence of tachycardia and resolution of hydrops is indicated. This may have an impact on timing of delivery.

Overview of Antiarrhythmic Drugs

1. *Digoxin:* Digoxin remains widely used as primary as well as second line drug for the management of fetal tachycardia given wide experience with this. Conversion rates approaching 50–60% of cases are reported in the absence of hydrops though this drops down to about 25% in setting of hydrops, due to poor transfer across the placenta in these states. Typical loading dose used, ranges from 1,000–1,500 µg/24 hours given IV in divided doses q 8 hours. Maintenance

dose of 375–500 μg/day divided q8–12 hours orally. Therapeutic dose range is from 0.7–2.0 ng/mL. A baseline Digoxin level is of benefit due to the presence of maternal Digoxin-like immunoreactive substances in some patients which can influence the level. Digoxin has a narrow therapeutic window and toxicity may manifest as significant nausea and vomiting, visual aberration including color distortion, arrhythmias including high grade atrioventricular block and both atrial and ventricular arrhythmias. It may also cause uterine irritability. Digoxin dosage should be adjusted if being used along with Amiodarone. Fetal intramuscular digoxin has been used in the setting of hydrops and persistent SVT.

2. *Sotalol:* It has been used as primary or secondary line therapy with Digoxin in management of fetal tachycardia. Conversion rates approaching 60–80% in fetal atrial flutter has been reported. It is a class III antiarrhythmic with β-blocking effects. Maternal dose of 160 mg/day orally in two divided doses and may be increased to a maximum of 480 mg/day in 3 divided doses. Toxicity includes maternal QTc prolongation >480 msec, bundle branch block, dizziness, nausea and vomiting and maternal and fetal proarrhythmia. Close monitoring of maternal EKG as well as electrolytes is recommended.

3. *Flecainide:* Demonstrates excellent transplacental transfer even in the setting of hydrops. It has been used as first line monotherapy as well as second line therapy with Digoxin in setting of fetal supraventricular tachycardia. Recent studies have shown up to 80% conversion in SVT with hydrops. Maternal dose is 100–400 mg/24 hours divided q 8–12 hours. Toxicity includes neurologic side effects, dizziness, conduction defects, maternal as well as fetal proarrhythmia may be seen. Therapeutic levels are 0.2–1 μg/mL.

4. *Amiodarone:* Given the long half-life and concerns over maternal and fetal toxicity, Amiodarone is used in most cases as third line therapy or second line in setting of severe hydrops. Toxicity includes maternal and fetal QT prolongation proarrhythmia fetal goiter and hypothyroidism and neurodevelopmental concerns in fetus. Several therapeutic regimens are reported. Current AHA guideline on fetal therapy recommends a loading dose of 1800–2400 mg per day divided every 6 hours for 48 hours orally, lower load of 800–1200 mg/day divided if prior antiarrhythmic therapy and a maintenance therapy of 200–600 mg/day oral. Therapy may be stopped once hydrops is resolved and rhythm controlled. Close neonatal monitoring is needed. Therapeutic levels 0.7–2.8 μg/mL.

5. *Propranolol:* Currently propranolol is used primarily for management of sustained as well as non-sustained ventricular tachycardia in the fetus. Though, it is also effective in the management of supraventricular tachycardia the risks of fetal intrauterine growth retardation, oligohydramnios and increased uterine tone associated with it, has limited its use in this setting. Dosing 60–320 mg PO divided q6 hours. Maternal side effects include bradycardia, hypotension and fatigue.

6. *Mexilitine:* It has been used in the management of fetal ventricular tachy-cardia. Oral dosing of 600–900 mg/day divided q12 hours. May cause pro-arrhythmia and nausea vomiting and tingling.

7. *Lidocaine:* It has been used as a continuous infusion in the setting of fetal torsade and persistent ventricular arrhythmias. Loading dose of 1–1.5 mg/kg/IV followed by a maintenance dose of 1–4 mg/min. Monitoring maternal levels is recommended.

8. Magnesium infusion may be used for 24–48 hours in the management of fetal

ventricular tachycardia. Monitoring levels (<6 mEq/L) and maternal patellar reflex to help guide therapy is essential.

Fetal Bradyarrhythmias

Fetal bradycardia is defined as persistent fetal heart rate below 100 BPM though persistent heart rates below 120 BPM or the 3rd percentile for gestational age merits an evaluation for cause and fetal well-being. Mild fetal bradycardia may be the only marker for ion channelopathy in the fetus and long QT syndrome. Persistent low fetal heart rates below 55 BPM have been associated with a high incidence of hydrops and adverse outcomes.

Sinus Bradycardia

Fetal bradycardia may be seen in the setting of fetal hypoxia and stress. In addition, sinus node dysfunction can be seen in a fetus with heterotaxy and associated congenital heart defects, fetal ion channelopathy, fetal myocarditis as well as maternal medications. In general, it is well-tolerated though close monitoring of fetal rhythm and neonatal evaluation is recommended in cases where LQTs is suspected. Ultrasound evaluation shows 1:1 atrioventricular conduction with a low atrial rate.

Blocked Bigeminy

Nonconducted atrial ectopic beats that occur in a bigeminal fashion results in an effective fetal heart rate of 75–90 BPM. This may be mistaken with 2:1 heart block however the atrial rate is irregular and every other atrial beat is premature and non-conducted. Monitoring and follow-up is similar to other irregular rhythms. Rarely ventricular bigeminy may be seen.

Atrioventricular Block

Abnormalities in impulse conduction from the atria to the ventricles may manifest as varying degrees of heart block in the fetus. Accurate diagnosis of mechanism and associated factors is essential for appropriate follow-up and management.

First degree AV block will not be apparent except with formal evaluation of the fetal rhythm and time intervals as the rhythm is regular. It is established by measuring the AV conduction time interval (AV interval), also called the 'mechanical PR interval', from the start of the 'a' wave on MV inflow to the start of ventricular ejection on the aortic Doppler or the beginning of the 'a' atrial flow reversal to beginning of flow in aorta on the SVC-AO Doppler (Figs 7.2B and D). Prolongation of this interval beyond +2 SD for gestational age signifies first degree heart block. There is however some variability in measurements and it also varies by gestational age, and is impacted by the electromechanical characteristics of the ventricle.

2:1 AV conduction or 2:1 block may be seen in the setting of Mobitz type II block with
- Maternal SSA and/or SSB antibodies
- Fetal LQTs or other ion channelopathies
- Fetal congenital heart disease including congenitally corrected transposition and complex CHD in setting of heterotaxy
- Idiopathic.

Close monitoring of fetus for progression and any other associated arrhythmias is recommended in idiopathic cases given that ultrasound cannot evaluate repolarization abnormalities and fMCG have limited availability. A neonatal ECG is recommended in these cases.

Immune-mediated conduction defects merit close follow-up for progression to complete heart block as well as signs of myocarditis. In utero progression as well as resumption of normal sinus rhythm or first degree heart block has been reported, both spontaneously as well as in the setting of steroid therapy. A brief trial of fluorinated steroids such as dexamethasone may be considered in this scenario especially if there is evidence for myocardial inflammation.

Complete Heart Block

Complete heart block results when the atrial impulses are unable to conduct to the ventricles resulting in slow ventricular escape rates usually in the 40–80 BPM range (Fig. 7.10). Diagnosis is made by documentation of:

- Regular atrial impulses with normal rate (mild sinus bradycardia may be noted).
- Slow ventricular rates <100 BPM
- AV dissociation.

Causes for complete heart block in a fetus, includes:

- Underlying congenital heart disease in about 50–55% of cases. Common diagnoses include left isomerism, congenitally corrected transposition of the great vessels, septal tumors as well as other congenital heart defects (Figs 7.10C and D).
- Immune-mediated complete heart block in about 40% of cases.
- Idiopathic in the remaining.

Idiopathic complete heart block may resolve in utero or after birth. However, late seroconversion has been reported in 8–10% of mothers with negative SSA/SSB antibodies on initial evaluation.

The combination of complex congenital heart disease with complete heart block is generally poorly tolerated and is associated with poor outcomes with in utero mortality of 60–90% being reported. Risk factors for

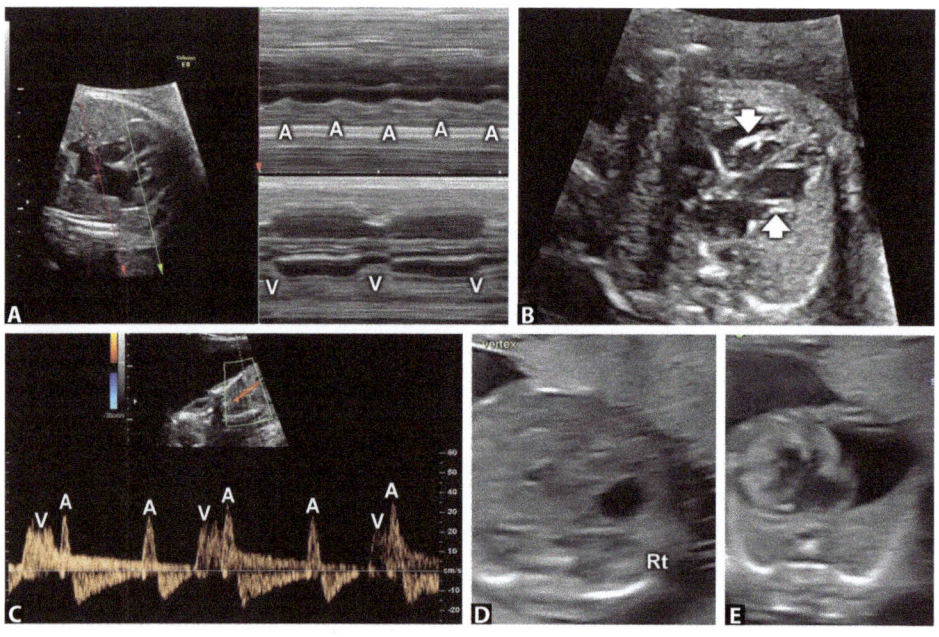

Figs 7.10A to E: Complete heart block in the fetus. (A) Anatomic M-mode demonstrating regular atrial contractions (A) on the top at a rate of 130 BPM and slower ventricular contractions (V) on the bottom with atrio-ventricular dissociation. Ventricular rate was 58 BPM; (B) 2D image of the fetal heart in isoimmune heart block demonstrating endocardial fibroelastosis of the atrioventricular valve chordal apparatus (bold arrow), (C and D) Fetus with complete heart block in setting of heterotaxy. Simultaneous Doppler signals from the descending aorta and azygous vein in setting of interruption of the inferior vena cava shows regular sinus bradycardia with prominent atrial flow reversal (A) demonstrating an atrial rate of about 110 BPM and a slower aortic flow signal or ventricular rate (V) of 65 BPM; (D) abdominal heterotaxy is noted with stomach to the right and levocardia is noted. There is a pericardial effusion; (E) and atrioventricular septal defect. The ventricular myocardium is thick

hydrops includes ventricular rates <55 BPM, ventricular dysfunction and slow sinus rates. Sympathomimetic therapy with maternal terbutaline therapy may be tried for fetal heart rates below 55 BPM but a survival benefit has not been shown.

Isoimmune complete heart block associated with maternal SSA/SSB antibodies occurs in about 1-3% of cases with positive antibodies. However, this risk increases to about 15% in the setting of a prior pregnancy with complete heart block or neonatal lupus. Risk factors for hydrops includes slow ventricular escape rates of <55 BPM, ventricular dysfunction and features of myocarditis. These cases may be associated with features of pan-myocarditis with associated endocardial fibroelastosis (EFE), valvular insufficiency, ventricular dysfunction, effusions as well as other tachyarrhythmias including junctional tachycardia, atrial tachycardia as well as ventricular ectopy. (Figs 7.10A and B) A slow sinus rate was associated with poorer outcomes. Late onset dilated cardiomyopathy is reported. Ultrasound plays an integral role in the evaluation and follow-up of these patients.

Screening

The period of maximal risk for heart block in the fetus appears to be between 17-26 weeks gestation with the risk decreasing beyond 30 weeks gestation, though late manifestation as well as late onset cardiomyopathy and onset of conduction defects after birth have been reported. Serial ultrasound evaluation either weekly or every other week between 17-26 or 30 weeks to assess the rhythm, conduction times and for evidence of myocarditis in the fetus is offered at many centers. It is important to recognize that fetal complete heart block may set in suddenly without evidence for prior conduction delay. Other findings such as new onset valve insufficiency, endocardial fibroelastosis and myocardial dysfunction may become apparent before conduction abnormalities.

Prophylactic steroid therapy or IV immunoglobulins (IVIG) was not shown to be benefit. Early data is suggestive for a protective role for hydroxychloroquin or Plaquenil in recurrence of heart block and is being evaluated systematically.

Management of Complete Heart Block

Currently, there are no standardized management protocols given small numbers. A recent European registry report suggested no benefit to therapy with survival in both treated and untreated cases of up to 90%. However, other studies have shown a survival benefit to in utero therapy for isoimmune heart block associated with signs of associated myocardial dysfunction and valvulitis. The recent American Heart Association guidelines of fetal therapy recommends a trial of fluorinated steroids for cases with isoimmune 2:1 block as well as complete heart block especially in the setting of associated ventricular dysfunction and inflammation. Dexamethasone is typically used in doses of 4-8 mg orally per day with a 4 mg per day dose being continued till there are signs of active inflammation or hydrops. The dose may be gradually tapered and stopped in later gestation in the absence of ongoing active inflammation and stable cardiovascular status or once gestational age is such that safe delivery is contemplated. Dexamethasone therapy has been associated with significant side maternal glucose intolerance, fluid retention, adrenal suppression in both mother and fetus if used for prolonged periods, as well as neurologic side effects in the baby, growth retardation as well as oligohydramnios and neurodevelopmental concerns have been reported, though some of this may be seen as a consequence of the disease process itself. However, given these significant concerns detailed counseling of pros and cons of therapy is advisable. Late diagnosis off CHB beyond 32 weeks may not merit therapy in the absence of hydrops and evidence for ongoing inflammation.

Intravenous immunoglobulin (IVIG) therapy, given initially in conjunction with steroids for evidence of inflammation may be of benefit. Repeat course in 3-4 weeks is given, if there is ongoing inflammation or progressive endocardial fibroelastosis in an effort to prevent cardiomyopathy. Progressive hydrops is associated with poor outcomes and may lead to premature delivery if the fetus is close to term β-sympathomimetics such as terbutaline or salbutamol may be used for fetal ventricular rates <55 BPM irrespective of etiology. Therapy is associated with maternal tachycardia and increased jitteriness. Rarely maternal arrhythmias may be noted. Maternal Terbutaline dose of 2.5-7.5 mg PO every 4 to 6 hours (total daily dose of 10-30 mg) or Salbutamol 10 mg PO q8 hours (max 40 mg per day) has been reported.

SUMMARY

Fetal rhythm abnormalities are commonly noted in obstetric practice. Transient ectopy is the most common and in general have a benign course and resolve spontaneously. In a small percentage of cases, they may serve as markers for underlying conduction abnormality or persistent arrhythmias and hence benefit from evaluation by personnel trained in higher evaluation of the fetal rhythm, especially if persistent. A small subset with persistent tachyarrhythmias or bradyarrhythmias will progress to hydrops and are associated with bad outcomes if unrecognized and untreated. Fetal echocardiography plays an important role in elucidating the etiology of the arrhythmia, associated findings, the impact on the fetus and in serial monitoring. A stepwise and systematic approach to the evaluation is essential to avoid misdiagnosis. In select cases in utero therapy for the management of the arrhythmia is indicated and can be successful. In such cases, a multidisciplinary approach is critical to minimize side effects to mother and fetus. The association of congenital heart disease with significant arrhythmia and hydrops in utero is associated with generally poor outcomes. Persistent mild variations from normal may be a marker for significant underlying fetal abnormalities associated with bad outcomes such as mild bradycardia seen with fetal long QT syndrome and mild tachycardia with fetal thyrotoxicosis and junctional tachycardia and merit close monitoring and a search for associated factors. Our ability to clinically detect repolarization abnormalities in fetuses is limited and a high index of suspicion is necessary in these cases.

SUGGESTED READING

1. Bettina F, Cuneo m, Strasburger Jf. Management strategy for fetal tachycardia. Obstetrics and Gynecology. 2000;96(4):575-81.
2. Breur JM, et al. Transient non-autoimmune fetal heart block. Fetal Diagnosis and Therapy. 2005;20(2):81-5.
3. Cuneo B, Strasburger J. We Only Find What We Look For: Fetal Heart Rate and the Diagnosis of Long-QT Syndrome. Circulation: Arrhythmia and Electrophysiology 2015. Volume 8, August. 2015;(4):760-2.
4. Cuneo BF, et al. A management strategy for fetal immune-mediated atrioventricular block. J Matern Fetal Neonatal Med. 2010;23(12):1400-5.
5. Cuneo BF, et al. An expanded phenotype of maternal SSA/SSB antibody-associated fetal cardiac disease. J Matern Fetal Neonatal Med. 2009;22(3):233-8.
6. Cuneo BF, et al. Atrial and ventricular rate response and patterns of heart rate acceleration during maternal-fetal terbutaline treatment of fetal complete heart block. American Journal of Cardiology. 2007;100(4):661-5.
7. Cuneo BF, et al. Prenatal diagnosis and in utero treatment of torsades de pointes associated with congenital long QT syndrome. American Journal of Cardiology. 2003;91(11):1395-8.

8. Cuneo BF, Strasburger JF, Wakai RT. Magnetocardiography in the evaluation of fetuses at risk for sudden cardiac death before birth. Journal of Electrocardiology. 2008;41(2):116 e1-6.
9. Cuneo BF. The beginnings of long QT syndrome. Curr Opin Cardiol. 2015;30(1):112-7.
10. Donofrio MT, et al. Diagnosis and treatment of fetal cardiac disease: a scientific statement from the American Heart Association. Circulation. 2014;129(21):2183-242.
11. Duke C, Stuart G, Simpson JM. Ventricular tachycardia secondary to prolongation of the QT interval in a fetus with autoimmune mediated congenital complete heart block. Cardiology in the Young. 2005;15(3):319-21.
12. Eliasson H, et al. Isolated atrioventricular block in the fetus: A retrospective, multinational, multicenter study of 175 patients. Circulation. 2011;124(18):1919-26.
13. Eliasson H, Wahren-Herlenius M, Sonesson SE. Mechanisms in fetal bradyarrhythmia: 65 cases in a single center analyzed by Doppler flow echocardiographic techniques. Ultrasound in Obstetrics and Gynecology. 2011;37(2):172-8.
14. Fouron JC, et al. Management of fetal tachyarrhythmia based on superior vena cava/aorta Doppler flow recordings. Heart. 2003;89(10):1211-6.
15. Fouron JC. Fetal arrhythmias: the Saint-Justine hospital experience. Prenat Diagn. 2004;24(13):1068-80.
16. Friedman DM, et al. Evaluation of fetuses in a study of intravenous immunoglobulin as preventive therapy for congenital heart block: Results of a multicenter, prospective, open-label clinical trial. Arthritis and Rheumatism. 2010;62(4):1138-46.
17. Friedman DM, et al. Prospective evaluation of fetuses with autoimmune-associated congenital heart block followed in the PR Interval and Dexamethasone Evaluation (PRIDE) Study. American Journal of Cardiology. 2009;103(8):1102-6.
18. Graatsma EM, et al. Fetal electrocardiography: feasibility of long-term fetal heart rate recordings. BJOG. 2009;116(2):334-7; discussion. 337-8.
19. Hahurij ND, et al. Perinatal management and long-term cardiac outcome in fetal arrhythmia. Early Human Development. 2011;87(2):83-7.
20. Ho A, et al. Isolated complete heart block in the fetus. Am J Cardiol. 2015;116(1):142-7.
21. Hunter LE, Simpson JM. Atrioventricular block during fetal life. J Saudi Heart Assoc. 2015;27(3):164-78.
22. Izmirly PM, et al. Maternal use of hydroxychloroquine is associated with a reduced risk of recurrent anti-SSA/Ro-antibody-associated cardiac manifestations of neonatal lupus. Circulation. 2012;126(1):76-82.
23. Jaeggi ET, et al. Comparison of transplacental treatment of fetal supraventricular tachyarrhythmias with digoxin, flecainide, and sotalol: Results of a nonrandomized multicenter study. Circulation. 2011;124(16):1747-54.
24. Jaeggi ET, et al. Prenatal diagnosis of complete atrioventricular block associated with structural heart disease: Combined experience of two tertiary care centers and review of the literature. Ultrasound in Obstetrics and Gynecology. 2005;26(1):16-21.
25. Jaeggi ET, et al. Prolongation of the atrioventricular conduction in fetuses exposed to maternal anti-Ro/SSA and anti-La/SSB antibodies did not predict progressive heart block. A prospective observational study on the effects of maternal antibodies on 165 fetuses. Journal of the American College of Cardiology. 2011;57(13):1487-92.
26. Jaeggi ET, et al. Transplacental fetal treatment improves the outcome of prenatally diagnosed complete atrioventricular block without structural heart disease. Circulation. 2004;110(12):1542-8.
27. Jaeggi ET, Nii M. Fetal brady- and tachyarrhythmias: new and accepted diagnostic and treatment methods. Semin Fetal Neonatal Med. 2005;10(6):504-14.
28. Joshua A, Copel M, Ren-Ing Liang, Demasio K, Ozeren S, Kleinman S. The clinical significance of the irregular fetal heart rhythm. Am J Obstet Gynecol. 2000;182:813-9.
29. Kelly EN, et al. Prenatal anti-Ro antibody exposure, congenital complete atrioventricular heart block, and high-dose

steroid therapy: impact on neurocognitive outcome in school-age children. Arthritis Rheumatol. 2014;66(8):2290-6.
30. Kleinman CS, Nehgme RA. Cardiac arrhythmias in the human fetus. Pediatr Cardiol. 2004; 25(3):234-51.
31. Krapp M, et al. Flecainide in the intrauterine treatment of fetal supraventricular tachycardia. Ultrasound in Obstetrics and Gynecology. 2002;19(2):158-64.
32. Krapp M, et al. Review of diagnosis, treatment, and outcome of fetal atrial flutter compared with supraventricular tachycardia. Heart. 2003;89(8):913-7.
33. Krishnan A, Pike JI, Donofrio MT. Prenatal Evaluation and Management of Fetuses Exposed to Anti-SSA/Ro Antibodies. Pediatric Cardiology. 2012.
34. Krishnan AN, Sable CA, Donofrio MT. Spectrum of fetal echocardiographic findings in fetuses of women with clinical or serologic evidence of systemic lupus erythematosus. J Matern Fetal Neonatal Med. 2008;21(11):776-82.
35. Lopes LM, et al. Perinatal outcome of fetal atrioventricular block: One-hundred-sixteen cases from a single institution. Circulation. 2008;118(12):1268-75.
36. Lopriore E, et al. Long-term neurodevelopmental outcome after fetal arrhythmia. Am J Obst Gyne. 2009;201(1):46 e1-5.
37. Macones GA, et al. The 2008 National Institute of Child Health and Human Development workshop report on electronic fetal monitoring: update on definitions, interpretation, and research guidelines. Obstet Gynecol. 2008;112(3):661-6.
38. Magee LA, et al. Neurodevelopment after in utero amiodarone exposure. Neurotoxicol Teratol. 1999;21(3):261-5.
39. Mikovic Z, et al. Developmental delay associated with normal thyroidal function and long-term amiodarone therapy during fetal and neonatal life. Biomed Pharmacother. 2010; 64(6):396-8.
40. Miyoshi T, et al. Fetal bradyarrhythmia associated with congenital heart defects—nationwide survey in Japan. Circ J. 2015;79(4):854-61.
41. Narayan HK, et al. Assessment of cardiac rate and rhythm in fetuses with arrhythmia via maternal abdominal fetal electrocardiography. AJP Rep. 2015;5(2):e176-82.
42. Nii M, et al. Assessment of fetal atrioventricular time intervals by tissue Doppler and pulse Doppler echocardiography: normal values and correlation with fetal electrocardiography. Heart. 2006;92(12):1831-7.
43. Ostensen M. Intravenous immunoglobulin does not prevent recurrence of congenital heart block in children of SSA/Ro-positive mothers. Arthritis and Rheumatism. 2010;62(4):911-4.
44. Oudijk MA, et al. Sotalol in the treatment of fetal dysrhythmias. Circulation. 2000;101(23):2721-6.
45. Pezard PG, et al. Fetal tachycardia: A role for amiodarone as first- or second-line therapy? Arch Cardiovasc Dis. 2008;101(10):619-27.
46. Phoon CK, et al. Finding the "PR-fect" solution: What is the best tool to measure fetal cardiac PR intervals for the detection and possible treatment of early conduction disease? Congenit Heart Dis. 2012;7(4):349-60.
47. Rasiah SV, et al. Prenatal diagnosis, management and outcome of fetal dysrhythmia: A tertiary fetal medicine centre experience over an eight-year period. Fetal Diagnosis and Therapy. 2011; 30(2):122-7.
48. Rein AJJT. Use of tissue velocity imaging in the diagnosis of fetal cardiac arrhythmias. Circulation. 2002;106(14):1827-33.
49. Saemundsson Y, et al. Hepatic venous Doppler in the evaluation of fetal extrasystoles. Ultrasound Obstet Gynecol. 2011;37(2):179-83.
50. Serra V, et al. Computerized analysis of normal fetal heart rate pattern throughout gestation. Ultrasound in Obstetrics and Gynecology. 2009;34(1):74-9.
51. Shah A, et al. Effectiveness of sotalol as first-line therapy for fetal supraventricular tachyarrhythmias. American Journal of Cardiology. 2012;109(11):1614-8.
52. Simpson JM, et al. Fetal ventricular tachycardia secondary to long QT syndrome treated with maternal intravenous magnesium: Case report and review of the literature. Ultrasound Obstet Gynecol. 2009;34(4):475-80.

53. Simpson JM, Sharland GK. Fetal tachycardias: Management and outcome of 127 consecutive cases. Heart. 1998;79(6):576-81.
54. Sonesson SE, Acharya G. Hemodynamics in fetal arrhythmia. Acta Obstet Gynecol Scand. 2015.
55. Sonesson SE, et al. Doppler echocardiographic isovolumetric time intervals in diagnosis of fetal blocked atrial bigeminy and 2:1 atrioventricular block. Ultrasound Obstet Gynecol. 2014;44(2): 171-5.
56. Srinivasan S, Strasburger J. Overview of fetal arrhythmias. Current Opinion in Pediatrics. 2008;20(5):522-31.
57. Strasburger JF, Cheulkar B, Wakai RT. Magnetocardiography for fetal arrhythmias. Heart Rhythm. 2008;5(7):1073-6.
58. Strasburger JF, Wakai RT. Fetal cardiac arrhythmia detection and in utero therapy. Nat Rev Cardiol. 2010;7(5):277-90.
59. Trucco SM, et al. Use of intravenous gamma globulin and corticosteroids in the treatment of maternal autoantibody-mediated cardiomyopathy. J Am Coll Cardiol. 2011;57(6): 715-23.
60. van den Heuvel F, et al. Drug management of fetal tachyarrhythmias: Are we ready for a systematic and evidence-based approach? Pacing and Clinical Electrophysiology. 2008;(31)1:S54-7.
61. Vergani P, et al. Fetal arrhythmias: natural history and management. Ultrasound in Medicine and Biology. 2005;31(1):1-6.
62. Vigneswaran TV, et al. Correlation of maternal flecainide concentrations and therapeutic effect in fetal supraventricular tachycardia. Heart Rhythm. 2014;11(11):2047-53.
63. Wiggins DL, et al. Magnetophysiologic and echocardiographic comparison of blocked atrial bigeminy and 2:1 atrioventricular block in the fetus. Heart Rhythm. 2013;10(8):1192-8.

CHAPTER 8

Fetal Heart Failure

Sejal Shah

ABSTRACT

This Chapter gives an overview of the etiopathogenesis of cardiac failure, step by step approach when cardiac failure is suspected including 2D and Doppler patterns and the prognosticating signs. Cardiac cause for fetal heart failure is less common. However, fetal echo does play a role in understanding the impact on the fetus and also monitoring pregnancy for an optimal outcome. Doppler patterns, generally less focused in fetal echo, are an important part of an overall understanding of hemodynamics. Normal Doppler patterns are shown along the side with the abnormal ones to help understand the physiology better. The fact that the ventricular compliance is poor, in addition to having a parallel circuit, makes the fetal heart more vulnerable to any stress and makes the fetal heart respond to any stress in a peculiar way.

INTRODUCTION

Fetal heart failure is a final common outcome of many diseases and may lead to mortality. It is defined as the inability of the heart to deliver adequate blood flow to the body organs. Fetal cardiac dysfunction may happen with a heart disease or without a heart disease. It is an uncommon event that typically occurs in presence of some condition which places a burden on the right ventricle. Congestive cardiac failure may present in prehydropic state or with hydrops. Hydrops fetalis is defined as accumulation of abnormal fluid in at least two different fetal compartments. Fetal echocardiogram not only helps diagnosing cardiac abnormality, but also enables diagnosing and prognosticating heart failure.

IS FETAL HEART DIFFERENT FROM ADULT HEART?

Fetal heart is different in some ways compared to an adult heart. Understanding these differences in terms of anatomy and physiology will help us understand the pathophysiology of fetal heart failure. Few peculiar points related to fetal circuit are summarized here.
- Fetal heart has parallel circuit due to presence of ductus arteriosus. Ductus arteriosus joins the pulmonary artery to aorta and has a diameter equivalent to these two major vessels.
- Oxygenated blood from umbilical vein passes through the ductus venosus, (along with left portion of inferior vena cava and

left hepatic veins) enters right atrium and then into left atrium through foramen ovale and is then directed into aorta to the head/brain.
- Deoxygenated blood from the superior vena cava (along with right portion of inferior vena cava and right hepatic veins) enters the right atrium, into the right ventricle and is then directed via ductus arteriosus down to the aorta and to the umbilical arteries.
- Right ventricular output is more compared to the left ventricular output. The ratio of right heart output: left heart output is 55%:45% at 20 weeks of gestation and 60%:40% in the last 10 weeks of gestation.
- As the fetal circuit is a parallel circuit, output from both the ventricles need to be added to get 'combined cardiac output' which is approximately 500 mL/kg/min. The pulmonary blood flow is only 13% of the combined cardiac output at 20 weeks and 25% at 30 weeks.
- The ventricular compliance is less in the fetus than in the neonate however the compliance improves with advancing gestational age.
- Any chronic stress in fetal life causes alteration in the right/left heart dominance. Alteration in the ventricular function leads to redistribution of cardiac output with preferential flow to the brain and coronaries.

PATHOPHYSIOLOGY

Any stimulus (like increase in preload or afterload to the heart) which can lead to chronic stress/hypoxia will cause altered ventricular function and redistribution of cardiac output. This in turn will lead to abnormal cardiac filling and increased venous pressure causing decompensation. This culminates in the evolution of fetal heart failure manifested as hydrops. Diastolic dysfunction may be less well-tolerated by the fetus compared to systolic dysfunction.

The mechanism of cardiogenic hydrops due to congestive cardiac failure is related to limited ventricular compliance and increase in ventricular end diastolic pressures. Occasionally in addition, contribution can be from lymphatic pulmonary edema secondary to left atrial hypertension (like in hypoplastic let heart syndrome with restrictive foramen ovale). Myocardial dysfunction may also affect the well-being of the fetus through the development of fetal hypoxia and acidosis secondary to altered umbilical venous return, reduced placental function and altered cardiac output which may result in fetal demise. Few still births are directly caused by fetal heart failure, however heart failure is likely a terminal event in many other causes.

Hydrops implies excess of total body water which is usually evident as extracellular accumulation of fluid in tissues and serous cavities. Hydrops can be due to intrauterine anemia or hypoproteinemia or heart failure or any structural anomaly interfering with fetoplacental circulation. The understanding of etiopathology of hydrops is complex. In fetus, the capillary membrane is more permeable for fluid and protein. The albumin concentration (which causes oncotic pressure) is lower in fetus (it increases with gestational age). In addition, small increase in venous pressures can alter the fetal organ function. All these reasons favor fluid movement out of the capillary into the tissue causing fluid accumulation in fetal tissue. Younger the fetus, higher is the extracellular water content and lower is the tissue pressure.

ETIOLOGY

Mechanisms that cause heart failure include increasing preload (e.g. atrioventricular valve regurgitation, twin transfusion), reducing preload (e.g. hemorrhage), decreased ventricular contractility (due to myocarditis, metabolic causes), increased afterload (e.g. aortic stenosis, pulmonary stenosis, placental insufficiency) and increasing peripheral demand (e.g. anemia, infection). Occasionally, multiple mechanisms may work together, e.g. in arrhythmias, premature ductal and foramen ovale closure. Any cause that can increase the right atrial pressure or increase the volume can cause hydrops.

Though etiology of hydrops can be predominantly divided into immune and non-immune hydrops, at times it may be multifactorial in origin. The prognosis differs markedly between different etiologies of hydrops. Immune hydrops is caused by maternal red cell immunization. Non-immune hydrops is considered in absence of maternal circulating red cell antibodies and it accounts for 85% of all cases of hydrops. Amongst non-immune hydrops, in 15–25% of cases etiology is not known. In the rest of the cases of non-immune hydrops, causes include cardiovascular (21%), hematological, chromosomal, syndromic, lymphatic dysplasia, inborn error of metabolism, infectious, thoracic, urinary tract malformations, extrathoracic tumors, twin-to-twin transfusion, gastrointestinal and miscellaneous. Though primary cardiovascular disorders account for 15–25% of cases, many noncardiac causes of non-immune hydrops alter cardiac loading and heart function eventually leading to fetal heart failure, also manifested as hydrops.

Cardiovascular causes of hydrops include atrioventricular septal defect with atrioventricular valve regurgitation, tetralogy of Fallot with absent pulmonary valve, severe aortic stenosis with mitral regurgitation, Ebstein's anomaly of tricuspid valve, hypoplastic left heart syndrome, cardiac tumors like rhabdomyomas or intrapericardial teratoma, premature closure of ductus arteriosus or foramen ovale, endocardial fibroelastosis with mitral regurgitation/aortic stenosis, myocardial dysfunction due to infection/inflammation/infarction with ventricular aneurysm/arterial calcification, arrhythmias: brady arrhythmias (especially when heart rate is less than 50 bpm) and tachyarrhythmias.

DIAGNOSIS

In fetal heart failure, fetal echocardiography by using 2D, color Doppler, pulsed Doppler and M-mode helps us in the following ways.
1. To assess cardiac anatomy: Diagnose congenital heart disease. Based on the heart disease, helps us consider syndromic association.
2. To assess cardiac function: Systolic and diastolic.
3. To check for cardiac rate and rhythm. To detect fetal arrhythmias and decide for fetal cardiac intervention.
4. To diagnose signs of cardiac failure and monitor treatment.

A systemic cardiac examination is mandatory for any case of heart failure to detect the cause and to see the effect.

Ventricular Disproportion

Both the ventricles in fetus are relatively of similar size. Using M-mode, the pulmonary artery: Aorta ratio can be calculated to see for any ventricular disproportion. Normal ratio is 1.06 to 1.11. Significant difference in the ventricular size may be due to structural heart disease or cardiac failure. Right heart dominance more than acceptable (Fig. 8.1) may be seen in cases with premature ductal or foramen ovale closure or primary tricuspid valve disease. Right heart dilatation may also be seen in presence of vein of Galen malformation or in agenesis of ductus venosus wherein the umbilical venous return preferentially streams to the right heart.

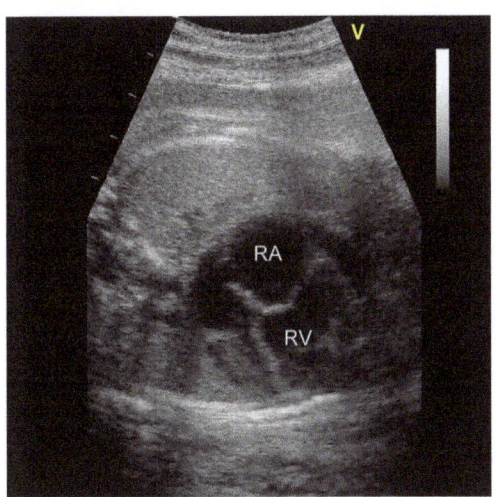

Fig. 8.1: Four-chamber view on 2D showing disproportionate right heart dilatation
Abbreviations: RA, right atrium; RV, right ventricle

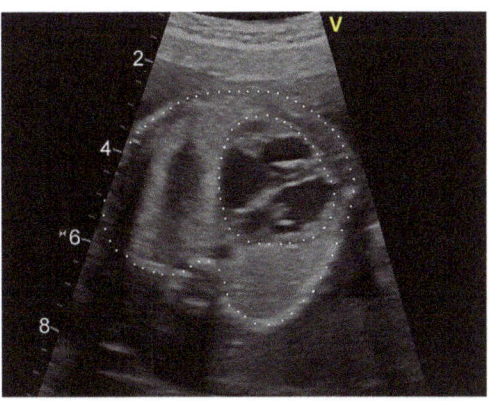

Fig. 8.2: Four-chamber view showing the ratio of the circumference of the heart to that of the chest being more than 0.5 indicating cardiomegaly

Cardiac Size

Cardiomegaly is a common and an important sign of altered cardiac function (Fig. 8.2). Roughly, the heart size should be one-third the size of the thorax. The cardiac size relative to thorax can be evaluated from cross sectional images through the fetal chest with measurements of cardiothoracic diameter, area and circumference ratios. The diameter of the heart can be compared to that of the thorax in the following way:

$$\frac{\text{Anteroposterior + transverse diameter of the heart}/2}{\text{Anteroposterior + transverse diameter of the thorax}/2}$$

Normal ratio is 45–55% and is independent of the gestation age.

The most common cardiac chamber to be enlarged as a sign of impending cardiac failure is the right atrium. This is may be due to the fact that right atrium is a final pathway for the blood returning to the heart (e.g. in cases of restrictive foramen ovale) or as the right ventricular end diastolic pressure is high.

Cardiomegaly also gives information regarding the duration of abnormality, e.g. in arrhythmias, if it is intermittent then the heart size is expected to be normal.

A small heart size (ratio of cardiac to thoracic area of under 0.20) which may be secondary to extrinsic compression or structurally small heart is also considered to have poor prognosis.

Doppler Imaging

Using color Doppler and pulse Doppler, the understanding of heart disease is refined. It can demonstrate normal flow patterns, show abnormal flow patterns like lack of flow across a valve/regurgitation or increased velocity across a valve and show reversal of normal flow in a vessel/foramen ovale. Pulse Doppler evaluation needs to be done in the heart and in the peripheral vessels. Pulsed Doppler evaluation gives information regarding the direction of flow, pattern of flow, velocity of flow and volume flow-function. Doppler study gives us information regarding the atrial and the ventricular filling, fetal arrhythmias and hemodynamic disturbances in severely compromised fetuses. In a way, it helps us understand the pathophysiology of developing heart failure. It may help identifying the failing ventricle prior to the onset of hydrops when fetal cardiac intervention may be more beneficial.

Pulse Doppler interrogation of the ventricular inflows, systemic and pulmonary veins, ductus venosus and umbilical vein provides clues to the diastolic properties and filling of the ventricles. Pulse Doppler study of ventricular outflows can be used to calculate ventricular stroke volumes and outputs and may be helpful in pregnancies at risk for high fetal cardiac output.

Peripheral Vessels

Angle independent indices like pulsatility index, resistance index and systolic/diastolic ratio are commonly used here.

Umbilical artery Doppler: The most common vessel used is umbilical artery (Fig. 8.3A). Changes in the Doppler waveform in umbilical artery would indicate placental insufficiency and may precede heart failure (absent or reversed end diastolic flow in umbilical artery indicates increased placental resistance) (Fig. 8.3B). Changes in the umbilical artery Doppler appear later than venous Doppler and cardiac function alterations. Other vessels are cerebral artery, carotid artery, aorta and renal arteries. Increased peak velocity of middle cerebral artery favors anemia in the fetus. The redistribution of flow to the brain is manifested by decrease in the pulsatility index in middle cerebral artery such that the diastolic flow is relatively increased. Umbilical and middle cerebral artery Doppler's do not change much in fetuses with congenital heart disease (except with severe outflow tract obstruction).

Umbilical vein Doppler: Sampling of the umbilical vein in the abdomen and the umbilical cord vein is needed (Fig. 8.4). Venous pulsations in the umbilical vein indicate increase in the reverse flow in the inferior vena cava which may be due to abnormal ventricular filling or arrhythmias.

Heart

Usually, the Doppler measurements done in the heart are absolute values where the angle of insonation should be less than 20°. Common parameters checked here are the peak velocity, acceleration time/time to peak velocity, time velocity integral and volume flow. The errors in Doppler velocity

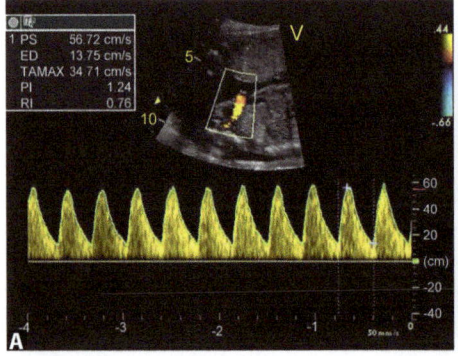 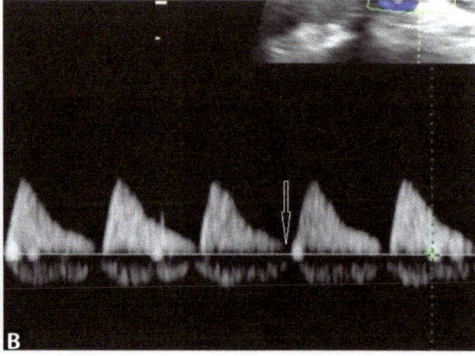

Figs 8.3A and B: (A) Normal pulse Doppler of umbilical artery showing saw tooth appearance and flow throughout the cycle; (B) Absent diastolic flow in the umbilical artery shown with an arrow indicating increased placental resistance

Fetal Heart Failure

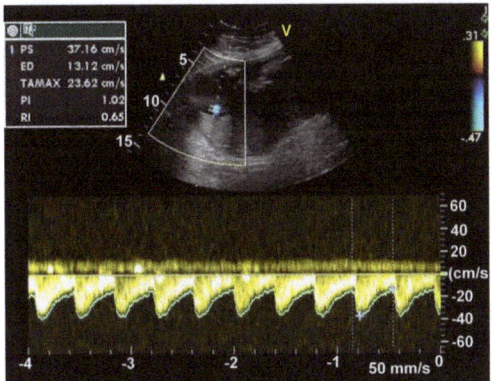

Fig. 8.4: Normal pulse Doppler of umbilical vein with linear forward flow throughout the cycle seen above the baseline. Below the baseline is the Doppler of the umbilical artery

calculations are primarily due to the angle of insonation being more than 20° and the lack of accuracy in measurement of the diameter of valve/vessel while calculating volume flow.

Ductus venosus: The flow across the ductus venosus can be seen as a turbulent flow throughout the cycle below the diaphragm which increases during respiration. Normally, there is a peak in systole flow (velocity of 65-75 cm/sec) followed by another peak in early diastole (nearly equal velocity) with continuous forward flow during atrial contraction (velocity of 35-45 cm/sec) (Fig. 8.5A and B). Abnormal waveform of ductus venosus identifies fetus at risk to have congenital heart disease and also predicts

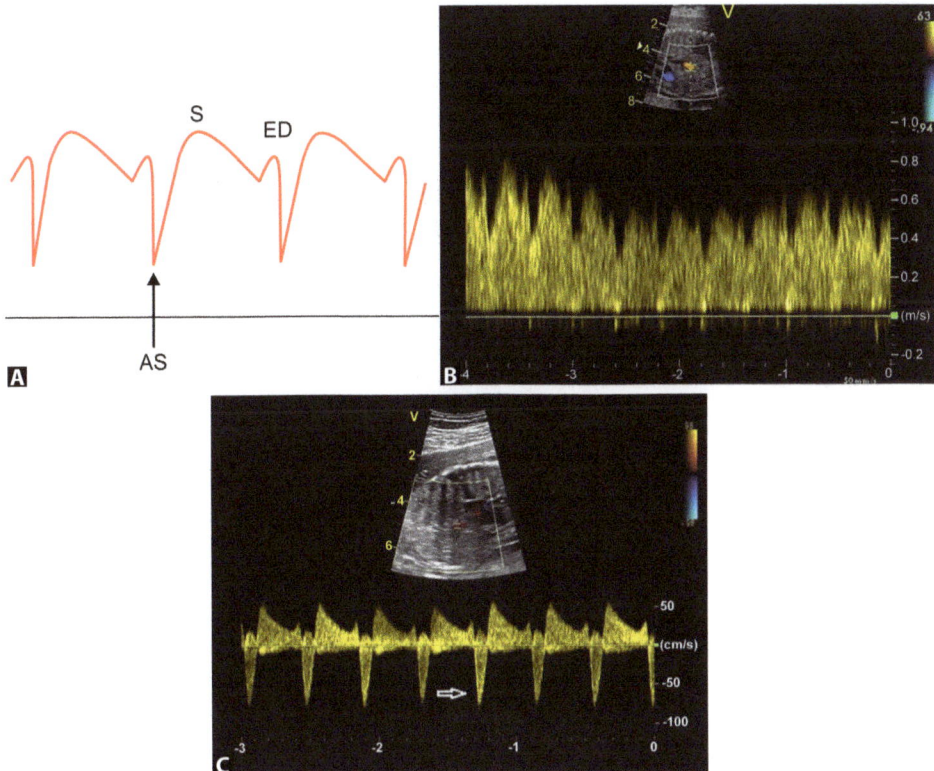

Figs 8.5A to C: (A) Diagrammatic representation of normal pulse Doppler of ductus venosus with two peaks in systole (S) and diastole (D) of nearly equal velocity with continuous flow in atrial systole (AS); (B) Shows the pulse Doppler with respiratory variation; (C) Shows abnormal reversal of "a" wave shown with an arrow

prognosis. Presence of any 'a' wave reversal in the ductus venosus suggests presence of increased central venous pressure (Fig. 8.5C). Hypoxia can cause abnormal flow pattern in the form of reduction or reversal of a wave. Reverse wave is also commonly seen in tricuspid atresia/pulmonary atresia intact ventricular septum with restrictive foramen ovale. Normally, the ratio of the area of the atrial reversal to the entire forward flow area should be less than 7%.

Inferior vena cava (IVC) Doppler: It has three components. The initial forward flow is with ventricular systole, the second forward flow is with ventricular diastole followed by the reverse flow in atrial contraction (Fig. 8.6A). In normal fetus, the peak velocity of the first wave of systole is greater than the early diastolic velocity. With advancing age, the S/D ratio do not change; however the flow reversal with atrial contraction decreases significantly related to change in the ventricular compliance.

An angle independent index which can be measured in IVC Doppler is PLI = Preload index. PLI = Reverse flow/Initial forward flow.

IVC/hepatic vein Doppler may show increased atrial reversal in congestive heart failure due to increased end diastolic pressures in the ventricles (Fig. 8.6B to D).

Pulmonary vein: The Doppler pattern in pulmonary veins reflect left atrium

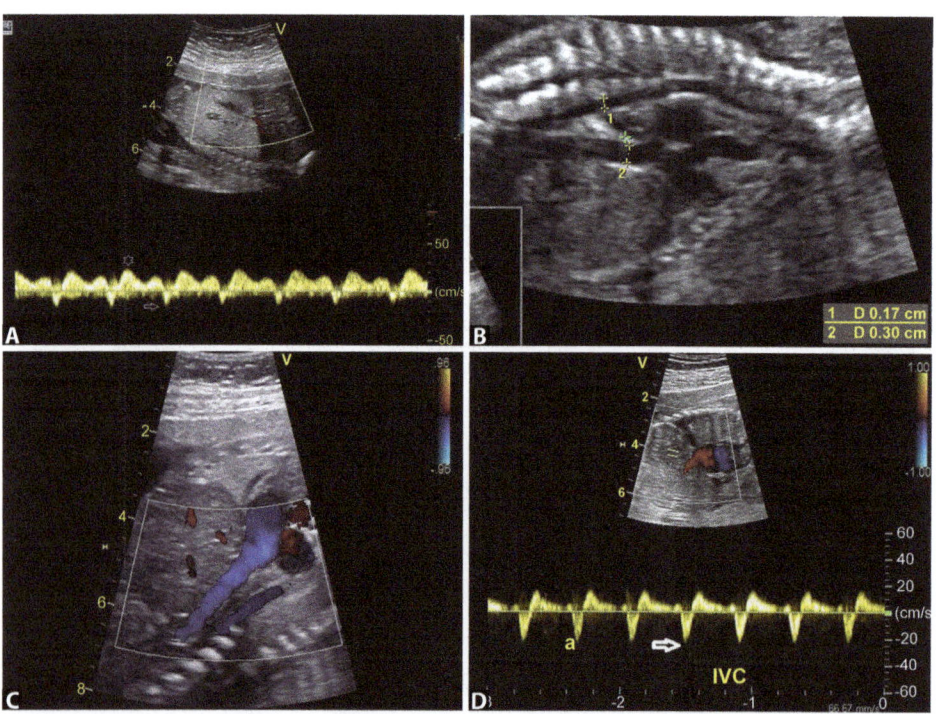

Figs 8.6A to D: (A) Normal pulse Doppler of IVC showing initial forward flow with ventricular systole, the second forward flow with ventricular diastole followed by the reverse flow in atrial contraction (arrow). Note that the peak velocity of the first wave of systole is greater (star) than the early diastolic velocity; (B) Shows IVC and SVC dilated (IVC compared to descending aorta); (C) Shows increased atrial reversal in congestive heart failure due to increased end diastolic pressures in the ventricles on color Doppler; (D) Shows atrial reversal (arrow) on pulse Doppler

hemodynamics and is not affected by respiration. Normally, there is a peak in ventricular systole (velocity of 10 cm/sec at 16 weeks of gestation to 40 cm/sec at term) which is due to suction effect of atrial relaxation followed by continuous flow due to descent of the mitral valve, followed by peak in early diastole due to opening of mitral valve and lastly cessation of flow/reverse flow in late diastole (velocity of less than 10 cm/sec) due to atrial contraction (Fig. 8.7). The volume of flow in systole is almost twice the volume in diastole. Doppler of the pulmonary vein may provide information regarding severity of left atrial hypertension, e.g. with hypoplastic left heart syndrome with restrictive foramen ovale.

Foramen ovale: It is important to reduce the color settings to demonstrate flow across the foramen ovale. Normally, there is R-L flow almost throughout the cardiac cycle with a peak in ventricular systole (velocity of 10 cm/sec at 16 weeks to 50 cm/sec at term) and a peak in diastole (due to mitral valve opening) followed by cessation of flow due to atrial contraction-closure of foramen ovale (Fig. 8.8). Narrow spike of L-R shunt may be seen at one point in cardiac cycle due to atrial

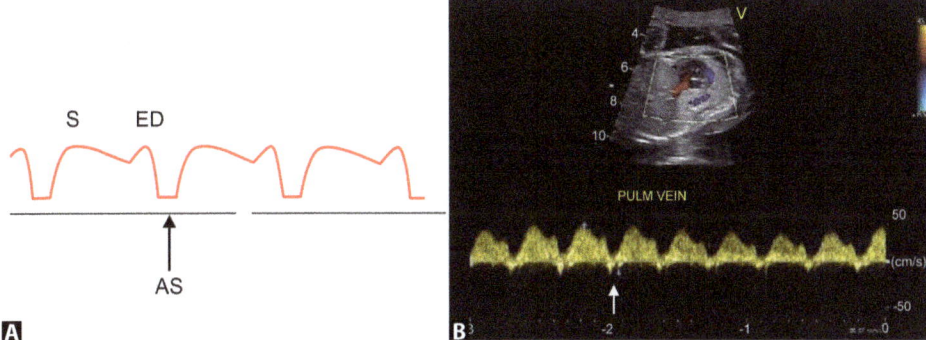

Figs 8.7A and B: Normal pulse Doppler of pulmonary vein: (A) Diagrammatic representation of the flow with systolic (S), diastolic (ED) flow with almost cessation of flow in atrial systole (AS); (B) Shows pulse Doppler in pulmonary vein which is low velocity with reverse flow in late diastole (arrow)

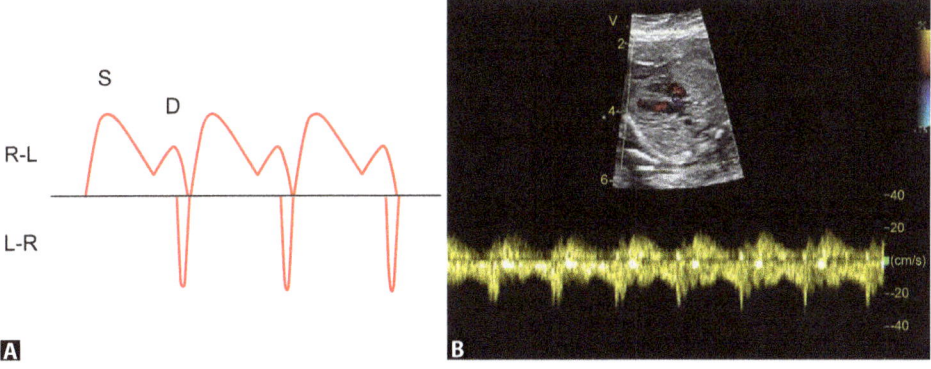

Figs 8.8A and B: Normal pulse Doppler of foramen ovale. (A) show a diagrammatic representation of the Doppler with right to left (R-L) flow almost throughout the cycle with two peaks S (systole) and D (diastole) followed by complete cessation of flow. Narrow spike of left to right (L-R) shunt is seen during atrial systole, (B) shows low velocity flow across foramen ovale

systole. L-R shunt across the foramen ovale may indicate increased left atrial pressures, e.g. in mitral stenosis or smallish left ventricle. For premature foramen ovale closure, see later in the chapter.

Atrioventricular valves: Mitral valve: Normally shows a typical biphasic pattern in diastole and no flow in systole. The velocity across the mitral valve increases during respiration. It has the early filling (E) wave and the late diastolic filling (A) wave. Unlike in the postnatal period, the E wave (velocity of 15 cm/sec at 12 weeks of gestation to 50 cm/sec at term) is lesser than the A wave (velocity of 35–65 cm/sec)(Fig. 8.9A). The E wave is passive filling which reflects the gradient between LA and LV and it increases during gestation due to better myocardial relaxation. A wave is due to atrial contraction, reflecting LV end diastolic pressure and remains constant during gestation. E/A ratio increases from 0.5 to 1 with advancing gestation.

Tricuspid valve: The pattern is similar to mitral valve, except that the velocities are higher as RV is the dominant ventricle. E wave velocity is 20 cm/sec at 12 weeks to 50 cm/sec at term and A wave velocity is 35–60 cm/sec (Fig. 8.10A). The shift from right to left ventricular dominance starts in utero towards the end of gestation. The Doppler pattern here reflects ventricular compliance and preload.

Diastolic function can be assessed by peak E velocity, peak A velocity, E/A ratio and velocity time integral. Increase in the A wave indicates increase in the right atrial pressures. Diastolic dysfunction shows shortened/

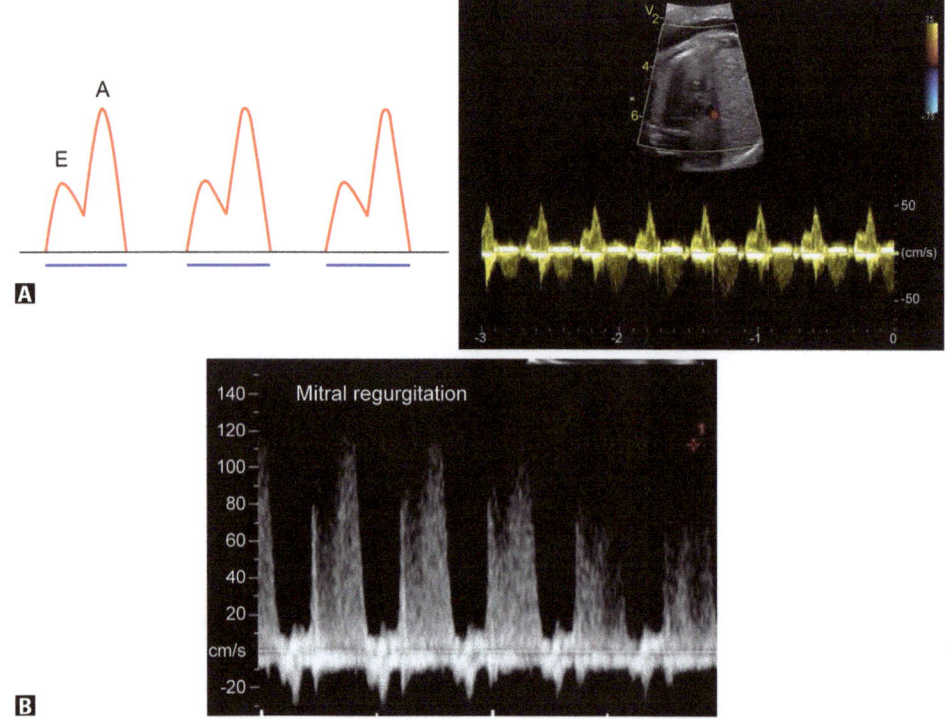

Figs 8.9A and B: (A) Normal pulse Doppler of mitral valve with diagrammatic representation with early filling (E) and late diastolic filling (A) waves, with E wave velocity lesser than the A wave; (B) Shows mitral regurgitation indicating increasing end diastolic pressures and severe myocardial failure

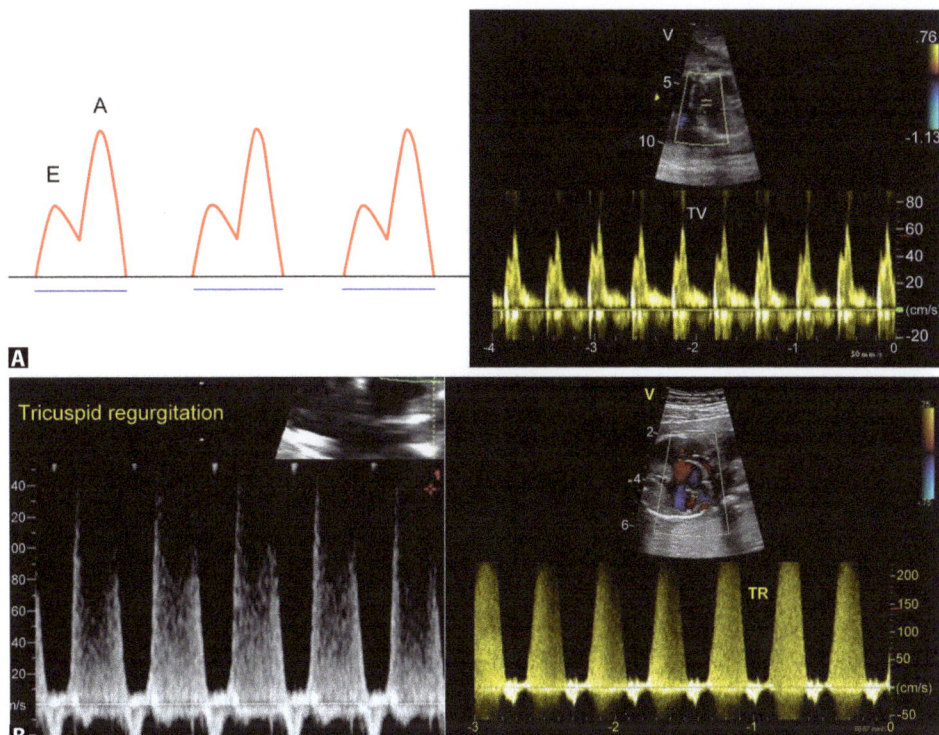

Figs 8.10A and B: (A) Normal pulse Doppler of tricuspid valve: Including the diagrammatic representation showing early filling (E) and late diastolic filling (A) waves, with E wave velocity lesser than the A wave. Note that the velocity is slightly higher than that of the mitral valve; (B) Shows holosystolic tricuspid regurgitation which is abnormal

normal isovolumic relaxation time, normal/increased but brief E wave and reduced A wave. Merging of E and A waves (uniphasic pattern) is not uncommon and may not signify any pathology. However, short duration monophasic ventricular inflow pattern is seen in fetal cardiomyopathies, ductus arteriosus constriction and severe semilunar valve stenosis. Abnormal myocardial function is seen as an increase in end diastolic pressure and increased wall stress causing atrioventricular valve regurgitation (Fig. 8.11). Tricuspid regurgitation when detected by color Doppler should be confirmed and graded by pulsed Doppler (Fig. 8.10B). Holosystolic tricuspid regurgitation is abnormal but could be a reversible sign of cardiac failure

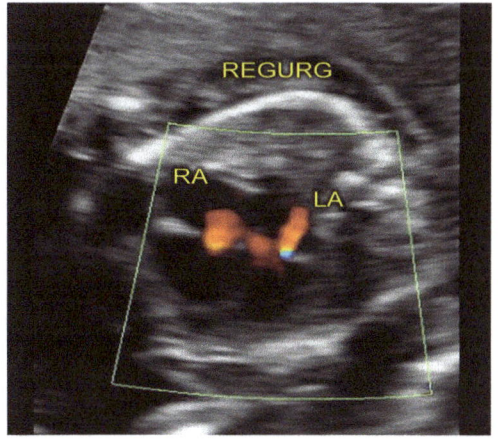

Fig. 8.11: Color Doppler showing regurgitation of both the atrioventricular valves indicating abnormal myocardial function

during treatment. Persistence of tricuspid regurgitation and progression to mitral regurgitation have been considered signs of more severe myocardial failure (Fig. 8.9B). Calculation of dP/dt (change of pressure over time) can predict fetal outcome. dP/dt of less than 800 mm Hg/sec is abnormal and less than 400 mm Hg/sec predicts poor outcome.

Ventricular outflows: Normally, they have a single forward flow in systole with no flow in diastole (Fig. 8.12A). The peak velocity is 30 cm/sec at 12 weeks of gestation to 80 cm/sec at term. The peak velocity is greater in the aorta than pulmonary artery due to decreased afterload and small diameter of aorta. Velocity time intergral and acceleration time can be measured on semilunar valve Dopplers. Acceleration time is longer in aorta than pulmonary artery as the resistance faced by LV is slightly lower than that faced by RV. The peak systolic velocity and acceleration time across the semilunar valves reflects ventricular contractility, arterial pressure and afterload.

Ventricular systolic function can be assessed by Doppler of the semilunar valve using peak velocity (Fig. 8.12B), acceleration time, stroke volume/cardiac output in addition to shortening fraction and myocardial perfusion index.

With severe myocardial failure, the aortic and pulmonary valves may also show

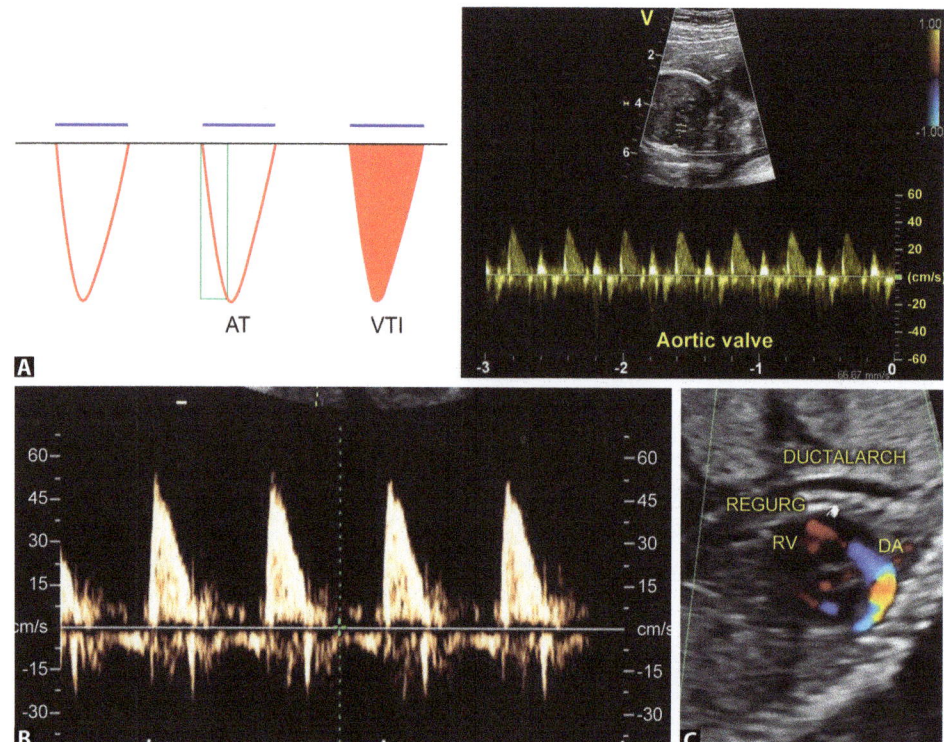

Figs 8.12A to C: (A) Pulse Doppler of semilunar valves: Showing a single forward flow in systole (diagrammatic representation). Panel A also shows the acceleration time (AT) and the velocity time integral (VTI); (B) Shows reduction in the peak velocity across the semilunar valve reflecting reduction in myocardial contractility; (C) Shows pulmonary regurgitation in myocarditis

regurgitation due to loss of support for semilunar valves (Fig. 8.12C).

Ductus arteriosus: It has a peak systolic flow (velocity of 50 cm/sec at 16 weeks to 1.8 m/sec at term) with a forward flow throughout diastole (peak velocity of 5-12 cm/sec) (Fig. 8.13A). There may be some reverse flow in early diastole in late gestation. The shape of diastolic peak is different from other fetal vessels as the duct is a conduit between two vascular systems and had different wall characteristics. The peak velocity in the duct is the highest in normal fetal heart (Fig. 8.13B). The acceleration time in duct is longer than that in AO and PA as the placental bed has low resistance. Reverse flow in the ductus may indicate pulmonary stenosis/atresia in Ebstein's anomaly of tricuspid valve. Doppler of the ductus arteriosus can detect premature ductal closure even in early stages (refer to premature ductal constriction).

Branch pulmonary arteries: They have a characteristic flow profile with sharp rise to peak (due to high vascular resistance and decreased capacitance) followed by slow decline and then a notch followed by low velocity forward flow in diastole (Fig. 8.14). There is often a short reverse wave in early diastole due to PV closure. The peak systolic velocity is 55 cm/sec at 18 weeks to 90 cm/sec at term. The origins of branch pulmonary arteries have high systolic velocity and less diastolic flow compared to distal branches.

Aortic isthmus: There is forward flow both in systole and diastole normally, however it changes with gestation (Fig. 8.15). There may be a small reverse flow in early diastole. Reversal of flow in diastole in the aortic isthmus may suggest significant vasodilatation of brain vessels.

Left ventricular inflow-outflow Doppler: Simultaneous Doppler study of left ventricular inflow and outflow can give information regarding the isovolumic relaxation (IRT) time of the left ventricle which is a measure of diastolic function (Fig. 8.16). Increased IRT is noticed in cardiomyopathies or with ventricular dysfunction.

Left/right ventricular function can also assessed by myocardial performance index

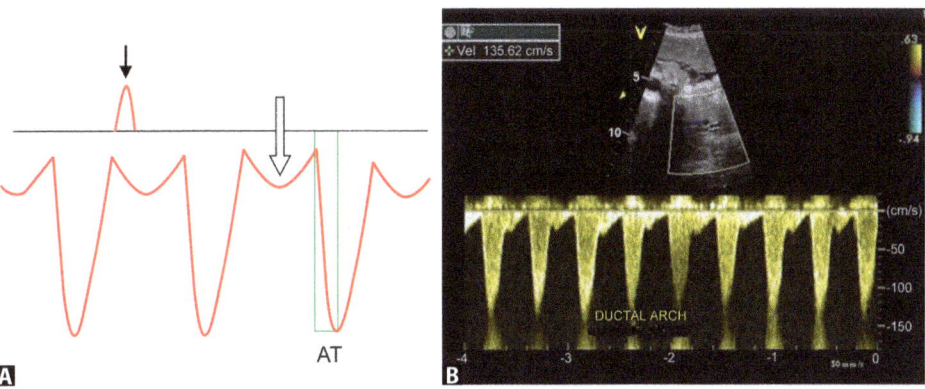

Figs 8.13A and B: (A) Normal pulse Doppler in the ductal arch (shows diagrammatic representation) with peak velocity in systole with a peculiar shape of the flow in diastole (wide arrow) and occasional reverse flow in early diastole (small arrow). It also shows acceleration time (AT); (B) Doppler across the ductal arch with peak velocity which is the highest in a normal fetal heart

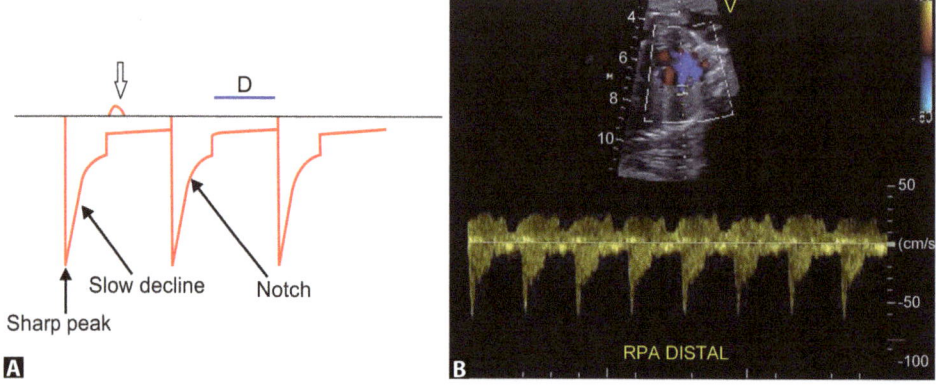

Figs 8.14A and B: Pulse Doppler in the branch pulmonary artery: (A) diagrammatic representation showing a sharp peak, slow decline and a notch: peculiar Doppler pattern seen in branches of pulmonary artery followed by forward flow in diastole (D). The wide arrow shows small reverse wave in early diastole. (B) Doppler waveform taken at distal right pulmonary artery (RPA) reveals the same peculiar Doppler pattern

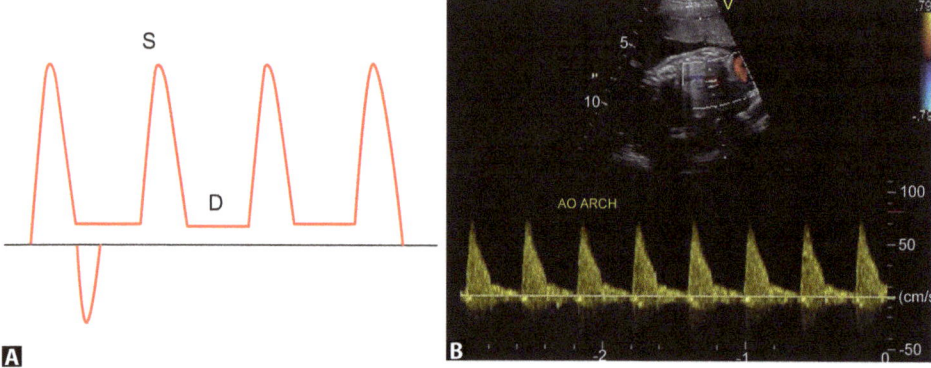

Figs 8.15A and B: Pulse Doppler in the aortic arch: with a peak in systole and some forward flow in diastole (A—diagrammatic representation). Occasional reverse flow may be seen in early diastole

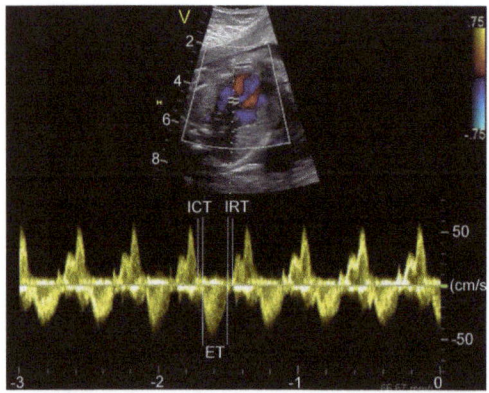

Fig. 8.16: Pulse Doppler waveform with the cursor on the lateral wall of the ascending aorta close to the mitral valve in an apical four-chamber view of the fetal heart showing the LV inflow tracing below the baseline and the LV outflow tracing above the baseline

Abbreviations: LA, left atrium; LV, left ventricle; AO, aorta; ICT, isovolumic contraction time; IRT, isovolumic relaxation time; ET, ejection time

(MPI) which is calculated by IRT + ICT/ ejection time (ICT = isovolumic contraction time). This is a load independent index of function.

Systolic Function

A qualitative assessment of both the ventricles' systolic function can be done by real time imaging. For quantitative evaluation of systolic function especially the left ventricle, we can measure the diameter of the ventricle in systole and diastole by M-mode or by 2D and calculate shortening fraction.

$$\text{Fractional shortening (FS)} = \frac{\text{End diastolic} - \text{End systolic ventricular diameter}}{\text{End diastolic diameter}}$$

Normal FS is more than 28%. Increase in the diastolic dimension may be due to decrease in the fractional shortening and needs close monitoring. Measurement of left ventricular wall thickness in diastole can give an understanding of ventricular hypertrophy. Left ventricular posterior wall measurement of more than 4 mm is abnormal.

Volume Flow

Velocity flow measurements can be obtained from number of sites in or near the heart using the following formula:

$$\text{Volume flow (mL/min)} = \pi/4 \times D^2 \times 1/\cos 0 \times FVI \times HR$$

Where D = Diameter in cm of any vessel
 0 = The angle between the ultrasound beam and the vessel
 FVI = Flow velocity integral
 HR = Heart rate

Volume of the left heart can be estimated at mitral and aortic valves and that of the right heart at tricuspid and pulmonary valves. The stroke volume of each ventricle increases by 10 folds between 20 to 40 weeks of gestation and most of this increase happens due to increase in the size of the valve orifice (the mean velocity remains relatively constant).

Signs of Developing Heart Failure

Signs of developing heart failure include low peak velocity in outflow tracts, exaggerated pulsations in inferior vena cava/ increased percentage of reverse flow in inferior vena cava, pulsations in umbilical vein (sign of fetal compromise) and tricuspid regurgitation. In advanced stages, would have cardiomegaly, valvular regurgitation, venous congestion, fetal edema/effusions (Figs 8.17A to C), oligohydramnios and preferential shunting of blood to brain/heart/adrenals. In presence of congenital heart disease and hydrops, abnormal hepatic vein and ductus venosus velocities and umbilical venous pulsations are strongly associated with fetal mortality.

A useful tool is cardiovascular profile score (CVP) (Table 8.1) which correlates ultrasound findings with cardiac function, helps in the prediction of cardiac failure in hydropic fetuses and helps predicting fetal outcome. Cardiovascular profile score is a composite of five signs: Hydrops, cardiomegaly, cardiac function, arterial Doppler and venous Doppler of umbilical vein and ductus venosus. Each is worth 2 points in a ten point scoring system wherein a score of 10 is normal. Abnormalities in the score may occur prior to clinical state of hydrops. The CVP score may be useful in baseline evaluation and then for serial evaluations for fetuses at risk for or with myocardial dysfunction.

MANAGEMENT

Tachyarrhythmia is the most treatable cardiac cause of hydrops. If fetal tachyarrhythmia is persistent or has evidence of cardiac compromise, then intrauterine therapy is indicated.

Maternal digoxin may be considered in some cases of heart failure (due to arrhythmias and high output states) as it is suppose to reduce the catecholamine response to congestive cardiac failure and

Fetal Echocardiography

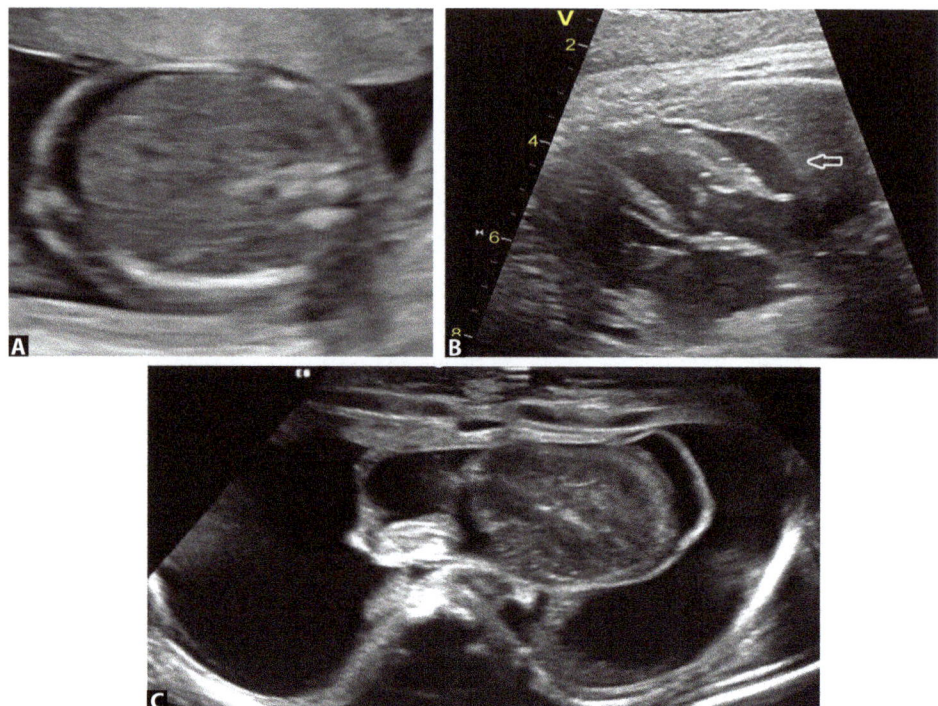

Figs 8.17A to C: Ascites, pericardial effusion and pleural effusion

Table 8.1: Fetal cardiovascular profile score

Category	Score 2	Score 1	Score 0
Hydrops	None	Ascites or pleural effusion or pericardial effusion	Skin edema
Cardiomegaly (cardiac area/thoracic area)	>0.20 and ≤0.35	0.35–0.50	>0.50 or <0.20
Cardiac function	Normal TV and MV, biphasic diastolic filling	Holosystolic TR	Holosystolic MR, monophasic diastolic filling
Arterial umbilical Doppler	Normal positive diastolic flow	Absent end diastolic flow	Reversed end diastolic flow
Venous Doppler UV DV	Normal • Non-pulsatile pattern • Low pulsatility	• No pulsations • Increase in pulsatility • Decreased velocity in atrial contraction (zero or reversed)	• Additional pulsations • Increase in pulsatility • Decreased velocity in atrial contraction (zero or reversed)

Abbreviations: TV, tricuspid valve; MV, mitral valve; TR, tricuspid regurgitation; MR, mitral regurgitation; UV, umbilical vein; DV, ductus venosus

improve filling and lower filling pressures in diastolic dysfunction. It may be useful in improving the cardiovascular profile score. If a maternal drug has caused heart failure, then the drug should be withdrawn, e.g. non-steroidal anti-inflammatory drugs causing ductal constriction.

PROGNOSIS

The outcome for fetal hydrops depends on the etiology (and whether the insult is reversible) and the gestational age at diagnosis. When the diagnosis is made prior to 20 weeks of gestation, it carries worse prognosis, with a mortality of 40–60% for non-immune hydrops. The abnormal venous Dopplers develop with increasing heart failure in the following order: Increased atrial reversal in the IVC, ductus venosus atrial reversal and umbilical venous atrial pulsations. The most useful predictor for perinatal death in hydrops is the presence of umbilical venous pulsations.

The two conditions needing a special mention here. They are premature ductal closure and premature foramen ovale closure.

Premature Ductal Closure

Premature ductal closure is a less recognized entity and may be subclinical in many cases. The closure of ductus though may happen due to many factors, including ingestion of non-steroidal anti-inflammatory drugs or polyphenol rich food; it is idiopathic in many cases. As ductus causes right ventricular unloading, closure of ductus causes profound effect on the cardiovascular system. It causes dilatation of right atrium, right ventricle, main pulmonary artery, right ventricular hypertrophy (seen in all the cases) and more than trivial tricuspid regurgitation (seen in all the cases) with suprasystemic gradients and pulmonary regurgitation (Figs 8.18A and B). Close monitoring to see for right heart failure is mandatory. 2D, color Doppler and pulsed

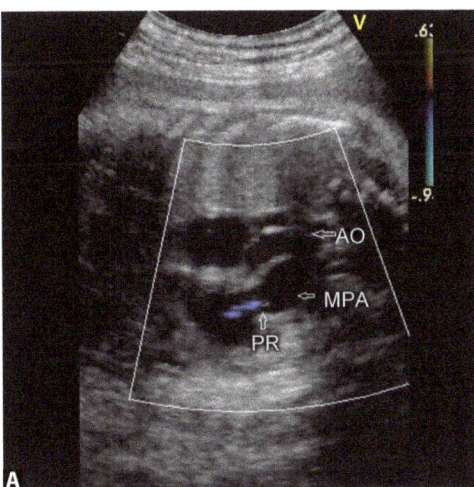 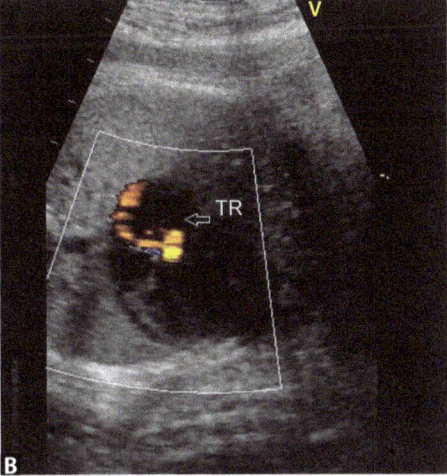

Figs 8.18A and B: (A) Pulmonary regurgitation with dilated main pulmonary artery in premature ductal closure; (B) The same fetus with significant tricuspid regurgitation, Note the right heart dilatation which is more than acceptable

Doppler on fetal echocardiography helps diagnosing ductal restriction or closure in pregnancy and assessing right heart failure. Criteria for ductal constriction include right and left ventricular enlargement, tricuspid valve regurgitation, reduced right ventricular ejection fraction, pulsatility index in the ductus of less than 1.9, peak systolic velocity of more than 1.4 m/sec, peak diastolic velocity of more than 0.3 m/sec and hourglass appearance of ductus on 2D (there is increase in both, the systolic and the diastolic velocity). Early delivery if feasible needs to be considered in selected cases as fall in pulmonary vascular resistance postnatally would unload the right ventricle. Intrauterine increase in the pulmonary pressures may cause hypertrophy of the media and cause pulmonary hypertension postnatally. After delivery, there can be right ventricular dysfunction, tricuspid regurgitation which can cause reduced pulmonary blood flow and atrial septal defect shunting R-L causing cyanosis and hypoxia. Management after delivery would include supplemental oxygen and occasional ventilation with vasodilators.

Premature Foramen Ovale Closure

Isolated premature foramen ovale closure can happen due to various reasons at any gestational age, the exact mechanism of which is debatable. It has been reported to be associated with transposition of great arteries, giant atrial septal aneurysm, aortic stenosis, mitral atresia, double outlet right ventricle, prenatal treatment with indomethacin and gene defects. Isolated foramen ovale closure may lead to sequence of event based on the amount of restriction and timing of the event. Reduced amount of flow to the left heart can cause hypoplasia of left-sided cardiac structures especially early in gestation. Excess amount of blood in the right ventricle can cause right-sided cardiac failure. Criteria for diagnosis of isolated foramen ovale closure include foramen ovale diameter of less than 2 mm with Doppler velocity of more than 120 cm/sec or foramen ovale diameter of less than 3 mm with doppler gradient of more than 5 mm Hg. There may be right heart dilatation, right heart failure, arrhythmias and hydrops. In presence of atrial septal aneurysm, this entity is difficult to diagnose. Isolated restriction of foramen ovale should be considered when there is unexplained disproportionate right ventricular dilatation. Once diagnosed, it is advisable to closely monitor for any signs of decompensation. Worsening of heart failure is an indication for early delivery if feasible. Maternal digoxin may offer some improvement. Postnatally, most of the babies improve, some may need ionotropic support. When in isolation, premature foramen ovale closure has a good prognosis.

ACKNOWLEDGMENT

I thank Dr Pradeep S for the contribution of some of the pictures in this Chapter.

KEY MESSAGES

- Fetal cardiac examination not only gives a clue to the etiology of heart failure but also helps diagnosing/prognosticating heart failure.
- Serial assessment is the key once cardiac failure is diagnosed.
- Prognosis depends on the etiology and the timing when diagnosis is made. The best predictor for adverse outcome is the venous Doppler of umbilical vein and ductus venosus.
- Timely intervention during pregnancy may be life-saving.

SUGGESTED READING

1. Allan LD, Cook AC, Huggon IC. Fetal echocardiography: a practical guide. Cambridge University Press:USA; 2009.pp.155-89.
2. Enzensberger C, Wienhard J, Weichert J, Kawecki A, Degenhardt J, Vogel M, et al. Idiopathic constriction of the fetal ductus arteriosus. Three cases and review of literature. J Ultrasound Med. 2012;31:1285-91.
3. Hofstaetter C, Hansmann M, Eik-Nes SH, Huhta JC, Luther SL. A cardiovascular profile score in the surveillance of fetal hydrops. J Matern Fetal Neonatal Med. 2006;19:407-13.
4. Huhta JC. Guidelines for the evaluation of heart failure in the fetus with or without hydrops. Ped Cardiol. 2004;25:274-86.
5. Li Yi-Dan, Li Zhi-An, He Yi-Hua. Premature closure or restriction of the foramen ovale. J Ultrasound Med. 2013;32:1291-4.
6. Ott WJ. Doppler echocardiographic assessment of fetal cardiac failure. 2005; Chapter 35 from the text book: Doppler Ultrasound in Obstetrics and Gynecology by Dev Maulik 2nd edition; Springer-Verlag GmbH and Co., Heidelberg: Pg. 517-33.

CHAPTER 9

Fetal Cardiac Interventions

Nageswara Rao Koneti, R Saileela

ABSTRACT

Fetal cardiac intervention has the potential to favorably alter the inutero course of some congenital heart defects, thus improving the natural history of those defects. Advancement in imaging modalities along with improvement in intervention techniques and inventory has resulted in major breakthrough in the field of fetal cardiac interventions in the last two decades. The complications of the procedure are usually manageable; however, the long-term results depend on variable factors like timing of intervention, fetal hemodynamics and requirement of postnatal procedure. This Chapter discusses the indications, procedural techniques and outcomes of inutero cardiac interventions.

INTRODUCTION

Fetal cardiac intervention has become an important therapy to prevent in utero progression of a simple lesion to a complex cardiac condition. Cardiac problems with risk of fetal demise (e.g. fetal tachyarrhythmia) and those causing impairment of organ development leading to significant postnatal mortality and morbidity (e.g. critical aortic stenosis) potentially benefit from in utero management.

Potential fetal cardiac therapy includes various modalities like (i) transplacental therapy (e.g. antiarrhythmic drugs to mother in tachyarrhythmia, maternal steroids in fetal heart block), (ii) fetal surgeries (e.g. tricuspid valve repair in severe Ebstein's anomaly, pulmonary arterioplasty in absent pulmonary valve) and (iii) fetal cardiac interventions (e.g. fetal balloon aortic valvotomy). This Chapter would restrict to the last category of the fetal cardiac interventions.

The first report of transplacental therapy dates back to 1975 when maternal propranolol was used for fetal tachycardia. The first percutaneous fetal intervention was an attempted in utero pacing in 1986. And most importantly, fetal balloon aortic valvotomy performed by Allan, Sharland and Tynan in 1989 in a fetus with critical aortic stenosis marked the beginning of a new era of in utero cardiac interventions. However, significant progress in this field occurred only in the last decade with advances in imaging modalities and refinement of the procedural technique. At present, nearly 25 centers across the world are enrolled in the fetal cardiac registry (IFCIR).

Established fetal cardiac interventions include:
- In utero management of fetal tachycardia/bradycardia.
- Fetal balloon aortic valvotomy for critical aortic stenosis (AS) with evolving hypoplastic left heart syndrome (HLHS).
- Atrial septal stenting in case of HLHS with intact atrial septum/restrictive foramen ovale.
- Balloon pulmonary valvotomy for pulmonary atresia with intact ventricular septum.

PROGRESSION OF CARDIAC LESIONS IN UTERO

Some primary cardiac defects may progress and evolve into more complex lesions with advancement of gestation. Lesions like critical AS and pulmonary stenosis progress to hypoplastic left and right heart syndromes respectively. Intervening at an appropriate stage can modify the evolution of disease and improve the postnatal outcome.

Critical Aortic Stenosis

The natural history of in utero critical AS is variable. Development of critical AS early in gestation may result in rapid progression to hypoplastic left ventricle (LV) with endocardial fibroelastosis. Critical AS in mid-gestation may result in dilatation of the left ventricle with subsequent progression to LV dysfunction. The elevated left atrial and left ventricular filling pressures result in reversal of flow across foramen ovale. This leads to redistribution of blood from the left atrium to right-sided chambers. Reduced blood flow across the mitral valve and left ventricle has a detrimental effect on left ventricular growth resulting in ventricular hypoplasia and endocardial fibroelastosis.

Fetal balloon aortic valvotomy at an appropriate stage would improve left ventricular filling and help to achieve biventricular circulation in postnatal life. The echocardiographic features suggesting potential progression to HLHS include narrow aortic jet >2 m/sec, dilated dysfunctional LV, neo-development of mitral regurgitation, monophasic mitral inflow Doppler, left to right shunt across the foramen ovale and reversal of flow in the aortic arch. Nevertheless, it is of utmost importance to identify the cases, which have a potential to achieve biventricular circulation following in utero relief of aortic stenosis. McElhinney et al. published a scoring system to predict biventricular circulation followed by fetal balloon aortic valvotomy (Table 9.1). Postnatal outcomes are not encouraging for those fetuses with a threshold score <4.

Hypoplastic Left Heart Syndrome with Intact Atrial Septum

Foramen ovale is essential to decompress the left atrium in HLHS and its variants. Restriction of foramen ovale or intact atrial septum may cause fetal pulmonary hypertension resulting in delayed regression

Table 9.1: Predictors of biventricular circulation

LV long axis Z-score	>0
LV short axis Z-score	>0
Aortic annulus Z-score	>−3.5
MV annulus Z-score	>−2
MR or AS maximum gradient	≥20 mm Hg

One point for each; threshold score >4 has 100% sensitivity and 53% specificity in predicting biventricular outcome.

or non-regression of pulmonary vascular resistance in the postnatal life. The interatrial septum and pulmonary venules become thickened and muscular (arterialization of pulmonary veins). The outcome of Norwood procedure in this subset is poor in view of pre-existing pulmonary venous hypertension. The neonatal mortality is reported to be as high as 48% in this subset despite early intervention and surgery.

Echocardiographic features of in utero pulmonary venous hypertension include restrictive foramen ovale flow or intact atrial septum and dilated pulmonary veins with prominent atrial reversal on pulmonary venous Doppler. In utero atrial stenting of interatrial septum to relieve left atrial hypertension in these fetuses may potentially prevent adverse pulmonary venous remodeling, thus improving the postnatal outcome.

Pulmonary Atresia with Intact Ventricular Septum

Hypoplastic right heart syndrome has relatively better prognosis compared to HLHS. In this condition, the pulmonary valve is atretic leading to redistribution of blood flow through foramen ovale to the left side. The resultant reduction of flow across the tricuspid valve leads to progressive hypoplasia of the right ventricle. Fetal pulmonary valve perforation/balloon pulmonary valvotomy in this subset helps to promote growth of right ventricle by improving the flow into the stiff hypertrophied ventricle, thus facilitating either biventricular circulation or at least 1.5 ventricular repair postnatally. Moreover, decompression of right ventricle reduces severity of tricuspid regurgitation thus preventing hydrops. Fetuses with membranous pulmonary atresia with tricuspid valve Z-score <-2 are ideal candidates for the procedure. Tricuspid to mitral valve ratio <0.7, right ventricle/left ventricle length ratio <0.6 and tricuspid inflow duration <31.5% of cardiac cycle length and presence of RV sinusoids are poor prognosticating features. Presence of three of the above four features predict non-biventricular outcome with a sensitivity of 100% and specificity of 75%.

DEVELOPMENT OF FETAL CARDIAC INTERVENTIONAL PROGRAM

Initiation and development of the fetal cardiac interventional program requires several prerequisites. Firstly, trained personnel to plan and perform the procedure are vital. Development of a multidisciplinary team is essential for a successful long-term program. Financial expenses appear to be a key factor, as the procedure is not covered by health insurance in some of the countries. Social and local governmental policies also play a role. Prenatal diagnosis and therapeutics act (PNDT) clearance may be needed in countries like India.

PROCEDURE

Case Selection

Postnatal outcome mainly depends on appropriate case selection. Planning the procedure at an appropriate gestational age is vital to allow ventricular growth antenatally. However, early procedure prior to 22 weeks is technically challenging in view of difficulties in imaging. A balance between the gestational age and the procedure time is crucial for a better outcome. The threshold scoring criteria for selection of patients for balloon valvotomy have already been discussed.

Counseling

Several social and cultural issues play a vital role in counseling. A balance between the maternal risk, fetal risk and procedural success should be drawn. The family has to be informed about the natural in utero progression of the lesion, possibility of procedural failure, the minimal risk of intrauterine death/premature labor and the need for postnatal procedures. The procedure-related maternal risk appears to be low and most centers now prefer to perform the procedure under intravenous sedation.

Team

Organizing the fetal interventional team is the crux of the program. The fetal cardiologist, fetal medicine specialist, obstetrician, anesthesiologist and perinatologist play a major role. Role of each individual person should be predefined. Prior discussion about the procedure, potential complications and physiology of the condition may give an insight to all the team members.

Hardware and Technical Aspects

The essentials apart from the team members are imaging equipment and catheterization material for the procedure.

Needle for Intramuscular Injection

Fetal anesthetic agents (Vecuronium, fentanyl) and antiarrhythmic drugs (e.g. digoxin in tachyarrhythmia) can be given as intramuscular injections to the fetal thigh. 21G or 22G spinal needle/aspiration needles are generally used for the intramuscular injection.

Needle for the Procedure

19G or 18G (12-15 cm long) Chiba needle, M3 coaxial or Hawkins Akins needle may be used for entry into ventricle for balloon valvotomy. 20G or 22G aspiration needle is used for fetal pericardiocentesis.

Guidewire

0.014" coronary guidewire (BMW, Whisper extra support or Galeo extra support wires) may be used based on the availability and individual preference.

Balloon for Valvotomy

Maverick, Hiryu and Relysis coronary balloons are ideal as they can be advanced through the 18G needle.

Procedure

Favorable fetal position is indispensable for a successful procedure. Anterior position of fetal heart with posterior spine is ideal for the procedure. The utero-ventriculo-outflow tract should be in line to coaxial the needle-balloon catheter assembly. Once the position is acceptable, fetal anesthesia (vecuronium and fentanyl) can be given using 21G spinal needle. Maternal general anesthesia may be initiated at the time of favorable fetal position. Most of the centers have now adopted maternal intravenous sedation without intubation anesthesia.

Good imaging is one of the key factors for the success of the procedure. Under ultrasound guidance, 18G long needle (12-15 cm) is used for the puncture of maternal abdomen, uterus and fetal chest wall to enter the ventricle. The fetal chest wall and ventricular entry may be difficult at times if baby is not immobile. An external counter support using hand may help to advance the needle without much effort. Site of ventricular entry should be in line with the outflow tract.

Fetal Balloon Aortic Valvotomy

The guidewire balloon assembly is prepared and premeasured (marked on the shaft of the balloon catheter) to give external guidance about the balloon position. Apical left ventricular puncture generally aligns well to left ventricular outflow tract. The dilated left ventricle usually gets collapsed after puncture. There may be transient bradycardia that generally improves on its own. After aligning the needle to the left ventricular outflow tract, the prepared guidewire balloon assembly is advanced through the needle. A gentle manipulation is needed to cross the aortic valve under ultrasound imaging. A balloon annulus size ratio of 1.0–1.2 usually gives adequate result. Semi-compliant balloons may be used to minimize the trauma to aortic valve. Immediate success may be defined by the demonstration of balloon inflation across the valve, appearance of aortic regurgitation and achievement of good antegrade flow across the aortic valve (Figs 9.1 and 9.2). The balloon catheter-wire assembly should be removed along with the needle to avoid balloon avulsion within the fetal heart. Inspection of the balloon integrity after removal is mandatory.

Fetal Pulmonary Valve Perforation and Balloon Dilatation

The puncture site should be at apico-infundibular free wall of the right ventricle, so that the needle will align to right ventricular outflow tract to perforate the

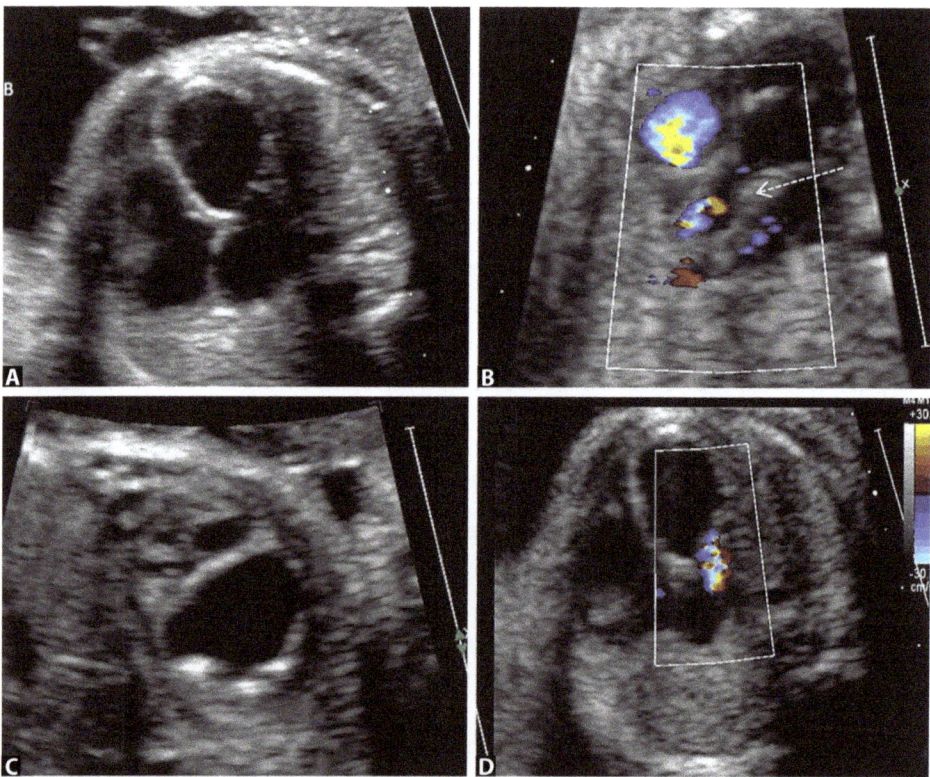

Figs 9.1A to D: Fetal echocardiographic images showing critical aortic stenosis with evidence of evolving hypoplastic left heart syndrome. (A) Four-chamber view showing dilated and dysfunctional left ventricle; (B) Color Doppler image showing left ventricular outflow tract and narrow jet of flow across the aortic valve (arrow); (C) Short axis view showing hyperechogenic endocardium suggestive of endocardial fibroelastosis of left ventricle; (D) Color Doppler showing mitral regurgitation

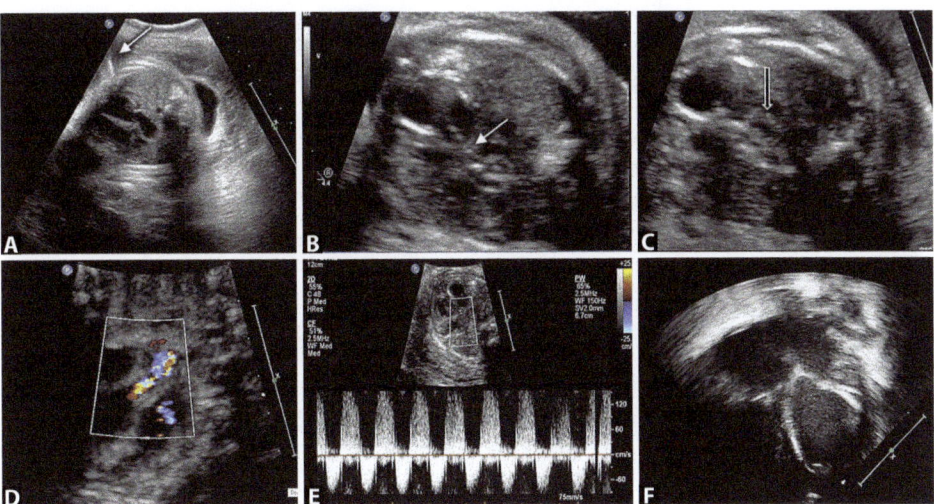

Figs 9.2A to F: Echocardiographic images during fetal aortic valvotomy. (A) Fetal echocardiographic image showing needle (arrow) entry into fetal chest wall; (B) Image showing needle aligned to left ventricular outflow tract and wire (arrow) across the aortic valve; (C) Image showing balloon inflation (open arrow) across the aortic valve; (D) Improved antegrade flow across the aortic valve following balloon valvotomy; (E) Pulsed wave Doppler showing development of aortic regurgitation following valvotomy; (F) Postnatal echocardiographic image of the child showing normal sized left ventricle (biventricular circulation)

atretic pulmonary valve. The needle should be positioned more anteriorly to conform to the anatomy of right ventricular outflow tract. The 18G needle can be directly advanced through the pulmonary valve for perforation. Alternately, a 22G Chiba needle can be advanced through the larger needle for valve perforation. The wire may be parked either in the pulmonary artery or in the descending aorta. The balloon-annulus ratio can be more (1.2 to 1.3) compared to aortic valve dilatation. Shorter balloon lengths of 8 mm or 10 mm may be used to prevent accidental dilatation of RV free wall.

Stenting of Foramen Ovale

The right atrium is punctured perpendicular to interatrial septum with a 18G/17G needle. The needle can directly be advanced to perforate the septum or a 22G Chiba needle may be advanced through it for perforation. The wire is placed in left atrium or advanced into the pulmonary vein. Short length stents of 3.5 × 13 mm can be easily passed through 17G needle and positioned across the septum under ultrasonic guidance. The stent should be kept in the center and dilated to maximum limits. The potential complications include stent malposition and embolization. There is only limited experience in this subset of cases in the world literature.

Fetal Tachyarrhythmia

Direct fetal therapy is adopted in hydropic fetuses with tachycardia which are resistant to transplacental therapy. There are reports of intraumbilical, intra-amniotic, intra-peritoneal, intramuscular and intracardiac administration of antiarrhythmic drugs in the literature. Intramuscular injections are most commonly adopted and is considered safe for the fetus.

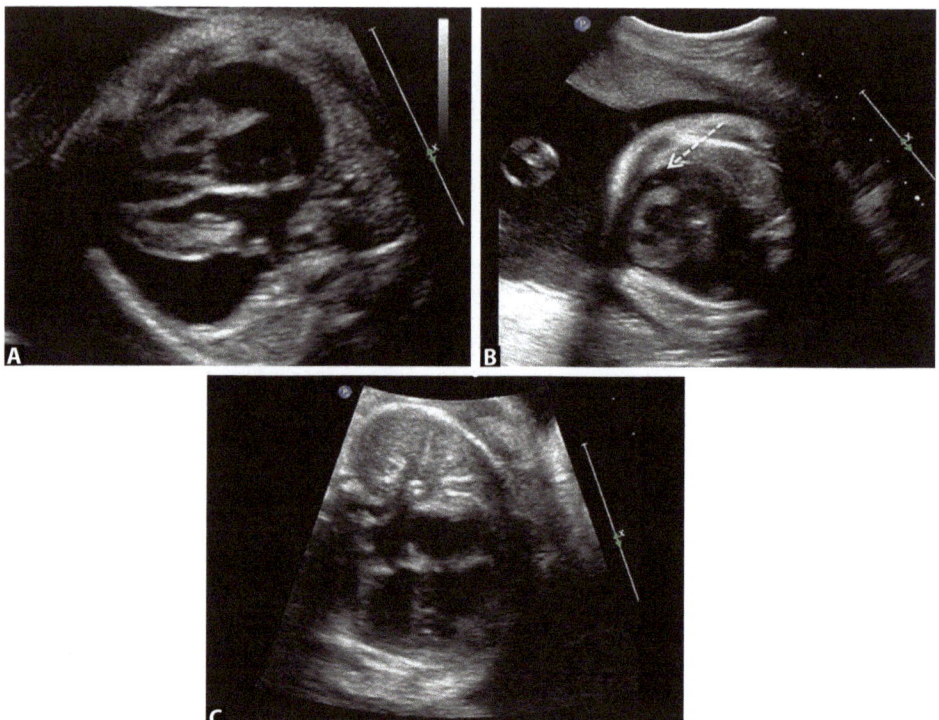

Figs 9.3A to C: Fetal pericardiocentesis. (A) Massive pericardial effusion in a fetus at 29 weeks gestation; (B) Image showing a 22G needle (arrow) in the pericardial space for aspiration; (C) Complete resolution of pericardial effusion following the procedure

Fetal Heart Block

Transplacental therapy with maternal steroids and sympathomimetic drugs are routinely used in fetal immune-mediated complete heart block. Presence of gross hydrops and fetal heart rate less than 55/min carries high risk of fetal demise. There are few reports of in utero pacing in such fetuses, with technical success but unfavorable outcome.

Fetal Pericardiocentesis

Pericardial effusion in a fetus can be isolated or associated with hydrops. Isolated pericardial effusion can be due to maternal lupus erythematosis, congenital infections, pericardial tumors, ventricular diverticuli, congenital hypothyroidism and idiopathic arterial calcification. Massive pericardial effusion can result in tamponade and impaired filling of ventricles. Moreover, it impairs the growth of lungs in utero and hence poses a grim postnatal prognosis. Pericardiocentesis can be performed using a 21G/22G aspiration needle (Fig. 9.3).

COMPLICATIONS OF FETAL CARDIAC INTERVENTIONS

- Pericardial effusion: Pericardial effusion is very common following fetal cardiac intervention. It is usually self-limiting and does not need any specific management and rarely may need aspiration.

- Persistent bradycardia: Fetal bradycardia is inevitable during entry into the ventricle. Usually, it is transient and needs no treatment. If it persists, it can be managed by intracardiac injection of atropine (20 µg/kg) and adrenaline (10 µg/kg) through the same needle.
- Placental hemorrhage
- Fetal loss/premature delivery: Fetal loss and premature delivery is reported in up to 11% of procedures. The incidence appears to be less in recent times with improvement of skills and technique.
- Valve regurgitation: Aortic valve regurgitation is reported in up to 40% of balloon aortic valvotomies. However, it is well tolerated in view of low systemic vascular resistance in the fetus (placenta) and high LV end diastolic pressure. It usually resolves in a few weeks.
- Avulsion of balloon and injury to other organs
- No maternal mortality or morbidity is reported so far.

Outcome and Prognosis

The outcome and prognosis depends on the severity of the cardiac lesion and timing of intervention. The technical success and long-term outcome has improved over the last decade with refinement of technique and patient selection.

Follow-up data of first 100 cases of fetal aortic valvuloplasty showed technical success in 77%; among them, 45% achieved biventricular circulation postnatally. The outcome depends on the severity of the disease at the time of intervention. Larger LV size and higher LV pressure at the time of intervention is more likely to be associated with biventricular outcome. Fetal intervention is never a standalone procedure, even when biventricular circulation is achieved. They usually need postnatal balloon valvuloplasty. Some of them require additional surgical procedures like Coarctation repair, Ross procedure, resection of endocardial fibroelastosis, aortic and mitral valve replacements during follow-up. However, the survival and morbidity is definitely superior to HLHS.

In their series of 10 cases of in utero pulmonary valvuloplasty, Tworetzky, et al. reported technical success in 6 cases; of which 4 could achieve biventricular circulation. Fetal tricuspid valve Z score below −3 were associated with univentricular outcome.

SUMMARY

Advancement in imaging and instrumentation has resulted in improved rates of technical success in fetal cardiac interventions. Proper patient selection and optimum timing of intervention can translate technical success into favorable postnatal outcome. Evidence is still evolving in this field and there is much to be learned. Evaluation of long-term outcome from various centers would help us to favorably alter the prenatal technique and perinatal management of this subset of patients.

SUGGESTED READING

1. Allan LD, Sharland G, Tynan MJ. The natural history of the hypoplasticleft heart syndrome. Int J Cardiol. 1989;25:341-3.
2. Assad RS, Zielinsky P, Kalil R, Lima G, Aramayo A, Santos A, et al. New lead for in utero pacing for fetal congenital heart block. J Thorac Cardiovasc Surg. 2003;126(1):300-2.
3. Carpenter R, Strasburger JF, Garson A, Smith RT, Deter RL, Englehardt H. Fetal ventricular pacing for hydrops secondary to complete atrioventricularblock. J Am Coll Cardiol. 1986;8:1434-6.
4. Eibschitz I, Abinader EG, Klein A, Sharf M. Intrauterine diagnosis andcontrol of fetal ventricular arrhythmia during labor. Am J Obstet Gynecol. 1975;122:597-600.
5. Freud LR, McElhinney DB, Marshall AC, Marx GR, Friedman KG, del Nido PJ, et al. Fetal

aortic valvuloplasty for evolving hypoplastic left heart syndrome: Postnatal outcomes of the first 100 patients. Circulation. 2014;130(8): 638-45.
6. Hallak M, Neerhof MG, Perry R, Nazir M, Huhta JC. Fetal supraventricular tachycardia and hydrops fetalis: combined intensive, direct, and transplacental therapy. Obstet Gynecol. 1991;78:523-5.
7. Hansmann M, Gembruch U, Bald R, Manz M, Redel DA. Fetal tachyarrhythmias: transplacental and direct treatment of the fetus. A report of 60 cases. Ultrasound Obstet Gynecol. 1991;1:162-70.
8. Kalish BT, Tworetzky W, Benson CB, Wilkins-Haug L, Mizrahi-Arnaud A, McElhinney DB, et al. Technical challenges of atrial septal stent placement in fetuses with hypoplastic left heart syndrome and intact atrial septum. Catheter Cardiovasc Interv. 2014;84(1): 77-85.
9. Marshall AC, van der Velde ME, Tworetzky W, Gomez CA, Wilkins-Haug L, Benson CB, et al. Creation of an atrial septal defect in utero for fetuses with hypoplastic left heart syndrome and intact or highly restrictive atrial septum. Circulation. 2004;110:253-8.
10. Maxwell D, Allan L, Tynan MJ. Balloon dilatation of the aortic valve in the fetus: a report of two cases. Br Heart J. 1991;65(5): 256-8.
11. McElhinney DB, Marshall AC, Wilkins-Haug LE, Brown DW, Benson CB, Silva V. Predictors of technical success and postnatal biventricular outcome after in utero aortic valvuloplasty for aortic stenosis with evolving hypoplastic left heart syndrome. Circulation. 2009;120(15):1482-90.
12. Parilla BV, Strasburger JF, Socol ML. Fetal supraventricular tachycardia complicated by hydrops fetalis: A role for direct fetal intramuscular therapy. Am J Perinatol. 1996;13:483-6.
13. Roman KS, Fouron JC, Nii M, Smallhorn JF, Chaturvedi R, Jaeggi ET. Determinants of outcome in fetal pulmonary valve stenosis or atresia with intact ventricular septum. Am J Cardiol. 2007;99:699-703.
14. Tworetzky W, McElhinney DB, Marx GR, Benson CB, Brusseau R, Morash D, et al. In utero valvuloplasty for pulmonary valve atresia with hypoplastic right ventricle: Techniques and outcomes. Pediatrics. 2009; 124(3):e510-e8.
15. Vlahos AP, Lock JE, McElhinney DB, Van der Velde ME. Hypoplastic left heart syndrome with intact or highly restrictive atrial septum: outcome afterneonatal transcatheter atrial septostomy. Circulation. 2004;109:2326-30.
16. Walkinshaw SA, Welch CR, McCormack J, Walsh K. In utero pacing for fetal congenital heart block. Fetal Diagn Ther. 1994;9(3):183-5.

CHAPTER 10

Genetics and Congenital Heart Disease

Pradeep S, SJ Patil, Meenakshi Bhat

Approach: To Evaluate for Extracardiac Malformations and Chromosome Anomalies After Diagnosis of Fetal Congenital Heart Disease

Pradeep S

ABSTRACT

- The scope of the chapter is to introduce to the reader about the association of findings in fetuses with cardiac anomalies.
- Cardiac anomalies can occur in isolation or in association with other anomalies. The associated anomalies may be chromosomal abnormalities or physical abnormalities or physical abnormalities constituting a genetic syndrome.
- When associated with chromosomal abnormalities the cardiac anomaly may be isolated or may be associated with other physical abnormalities.
- Among various genetic syndromes commonest few are described in this Chapter.
- Extracardiac abnormalities in association with cardiac anomalies can involve gastrointestinal system, genitourinary system, respiratory system, musculoskeletal system, craniofacial and central nervous system.
- Among various chromosomal abnormalities, Trisomy 21, Trisomy 18, Trisomy 13, Trisomy 22, 22Q deletion, Turner's 45 × and triploidy are common associations in fetuses with cardiac anomalies and are described in the text.
- When cardiac anomalies are encountered, attempt should be made to evaluate the entire fetus to detect all other associated abnormalities in extracardiac systems. Invasive testing by chorion villous sampling, amniocentesis or cordocentesis has to be done to exclude associated aneuploidy (Tables 10.1 and 10.2). Noninvasive prenatal cell free DNA analysis may be selectively used in certain appropriate circumstances for aneuploidy and single gene disorder detections.
- History of known genetic disorders in family or siblings can help in exclusion of the same in the fetus.
- Prognosis and counseling can be complete with knowledge of presence of associated extracardiac anomalies and chromosomal/genetic abnormalities.

INTRODUCTION

Cardiac anomalies are frequently encountered during antenatal sonography. Advanced equipment, high frequency transducers, transvaginal ultrasound, fetal echosonography settings, volume cardiac acquisition, sectional planes and post-processing better training and experienced hands have made detection of cardiac anomalies a reality in the first trimester from 14 weeks onwards.

With such capabilities and early diagnosis of cardiac anomalies, it is very important to complete the analysis by determining the presence or absence of extracardiac associated anomalies. This can be achieved by performing a detailed targeted imaging for fetal anomalies (TIFFA) in a systematic manner, system wise with documentation of a minimum of 40 pictures and a minimum of 15 measurements called as the extended biometry. Extended biometry includes the following measurements—biparietal diameter, head circumference, occipitofrontal diameter, interorbital distance, binocular diameter, nasal bone length, ear length, cerebral lateral ventricle, transcerebellar diameter, cisterna magna, intracranial lucency, facial angle, prenasal thickness, nuchal lucency, nuchal fold thickness, thoracic circumference, kidney bipolar lengths, femur length, tibia length, foot length, humerus length, radius length. From the above measurements, cephalic index, FL/foot ratio, BPD/FL ratio, AC/FL ratio, etc. can be calculated.

In the first trimester, aneuploidy markers are increased nuchal lucency thickness, nasal bone absence, increased prenasal thickness, abnormal intracranial lucency, tricuspid regurgitation, ductus venosus with 'a' wave reversal and abnormal facial angle. In the 2nd trimester, sonographic markers of fetal aneuploidy (SMFA) are thickened nuchal fold, absent nasal bone, ventriculomegaly, aberrant right subclavian artery, echogenic bowel, pyelectasia, echogenic intracardiac focus, short humerus, short femur. Each of the above SMFA has a numerical likelihood ratio (LR).

Every fetus based on maternal age has an a prior risk or background risk for aneuploidy. This risk gets altered into low-risk or high-risk based on the presence or absence of 1st and 2nd trimester markers of aneuploidy.

Maternal biochemical analysis in 1st trimester—double marker test (Beta-hCG and pregnancy-related plasma protein A) and in 2nd trimester—triple marker test (Alpha fetoprotein, estradiol, beta hCG) and quadruple marker test (Beta-hCG, estradiol, Alpha fetoprotein and inhibin) will alter the above risk of aneuploidy and then arrive at a combined risk which is the best method of determining the risk for aneuploidy.

Cardiac anomaly detection qualifies as major abnormality and will increase the risk of aneuploidy irrespective of presence or absence of other abnormalities and hence will indicate requirement of karyotype analysis by invasive or noninvasive methods. Thus, detection of extracardiac anomalies and associated genetic/chromosomal abnormalities in a case of cardiac anomaly helps in counseling regarding severity of the situation and further course of action.

The following text will help the reader to understand the spectrum of disorders that may be associated with cardiac anomalies.

CARDIAC ANOMALIES AND GENETIC SYNDROMES

Cardiac anomalies can be isolated or can be associated with aneuploidy and when associated with aneuploidy they can be part of a genetic syndrome. If a cardiac anomaly is detected, then a detailed targeted imaging of the fetus is advised to look for any other anomalies. The list of genetic syndromes

associated with cardiac anomalies is exhaustive and hence, it is not important to know about all the genetic and chromosomal syndromes, but it is important to understand certain principles to be followed when a cardiac anomaly is identified:
- History taking is very important.
  - Detailed medical history of both parents and family for any autosomal dominant or recessive conditions.
  - History of consanguinity.
  - Sibling history of cardiac anomaly or genetic disorder.
  - History of teratogenic or anticonvulsant medications.
- Targeted imaging for fetal anomalies (TIFFA) scan increases the detection rate of anomalies.
- Maternal biochemistry helps in risk analysis and increases detection rate of aneuploidy.
- Chorionic villus sampling (CVS), amniocentesis, cordocentesis with FISH for 22q11 deletion, karyotype will be helpful in identifying aneuploidies.

The common genetic syndromes are:
- Holt-Oram syndrome
- Short rib polydactyly syndrome
- Ellis-van Creveld syndrome
- VACTERL syndrome
- Thrombocytopenia-absent radius syndrome (TAR)
- Cornelia de Lange syndrome
- Campomelic dysplasia
- Smith-Lemli-Opitz syndrome
- Noonan's syndrome
- Heterotaxy syndromes
- Anticonvulsant syndrome
- Goldenhar syndrome/hemifacial syndrome
- CHARGE syndrome
- Tuberous sclerosis
- Marfan's syndrome
- Alagille syndrome
- Williams syndrome.

Holt-Oram Syndrome

This condition is inherited as autosomal dominant fashion with high penetrance and variable expression.

Some cases are caused by mutations on the TB × 5 gene on 12q2 chromosome. ASD occurs in 90% cases. Hence, it is also called Atriodigital dysplasia. Conduction disorders, VSD, aortic coarctation, truncus arteriosus, PDA, mitral valve defects can occur.

Skeletal anomalies include thumb aplasia, hypoplasia, triphalangeal thumb, radial dysplasia, hypoplasia, radial fusion, phocomelia, clavicle, humerus and ulnar hypoplasia.

Short Rib Polydactyly Syndrome

These are a group of autosomal recessive lethal skeletal dysplasia distinguished by the presence of thoracic hypoplasia, short ribs, short limbs, post-axial polydactyly, gastrointestinal anomalies and other internal organ anomalies.

The potentially surviving conditions are:
- Thoracic asphyxiating syndrome (Jeune's syndrome).
- Ellis-van Creveld syndrome (chondroectodermal dysplasia).

A wide variety of cardiac malformations may occur including atrioventricular septal defect (AVSD), persistent left superior vena cava (LSVC), situs inversus, transposition of great arteries (TGA), aortic coarctation, hypoplastic ventricle and ventricular septal defect (VSD). Recurrence risk is about 25%.

Ellis-van Creveld Syndrome (Chondroectodermal Dysplasia)

This condition is inherited as an autosomal recessive fashion and is characterized by short limbs, short ribs, post-axial polydactyly, cardiac-renal anomalies, dysplastic nails and teeth. Characteristic tetrad include chondrodysplasia, ectodermal dysplasia, post-axial polydactyly, congenital cardiac anomalies. It is caused by mutation on 4p16. Cardiac anomalies include atrial septal defect (ASD), ventricular septal defect (VSD), common atrium, AVSD and situs inversus.

VACTERL Syndrome

These are a group of disorders arising due to defect in mesodermal development in the primitive streak. It is a mitochondrial disorder with a recurrence rate of 1 to 50%. It is inherited as an autosomal recessive and X-linked disorder. Conditions with a spectrum of disorders like, vertebral anomalies (Fig. 10.1), anal atresia, cardiac anomalies, tracheoesophageal fistula, esophageal atresia, radial dysplasia, renal and limb anomalies have been grouped under the name VACTERL. Cardiac anomalies are a frequent occurrence.

Thrombocytopenia Absent Radius (TAR) Syndrome

It is an autosomal dominant condition with variable penetration. This is characterized by the absence of both radius and preservation of both thumbs and thrombocytopenia. In 50% of case, there can be absent ulna or humerus. In 40% of cases, there may be lower limb anomalies. In 23% of cases, there may be renal anomalies. Cardiac anomalies are seen in 20–33% cases and can be tetralogy of Fallot (TOF), ASD (>50%), VSD, AVSD (atrio-ventricular septal defect) and PDA in 15% cases.

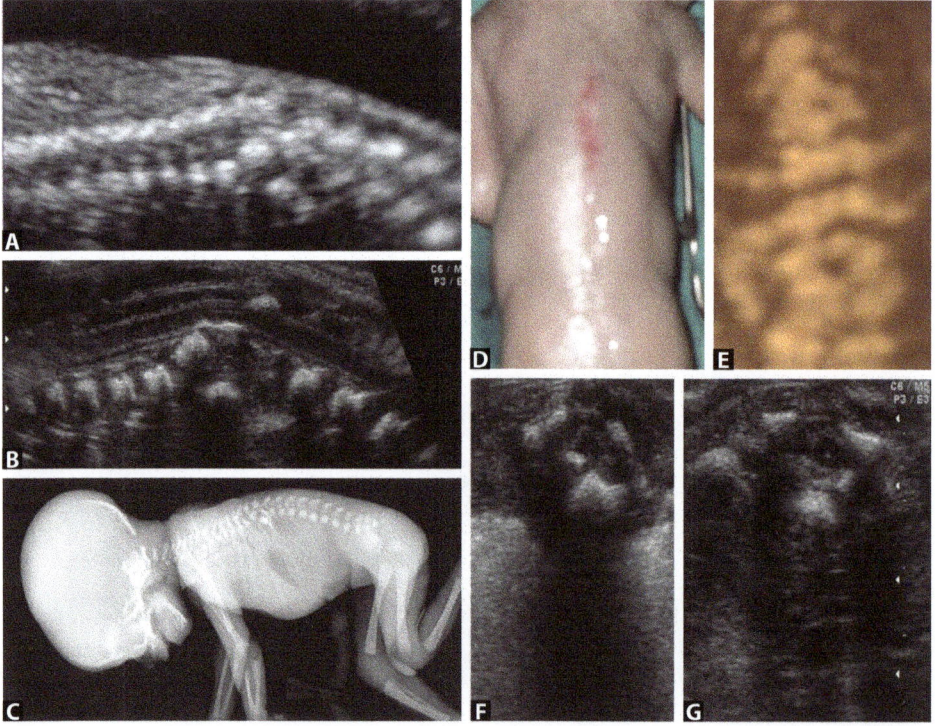

Figs 10.1A to F: Fetus with hemi vertebrae. (A) Fetal ultrasound showing spinal hemi vertebrae; (B) Abortus ultrasound showing hemi vertebrae; (C) Abortus X-ray showing hemi vertebrae; (D) Abortus photo of the spine; (E) 3D ultrasound of spine; (F and G) Axial ultrasound of abortus showing the same

Cordocentesis may detect thrombocytopenia. Intrauterine platelet transfer prior to delivery can be helpful. Chromosomal analysis may show 22q11 deletion.

Cornelia De Lange Syndrome

Inherited as an autosomal dominant or X-linked disorder. There is a 50% chance of passing the disorder to the offspring. This condition is characterized by limb abnormalities, IUGR, hearing loss, microcephaly, hirsutism, synophrys, thick eyelashes, low frontal hairline, anteverted nostrils, long philtrum, thin lips, retrognathia and low ears. It is an autosomal dominant condition and 99% of cases are sporadic. Upper limb anomalies include oligodactyly, thumb and first metacarpal hypoplasia, clinodactyly of 5th finger, aplasia of ulna and elbow fusion. Other features include diaphragmatic hernia, nuchal webbing, duodenal atresia, renal dysplasia, cleft palate and genital anomalies. Cardiac anomalies include VSD, ASD, pulmonary stenosis, TOF, mitral atresia, coarctation of aorta, AVSD and single ventricle. Clues to the condition are oligodactyly, late onset IUGR and microcephaly and low PAPPA.

Campomelic Dysplasia

Also called as Campomelic dwarfism. This condition is seen frequently and is caused by a severe defect in cartilage development causing bowing of femur and tibia, talipes, hypoplastic scapulae, 11 pairs of ribs, micrognathia and a small chest. One-third have cardiac malformations including VSD, ASD and TOF. Hypospadiasis and bifid scrotum can occur. Neonatal death occurs due to pulmonary hypoplasia. Heterozygous mutation of 50 × 9 located on 17q24 is the cause.

Cardiac Anomalies and Nuchal Edema/Hydrops

Accumulation of subcutaneous fluid may range from increase in nuchal translucency to nuchal fold to cystic hygroma to hydrops. Hydrops is characterized by accumulation of fluid in causing ascites, pleural or pericardial effusion. Cardiac conditions associated with nonimmune hydrops include tachyarrhythmias, congenital heart block, cardiomyopathy, myocarditis (Coxsackie virus and cytomegalovirus).

Associated genetic syndromes are:

Smith-Lemli-Opitz Syndrome

This condition is an autosomal recessive condition caused by a mutation in 7-dehydrocholesterol reduction gene on 11q13. This causes elevated levels of 7-dehydrocholesterol, which causes teratogenic effects. Polydactyly, 3 toe syndactyly, thickened NT, cataract, renal anomalies, ambiguous male genetalia and holoprosencephaly can occur. Cardiac anomalies include AVSD, ASD, TOF, PDA, aortic coarctation, hypoplastic left heart syndrome (HLHS), pulmonary stenosis, tricuspid atresia. CVS can be used to detect 7-dehydrocholesterol reductase activity. Material urine testing can also detect the condition.

Noonan's Syndrome

This is an autosomal dominant condition caused by mutation in PTPN11. It is characterized by short stature, facial dysmorphism, webbed neck and cardiac anomalies. Cardiac anomalies include left ventricular hypertrophy, dysplastic pulmonary valve, pulmonary stenosis and

ASD. Hydrops, short femur and cardiac anomaly should alert the condition.

Heterotaxy and Isomerism

These are conditions associated with characteristic cardiac and abdomino-respiratory anomalies. Also referred to as isomerism of the atrial appendages. It is defined as an abnormal arrangement of thoracic and abdominal organs from the normal situs solitus arrangement caused by a disruption of the left right arrangement during embryonic development. Cardiac anomalies are a major component. There can be paired right atria resulting in right atrial isomerism or paired left atria resulting in left atrial isomerism.

Right Atrial Isomerism

This condition has paired right-sided viscera, bilateral trilobed lungs, tracheal atresia and enlarged obstructed echogenic lungs, esophageal atresia (Figs 10.2 and 10.3) midline liver, absent spleen, dextrocardia, DORV (Fig. 10.4), total anomalous pulmonary venous connection (TAPVC), AVSD, TGA, pulmonary

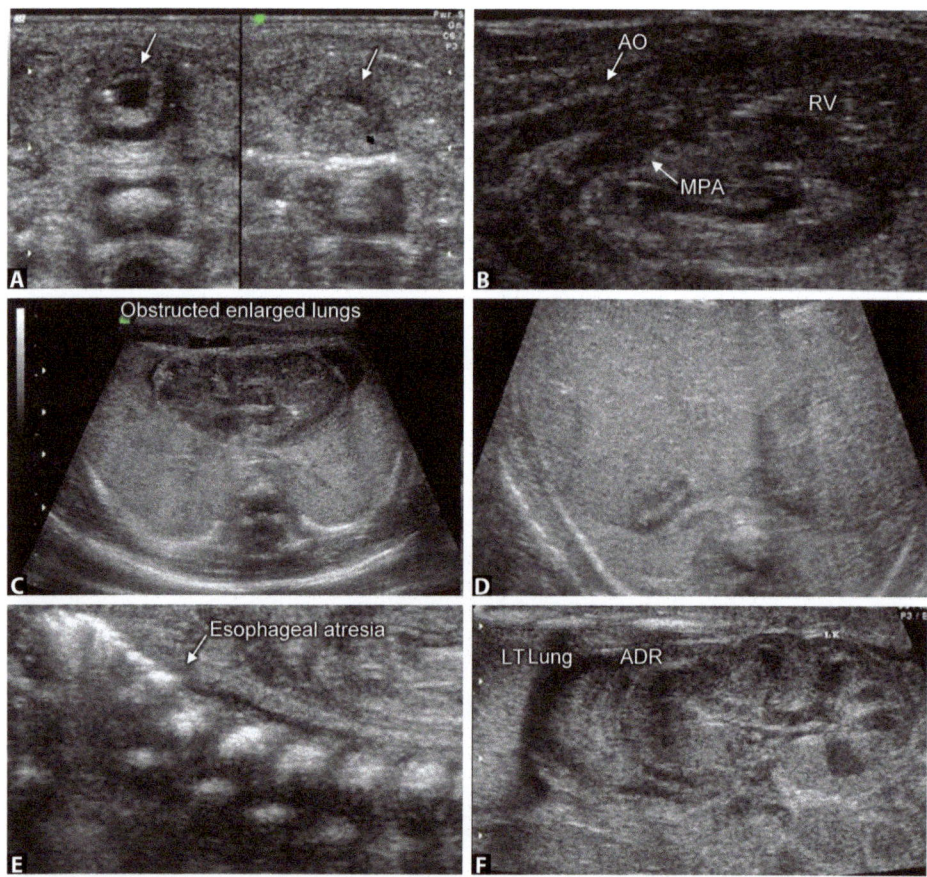

Figs 10.2A to F: Ultrasound of abortus with right atrial isomerism; (A) Tracheal stenosis; (B) DORV showing anterior aorta and posterior pulmonary artery arising from RV; (C) Echogenic enlarged lungs; (D) Central liver and absent spleen; (E) Esophageal atresia with blind ending air column; (F) Absent spleen in left sub-diaphragmatic area

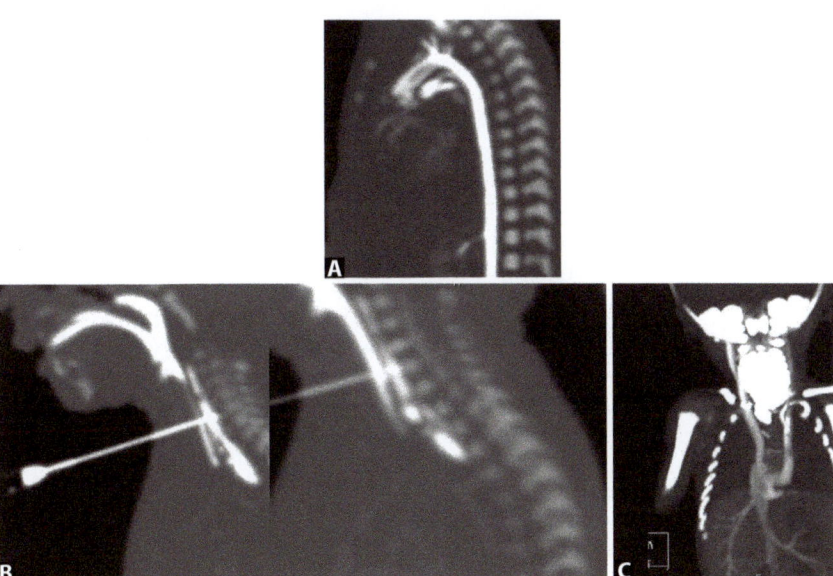

Figs 10.3A and B: Contrast injected into right ventricle of abortus shows both aorta and pulmonary artery filling from RV. *Note-* Transposed anterior aorta and posterior pulmonary artery; (B) CT tracheogram and esophagogram of abortus-contrast injected into trachea and esophagus show blind ends—Atresia; (C) Contrast injected into right atrium shows two SVC and one IVC

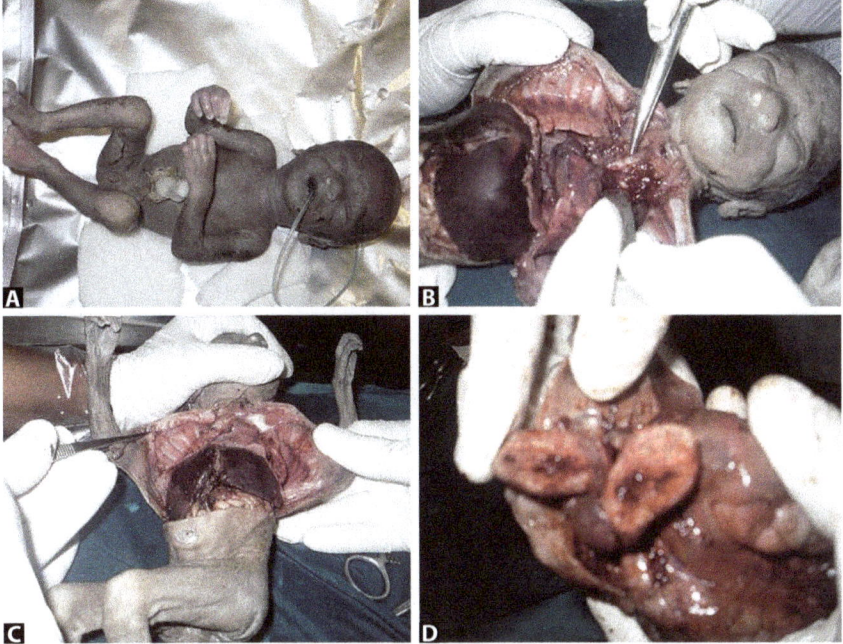

Figs 10.4A and B: Dissection of abortus with right atrial isomerism. (A) Abortus; (B) Esophageal atresia; (C) Central liver and absent spleen; (D) DORV with transposed great vessels

atresia. Asplenia is associated with serious cardiac anomalies (IVEMARK syndrome). CNS and renal anomalies can occur.

Left Atrial Isomerism

This condition has bilateral bilobed lungs, malpositioned stomach, polysplenia.

AVSD, IVC interruption with azygos continuation and bilateral SVC are common. About 5-10% sibling risk is implied in nonconsanguinity (Fig. 10.5).

Cardiac anomalies in heterotaxy syndromes include dextrocardia, single atrium/ASD, single ventricle/VSD, TGA, common AV valve, total or partial anomalous pulmonary return, endocardial cushion defect, aortic coarctation, pulmonary atresia, DORV.

Teratogens

Women taking anticonvulsants have a 2-7 fold increase in risk for malformations.

Neural tube defects (Fig. 10.6), genital, cardiac and musculoskeletal anomalies may occur. VSD, ASD, pulmonary stenosis and aortic stenosis may occur.

Goldenhar Syndrome/Hemifacial Microsomia

This condition is also called facio-auriculovertebral syndrome. It involves anomalies of the 1st and 2nd branchial arches. Asymmetric facial deformities include ear deformities, (preauricular tags, ear dystopia), epibulbar dermoids, upper eyelid colobomas, facial clefting and hemifacial microsomia. Vertebral, thoracic, renal anomalies may occur. Cardiac anomalies include TOF and VSD. Unilateral microphthalmia (Fig. 10.7), orbital hypoplasia and cleft lip must alert the condition.

CHARGE Syndrome

This condition encompasses coloboma of iris or retina, heart defects, atresia of choanae, retardation of mental and somatic development, genital anomalies, ear abnormalities and deafness. Cardiac anomalies include conotruncal malformation, TOF, AVSD, PDA, outflow anomaly, arch anomalies and VSD.

Tuberous Sclerosis

This condition has a prevalence is 1:6,000. It is inherited as autosomal dominant fashion. Many cases are sporadic. Changes occur in TSCI and TSC2 gene of 9q34 and 16p. Features include depigmented macules, facial angiofibromas, ungual fibromas, cranial subependymal nodules, renal angiomyolipomas, renal cysts, cardiac rhabdomyomas. Cardiac rhabdomyomas grow till 32 weeks and stabilize with excellent resolution postnatally. Fetal MRI may be helpful to detect subependymal nodules (Fig. 10.8).

Marfan's Syndrome

This condition comprises of connective tissue disorders and cardiac malformations.

It is an autosomal dominant multisystem disorder. Abnormalities are expressed in musculoskeletal system, ocular system and cardiovascular system predominantly.

The gene for fibrillin undergoes mutation. Cardiovascular abnormalities include aortic root dilatation and mitral valve prolapse. This condition is seldom diagnosed antenatally.

Alagille Syndrome

This condition is an autosomal dominant disorder with intrahepatic cholestasis, facial abnormalities (prominent forehead, deep set eyes, long nose) ocular posterior embryotoxon and hemivertebrae. Cardiac anomalies include TOF, peripheral pulmonary artery stenosis. Mutation or deletion of Jagged 1 gene is observed.

Genetics and Congenital Heart Disease

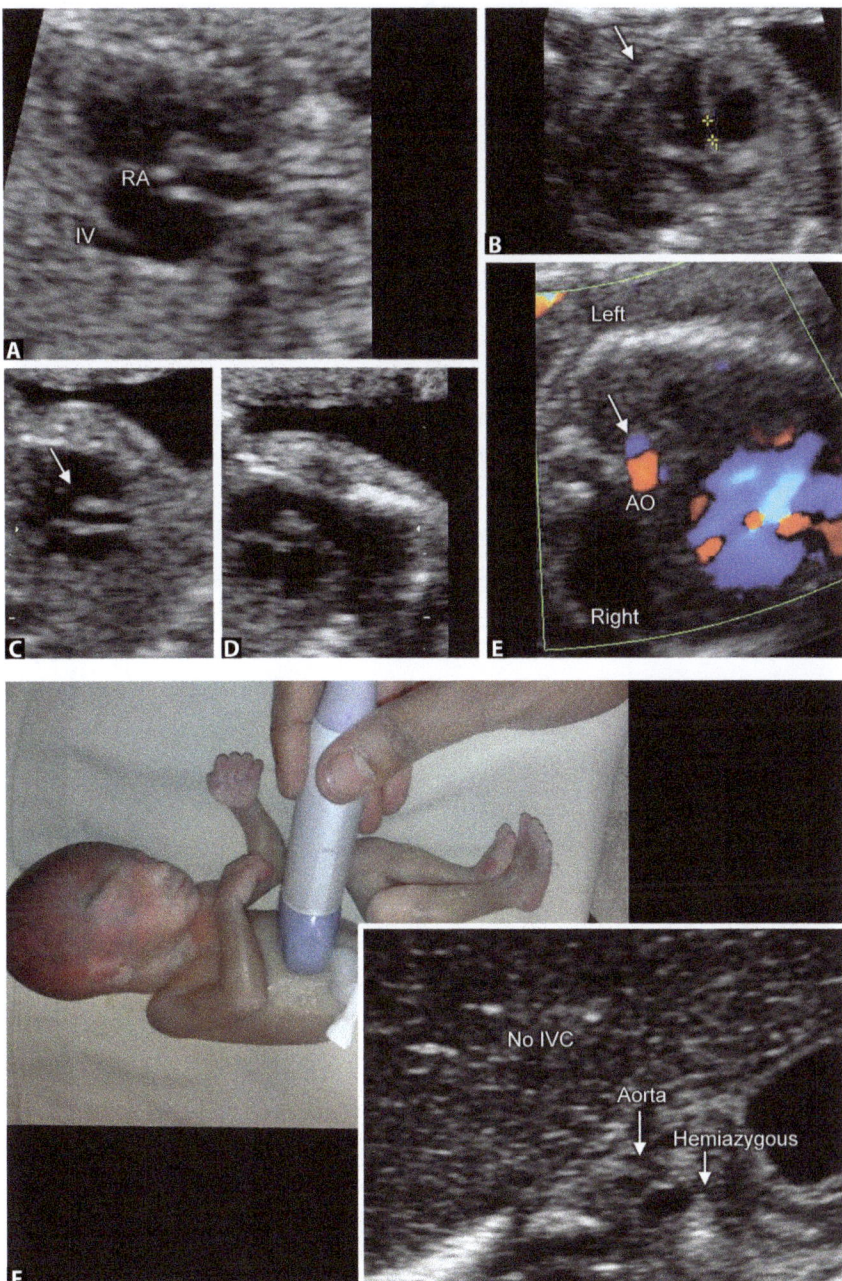

Figs 10.5A to F: Fetal echo of left atrial isomerism. (A) IVC interruption; (B) VSD with mesocardia; (C) VSD in long axis view with small size aorta; (D) RVOT view showing normal sized pulmonary artery; (E) Hemiazygos vein to the left of aorta and absent IVC; (F) Ultrasound of abortus of left atrial isomerism showing absent IVC and hemiazygos vein to the left of aorta

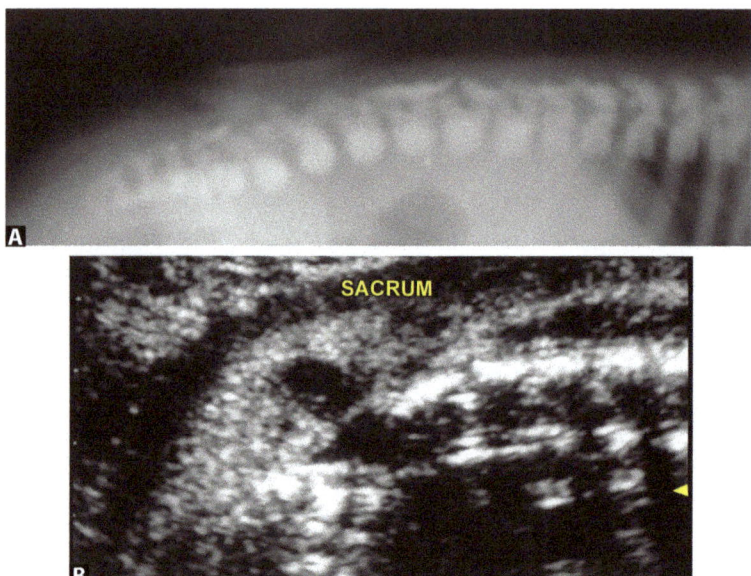

Figs 10.6A and B: Lateral spine X-ray of abortus showing spina bifida at L5 level; (B) Fetal ultrasound showing L5 spina bifida with small posterior meningocele

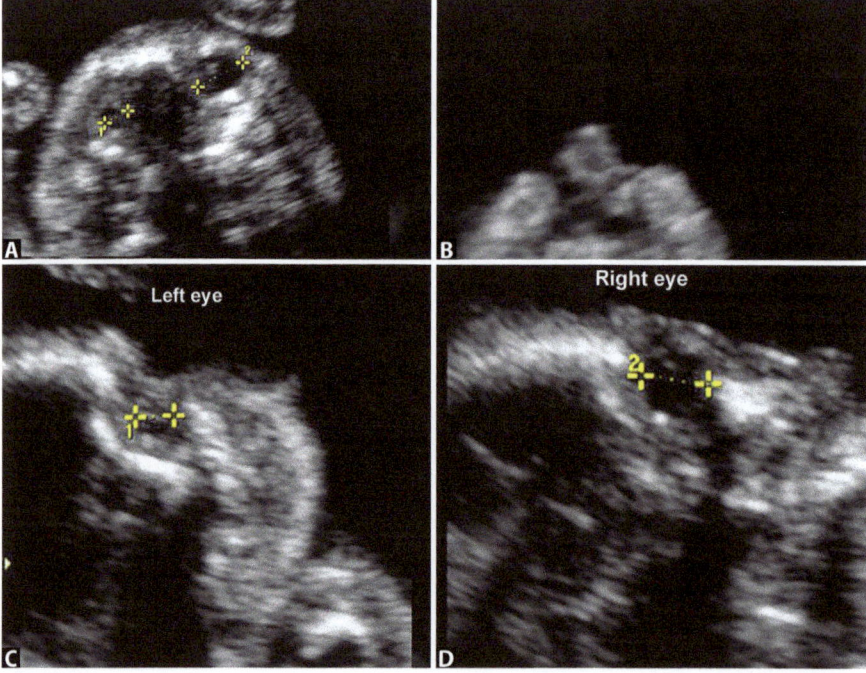

Figs 10.7A to D: (A, C and D) Sonography of left hemifacial microphthalmia. (A) Axial scan showing small sized left globe and normal right globe left microphthalmia; (C) Sagittal scan showing small left globe; (D) Sagittal scan showing normal sized right globe; (B) Axial scan of lips showing bilateral cleft lip

Genetics and Congenital Heart Disease

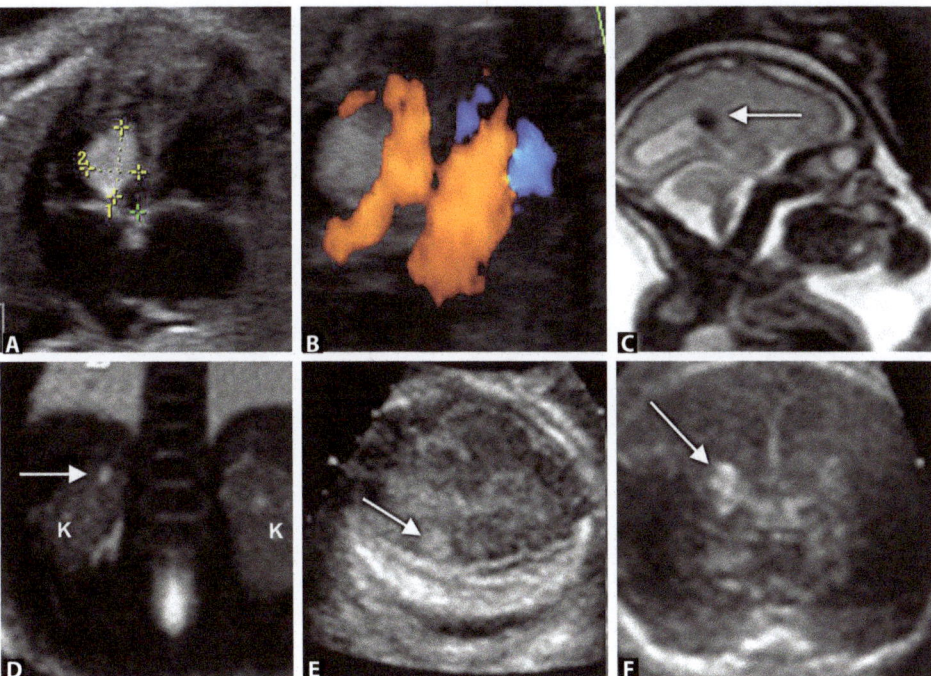

Figs 10.8A to F: Fetus with tuberous sclerosis. (A and B) 4-chamber view showing left ventricular echogenic well-defined solid mass—Rhabdomyoma; (C) Cerebral tuber in T2w MRI; (D) Renal cyst in fetal MRI; (E and F) Echogenic periventricular nodules—Cerebral tubers

Williams Syndrome

This condition is a contiguous gene deletion syndrome with 1–2 megabase deletion on long arm of chromosome 7. This results in defective elastin. Cardiac anomaly is characteristically supravalvular aortic stenosis. Other abnormalities include periorbital fullness, short anteverted nose and long philtrum.

EXTRACARDIAC ANOMALIES AND CHROMOSOMAL ABERRATION IN CARDIAC MALFORMATIONS

Congenital heart defects account for 1% of malformations. Cardiac malformations can be isolated. In approximately, 30% of cardiac malformations chromosomal aberrations occur. Incidence of cardiac malformation as per various studies is between 4 and 8 per 1,000 live births. In still births and fetal life, the incidence in about 10 times more and associated extracardiac malformations and chromosomal aberrations are also more.

Extracardiac abnormalities can involve central nervous system, kidneys, urinary tract and genital system, gastrointestinal system, respiratory system and skeletal system.

The incidence of abnormal karyotype association increases with the number of anomalies detected. There is a 50% chance of abnormal karyotype in fetuses with more than 3 anomalies and a 90% chance of abnormal karyotype is seen in fetuses with more than 8 anomalies.

Chromosomal aberrations can involve the following chromosomes commonly:

- Trisomy 21.
- Trisomy 18.
- Trisomy 13.
- x-45 x
- All chromosomes—triploidy (Fig. 10.9).
- Trisomy 22.
- 22q11 microdeletion.

Common cardiac abnormalities seen in chromosomally abnormal fetuses are:
- Atrioventricular septal defect
- Ventricular septal defect
- Tetralogy of Fallot
- Double outlet right ventricle (Figs 10.10 and 10.11)
- Coarctation of aorta
- Truncus arteriosus
- Aortic valve stenosis
- Hypoplastic left heart syndrome
- Atrial septal defect

Most common cardiac abnormalities in Trisomy 21 and 18 are atrioventricular septal defect and VSD. Less common cardiac abnormalities are hypoplastic left heart, double outlet right ventricle, coarctation of aorta, tetralogy of Fallot.

In aneuploid fetuses with cardiac anomalies, the incidence of extracardiac anomalies are higher than in euploid fetuses with cardiac anomalies.

Cardiac anomalies are seen in 30% of fetuses with omphalocele, 20% of fetuses with duodenal atresias, 30% fetuses with diaphragmatic hernias, 5% of fetuses with CNS malformation and 30% of fetuses with genitourinary tract anomalies. Every case of cardiac anomaly should have a chromosome analysis. If the karyotype is normal, mosaicism and microdeletions have to be ruled out. Conotruncal anomalies such as TOF, TGA, DORV, truncus arteriosus together with various types of VSD are associated strongly with microdeletion on chromosome 22. Other causes of cardiac anomalies are deletion in 7q11.23, 10p13 and 8p.

Extracardiac malformations are rare with pulmonary atresia with intact ventricular septum, Ebstein's anomaly and mitral stenosis. Splenic malformation are high with single ventricle. Conotruncal defects are associated with GIT and GUT abnormalities.

Well-known associations are:
- Trisomy 21 and endocardial cushion defects and ventricular septal defects.
- Splenic agenesis and conotruncal anomalies.
- Limb anomalies and septal defects (Holt-Oram).

Extracardiac malformation can be categorized in seven groups:
1. Central nervous system anomalies include:
   - Microcephaly
   - Hydrocephaly
   - Agenesis of corpus callosum
   - Meningomyclocele
   - Encephalocele
   - Olfactory nerve agenesis
   - Dandy-Walker malformation (Fig. 10.12)
   - Lissencephaly
   - Holoprosencephaly
2. Craniofacial anomalies include:
   - Microphthalmia
   - Anophthalmia
   - Optic nerve agenesis/hypoplasia
   - Coloboma
   - Corneal opacity
   - Low set ears
   - Malformed ears
   - Facial dysmorphism
   - Cleft lip (Fig. 10.7)/palate/high arched palate
   - Skin defects.
3. Respiratory anomalies include:
   - Congenital diaphragmatic hernia (Figs 10.13 and 10.14)
   - Lung hypoplasia/agenesis
   - Tracheoesophageal fistula
   - Thymic anomalies.

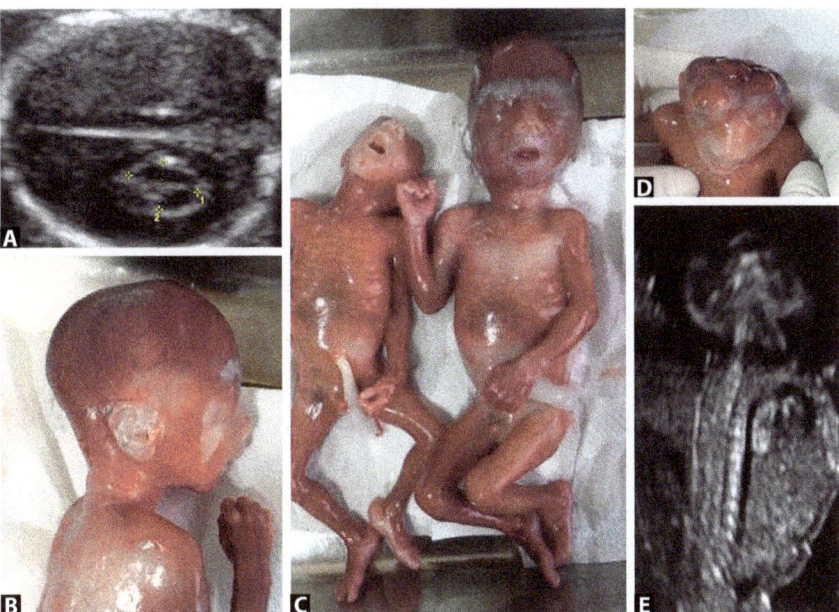

Figs 10.9A to E: (A) Choroid plexus cyst in triploidy fetus; (B) Triploioy abortus picture; (C) Twin with discordant growth; (D) Anencephaly abortus picture; (E) Anencephaly fetus ultrasound

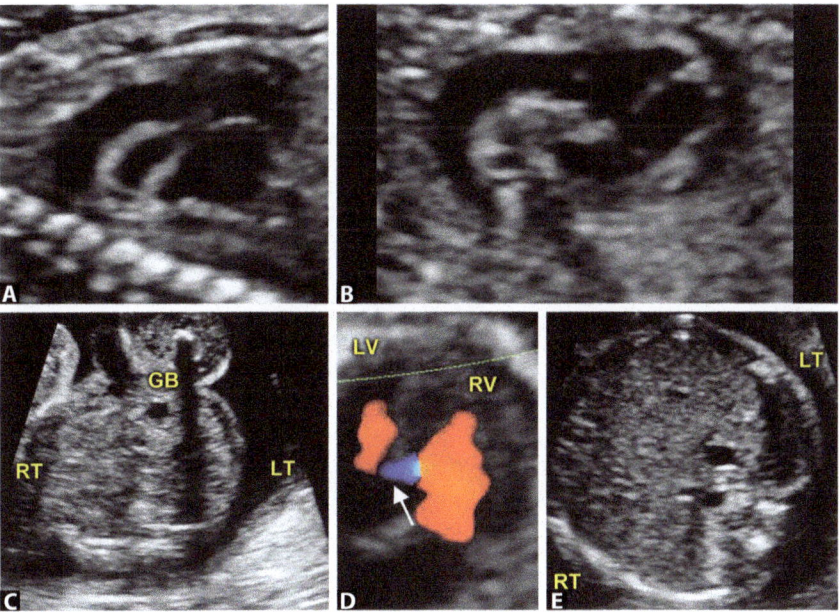

Figs 10.10 A to E: Fetus with double outlet right ventricle. (A) Fetal echo showing anterior aorta and posterior pulmonary artery arising from right ventricle; (B) Aorta rising from right ventricle; (C) Left sided gallbladder and liver—situs inversus; (D) Fetal echo showing membranous VSD; (E) Left sided liver and IVC

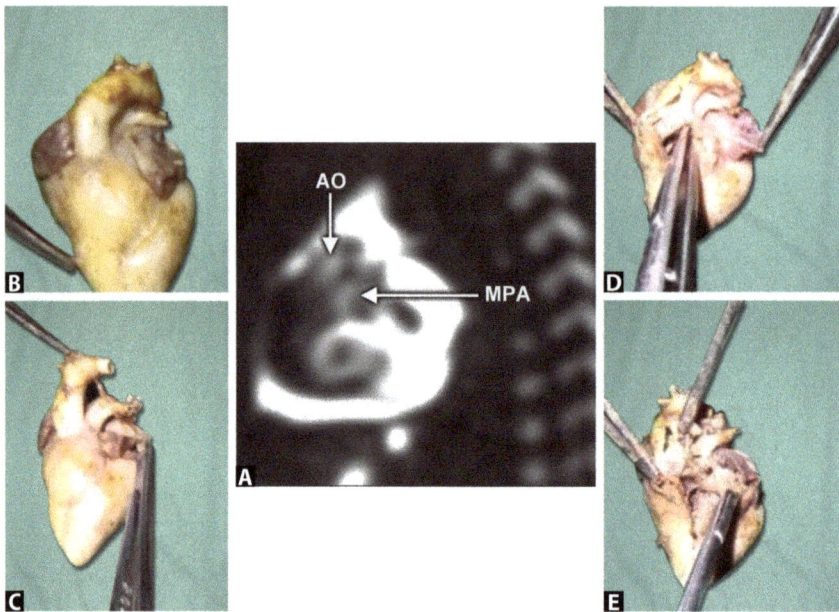

Figs 10.11A to E: Cardiac specimen of DORV with transposition: (A) Abortus CT angiogram showing anterior aorta and posterior pulmonary artery arising from right ventricle; (B to E) Cardiac dissection showing double outlet right ventricle and transposition

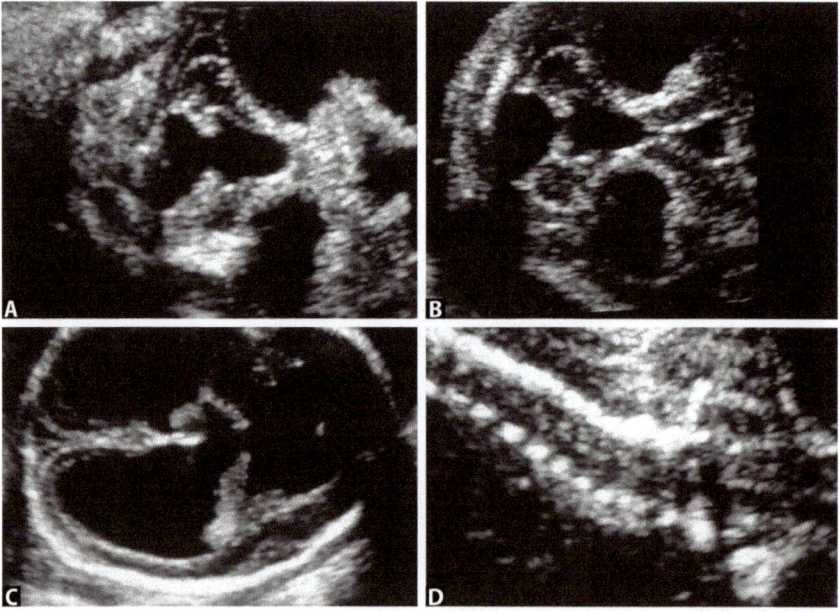

Figs 10.12A to D: Fetal neuro sonogram. (A and B) Vermian agenesis with 4th ventricle broadly communicating with cisterna magna; (C) Hydrocephalus; (D) Spine of the same fetus

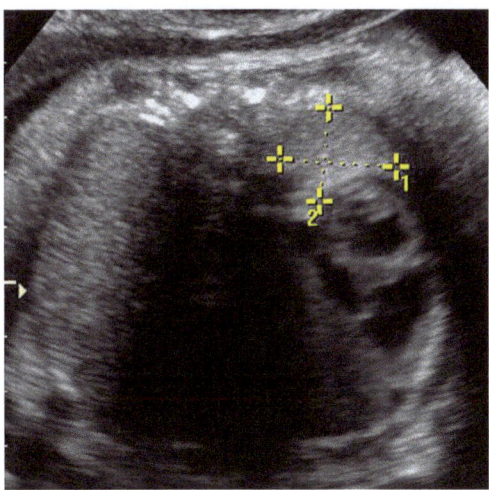

Fig. 10.13: Axial section of the chest showing cardiac displacement of intrathoracic right sided liver. Compressed left lung is marked by calipers

4. Gastrointestinal malformations include:
   - Meckel's diverticulum
   - Duodenal (Fig. 10.15)/jejunal atresia (Fig. 10.16)
   - Omphloocele (Fig. 10.17)
   - Malrotation
   - Duplication
   - Biliary atresia/choledochal cyst
   - Anal atresia
5. Splenic anomalies include:
   - Asplenia (right isomerism)
   - Polysplenia (left isomerism)
6. Genitourinary anomalies include:
   - Renal hypoplasia/agenesis
   - Renal cortical cysts
   - Dysplastic kidney
   - Uteropelvic junction stenosis/hydronephrosis

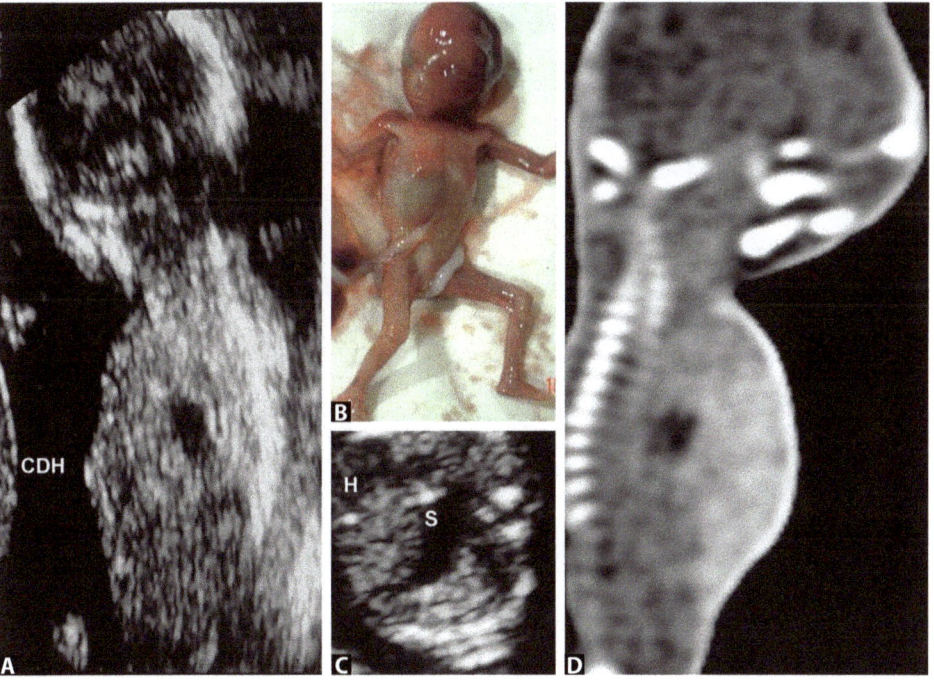

Figs 10.14A to D: Trisomy 18 fetus with left diaphragmatic hernia. (A) Sagittal USG CT of abortus showing intrathoracic stomach, congenital diaphragmatic hernia (CHD); (B) Photograph of abortus; (C) Atrial ultrasound of fetus showing intrathoracic stomach with cardiac displacement to the right, H (hernia), S (stomach); (D) CT of fetus showing intrathoracic stomach

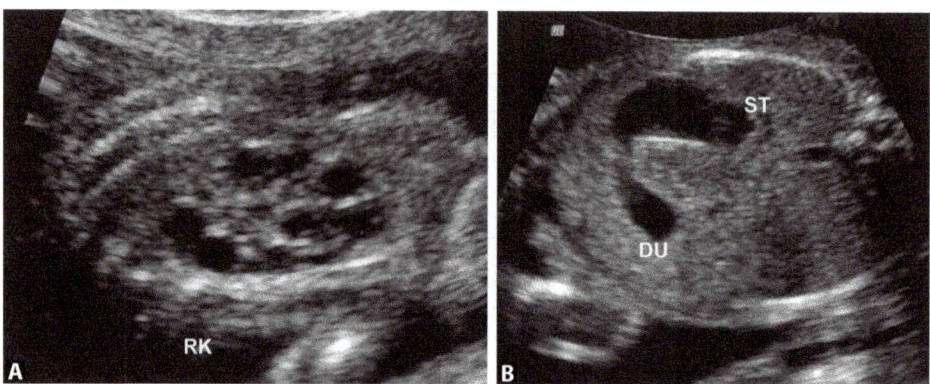

Figs 10.15A and B: Down's fetus showing renal and gastrointestinal tract anomaly. (A) Ultrasound showing cystic kidney; (B) Ultrasound showing double bubble sign—Duodenal atresia

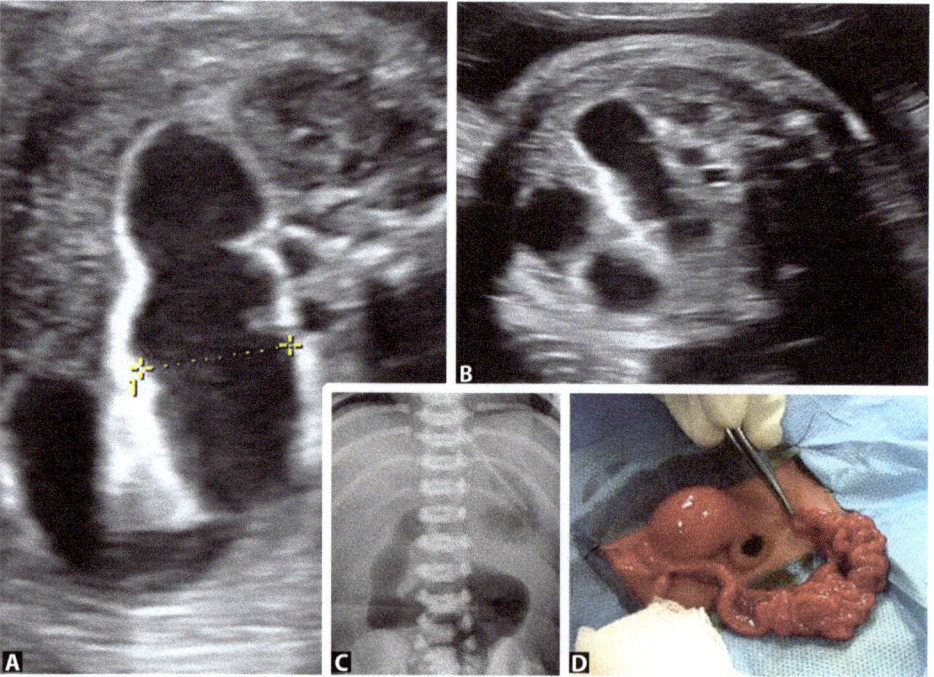

Figs 10.16A to D: Fetus with dilated proximal small bowel 3rd trimester: (A and B) Dilated jejunal loops in ultrasound; (C) X-ray of infant showing dilated jejunum; (D) Intraoperative picture of Jejunal atresia and micro colon

- Double ureters/collecting system
- Hypospadias
- Horseshoe kidney
- Genital agenesis/micropenis/uterus bicornis

7. Musculoskeletal anomalies include:
   - Anomalies of upper and lower limbs
   - Vertebral anomalies
   - Joint dislocation
   - Meningomyelocele

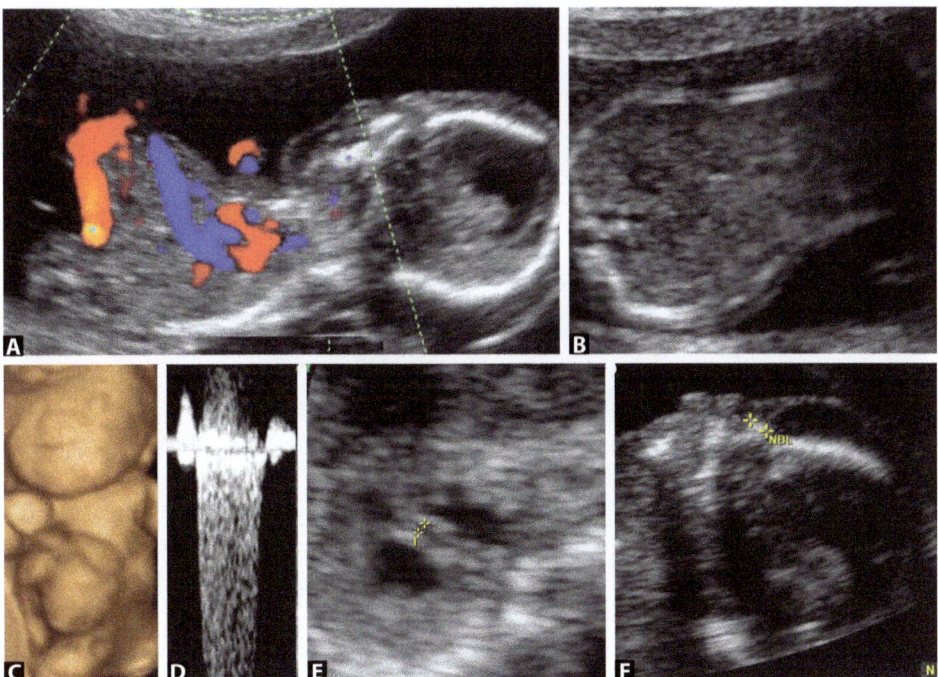

Figs 10.17A to F: Down fetus with omphalocele and aortic atresia: (A) Sagittal ultrasound showing omphalocele with liver; (B) Axial ultrasound showing the same; (C) 3D of fetus showing omphalocele; (D) Doppler showing tricuspid regurgitation; (E) Fetal Echo showing aortic atresia; (F) Facial profile showing flat face and hypoplastic nasal bone

Some common chromosomal abnormalities associated with cardiac anomalies and their phenotypic abnormalities are described below.

TRISOMY 13 (PATAU SYNDROME)

This condition is characterized by the presence of 3 copies of the 13th chromosome summing up to a total of 47 chromosomes. It is a numerical abnormality and an aneuploidy. Three types can occur.
1. Full trisomy 13
2. Mosaicism
3. Unbalanced Robertsonian translocation– 13/14.

CRL may be <5th percentile in 22% of T13 fetuses. FHR may be >95th percentile in 70% of the T13 fetuses the reason being that the heart attempts to increase cardiac output in left heart obstructions. Thickened NT is seen in >70% T13 fetuses. Absent NB seen in 32% of T13 fetuses. Common anomalies seen in 50% of T13 are omphalocele, holoprosencephaly, megacystis and SUA (single umbilical artery seen in 25% of T13).

Anomalies in T13 fetuses may involve the following systems:

Central Nervous System (58%)

- Holoprosencephaly (20-30%)
- Cerebellar hypoplasia
- Microcephaly
- Ventriculomegaly
- Choroid plexus cyst
- Neural tube defect.

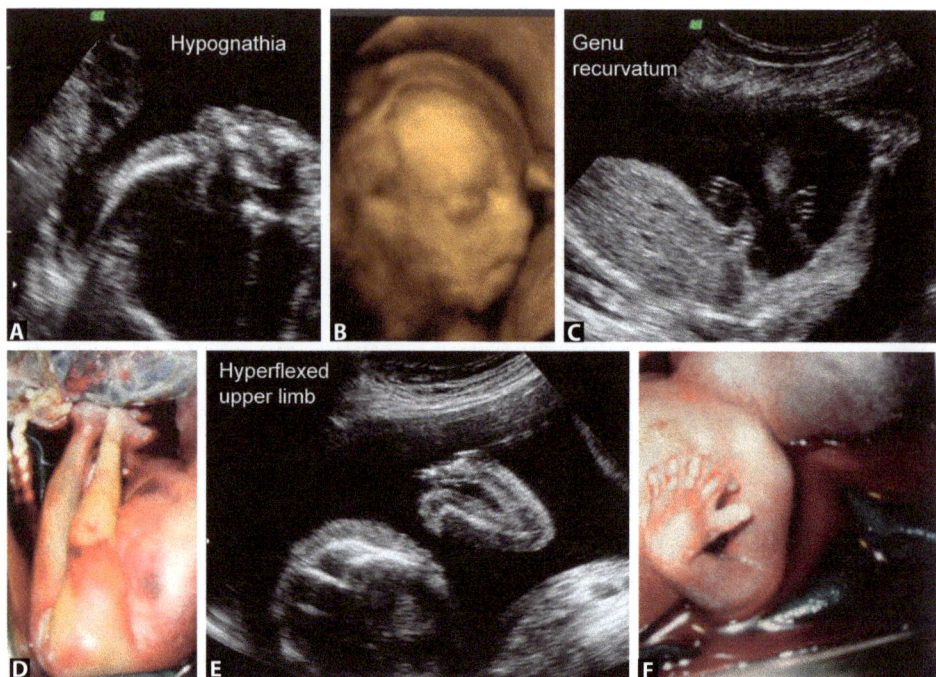

Figs 10.18A to F: Ultrasound of trisomy 18 fetal musculoskeletal and facial anomalies. (A) Sagittal facial view showing in drawn jaw; (B) 3D of the same finding; (C) Lower limb showing hyperextension at the knee genu recurvatum; (D) Abortus photo of the same; (E) Hyperflexed elbow and wrist; (F) Abortus photograph of the same

Face (48%)

Cleft lip/palate, hypotelorism, cyclopia, cystic hygroma, nuchal edema, hypognathia (Fig. 10.18).

Gastrointestinal System

Omphalocele, echogenic bowel, diaphragmatic hernia.

Genitourinary System

Enlarged echogenic kidneys and pyelocaliectasis.

Extremities

Polydactyly, clenched hands, short femur and humerus, clubbed foot.

Cardia

- ASD, VSD, HLHS, EIF, TOF, pulmonary atresia, DORV, aortic atresia (Figs 10.28 and 10.29)
- Hydrops
- SUA.

TRISOMY 18 (EDWARD'S SYNDROME)

This condition is seen in fetuses with 3 copies of 18th chromosome summing up to 47 chromosomes. It is a numerical abnormality and an aneuploidy.

The following systems may be involved. Cardia—84%, central nervous system—87%, upper limb—95%, lower limb—63%, Face—

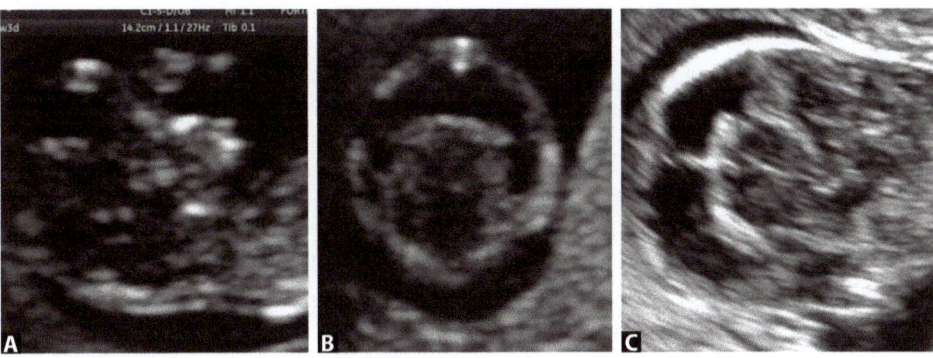

Figs 10.19A to C: Trisomy 18 fetus with holoprosencephaly. (A) Flat face, absent nasal bone, absent nose, cystic space in the anterior cranial area; (B) Univentricle; (C) Fused thalami

53%, choroid plexus cyst —50%, GIT—26%, GUT—16%, Short ear—10%.

Cardia

Atrioventricular canal defect, pulmonary stenosis, TGA, VSD, HLHS, coarctation.

Central Nervous System

Choroid plexus cysts, holoprosencephaly (Figs 10.19 to 10.22), Banana sign, cerebellar hypoplasia, Dandy-Walker syndrome (Fig. 10.12), dilated cavum septum pellucidum, enlarged cisterna magna, arachnoid cyst, dysplastic brain, absent cavum, strawberry head, lemon head.

Genitourinary Tract

Enlarged echogenic kidneys, small bladder, small kidneys, hypospadias.

Upper extremity, posterior urethral valve (Figs 10.23 and 10.24).

Clenched hands (Fig. 10.25), unilateral radial aplasia, absent thumb, overlapping digits, wrist contraction.

Lower Limbs

Rocker bottom feet, laterally deviated toes, club feet (Fig. 10.25).

Gastrointestinal Tract

Omphalocele (Fig. 10.17), diaphragmatic hernia (Fig. 10.14), absent stomach, anorectal atresia.

Face

Abnormal profile, cleft lip/palate, hypotelorism, micrognathia (Fig. 10.18).

Ear

Short ear may be seen.

TRISOMY 21

This condition is seen in fetuses with 3 copies of 21st chromosome (Figs 10.26 and 10.27) summing up to 47 chromosomes. It is a numerical abnormality and aneuploidy. The following anomalies can be seen in T21.

Cardiac Defects

Atrioventricular septal defect, (Fig. 10.30) ASD, VSD, tricuspid regurgitation, TOF, pulmonary atresia (Fig. 10.30).

Gastrointestinal Tract

Duodenal atresia (Fig. 10.15), esophageal atresia, jejunal atresia (Fig. 10.16) omphalocele (Fig. 10.31), echogenic bowel (Fig. 10.35).

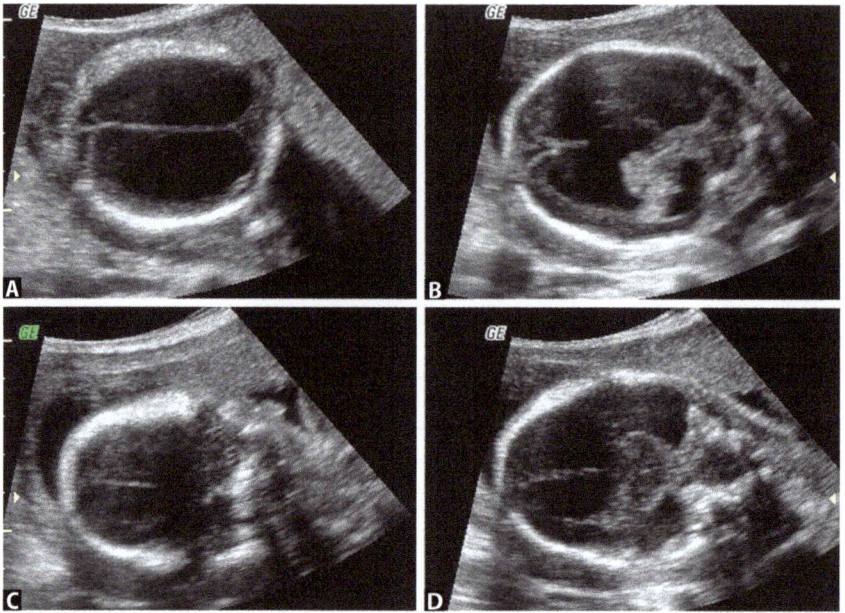

Figs 10.20A to D: Ultrasound of trisomy 18 fetal brain showing semilobar holoprosencephaly. (A) Dilated lateral ventricle; (B) Absent corpus callosum; (C and D) Fused thalami

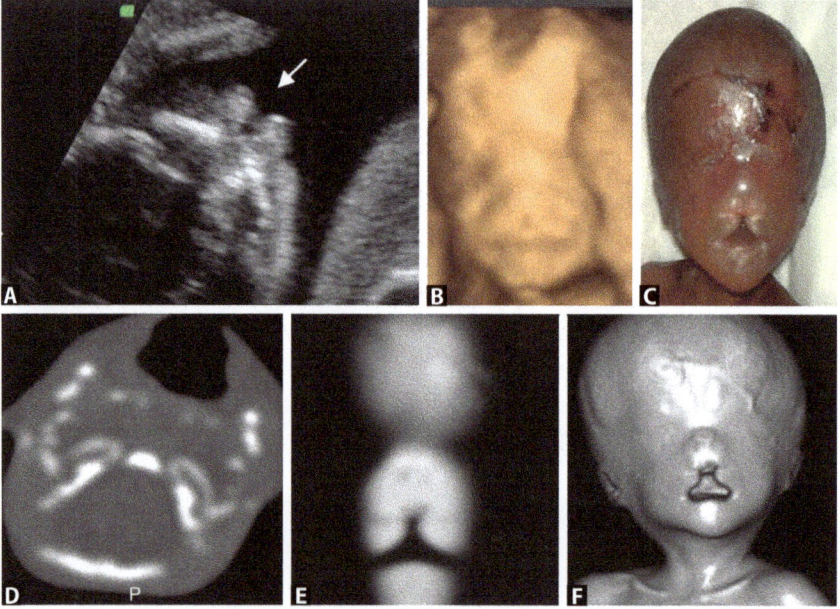

Figs 10.21A to F: Trisomy 18 fetal anomalies. (A) Ultrasound of fetus showing cleft lip; (B) 3D ultrasound of fetus showing cleft lip; (C) Abortus photo showing midline cleft lip and hypotelorism; (D) CT of abortus showing cleft lip; (E) Coronal CT of abortus showing medline cleft; (F) 3D CT showing the same

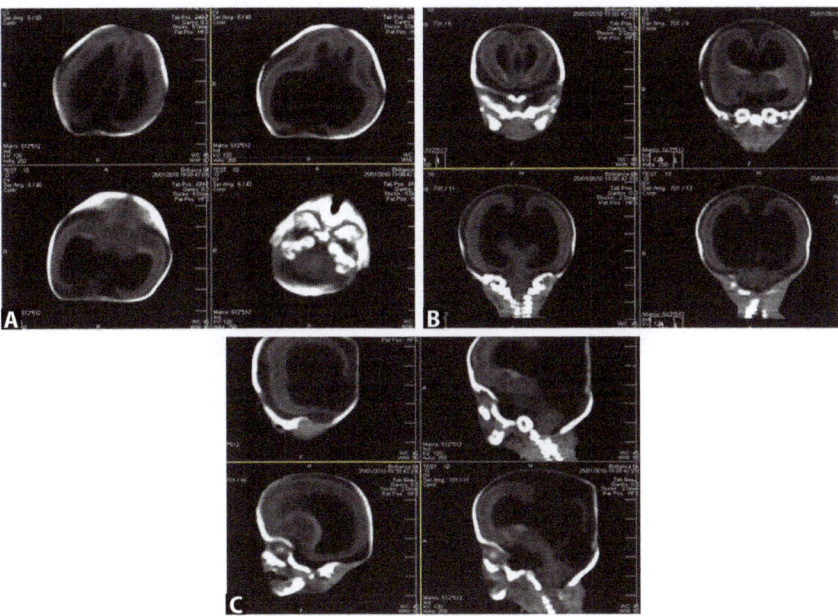

Figs 10.22A to C: CT of abortus of lobar holoprosencephaly: (A) Axial CT scan showing dilated ventricle; (B) Coronal CT scan showing absent corpus callosum fused thalami, dilated ventricles; (C) Sagittal CT of aborto showing the same

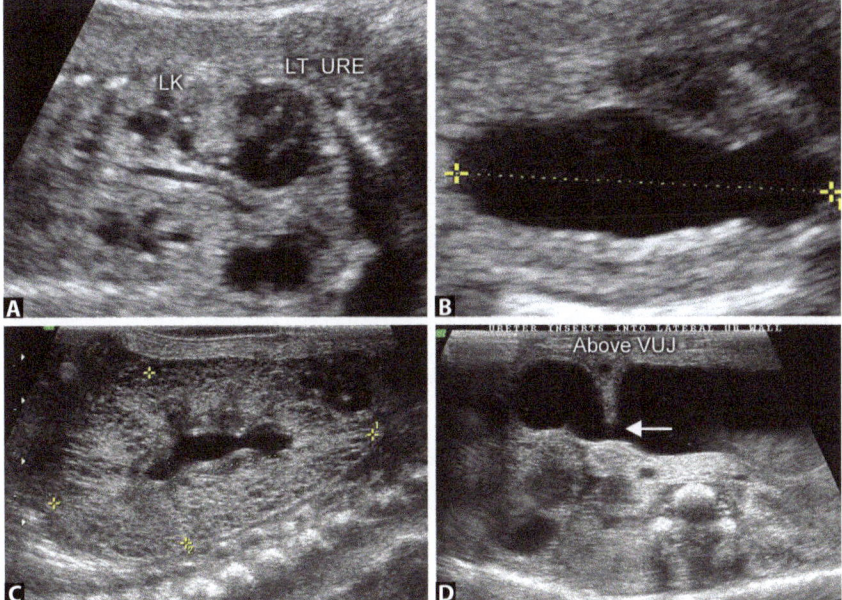

Figs 10.23A to D: Ultrasound of fetus with posterior urethral valves. (A) Bilateral echogenic kidneys with bilateral hydroureter LK, Left kidney; LT URE, Left uterus; (B) Dilated urinary bladder; (C) Abortus ultrasound shows echogenic kidney with cystic changes and hydroneprosis; (D) Abortus ultrasound showing dilated ureter and bladder

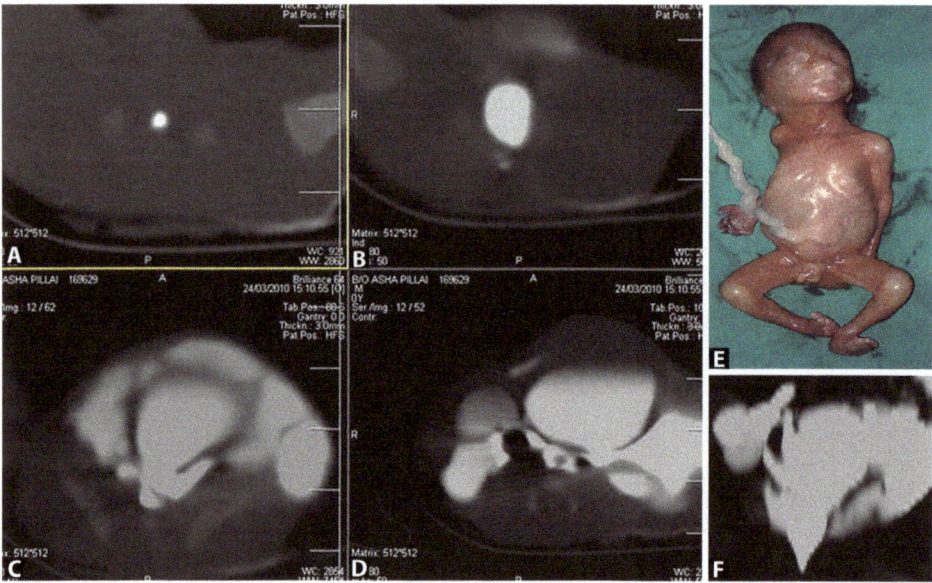

Figs 10.24A to F: CT urography of abortus with posterior urethral valves. (A to D and F) CT urogram showing dilated posterior urethra, bladder and lower ureters; (E) Abortus showing distended abdomen due to dilated urinary bladder and ureter

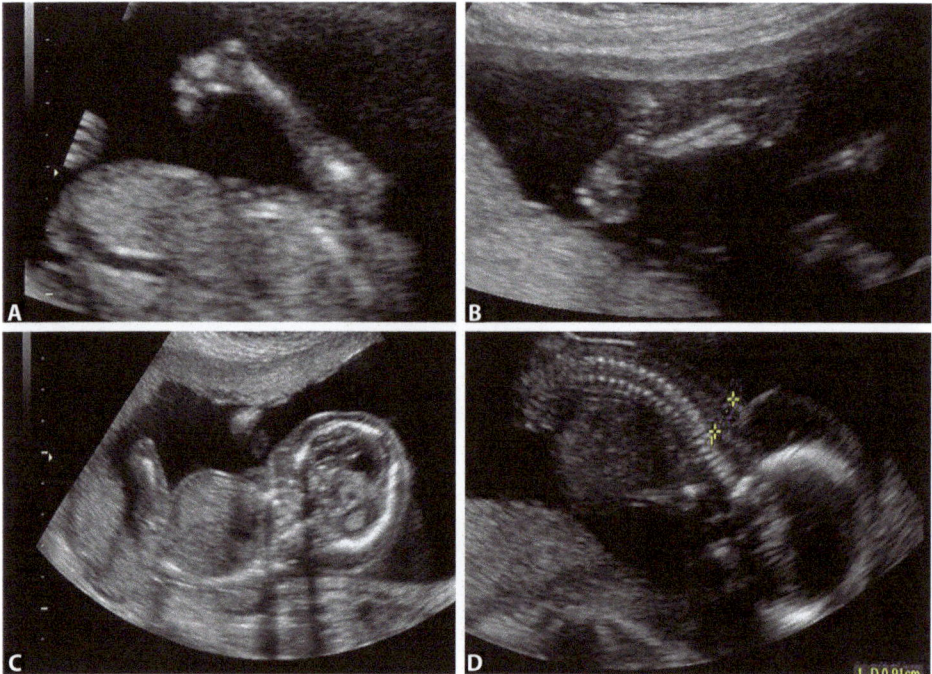

Figs 10.25A to D: Sonography of 20 weeks fetus showing musculoskeletal and cutaneous anomalies in trisomy 18. (A) Persistently flexed wrist; (B) Talipes; (C) Head and neck edema; (D) Nuchal edema

Genetics and Congenital Heart Disease

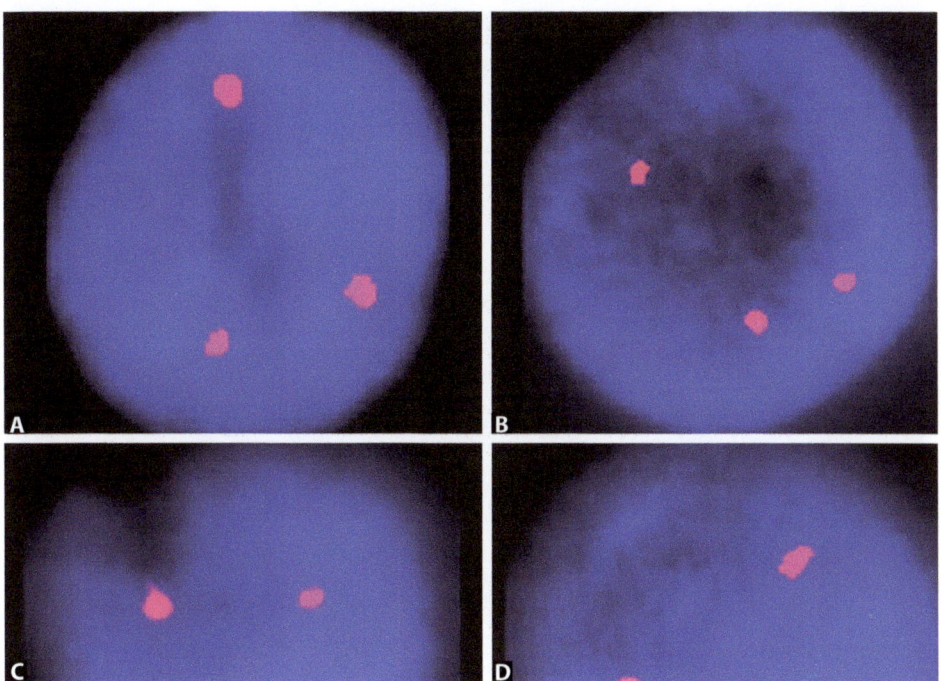

Figs 10.26A to D: Fluroscence insitu hybridization result of 21st chromosome. (A to D) 3 chromosomes (signals) in 21st chromosome

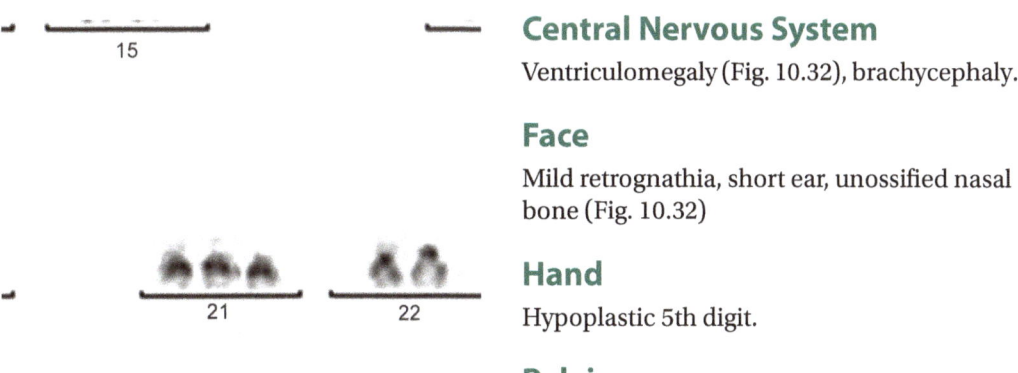

Fig. 10.27: Karyotype result of 21st chromosome. 3 chromosomes seen in 21st chromosome, 2 chromosomes seen in 22nd chromosome

Central Nervous System

Ventriculomegaly (Fig. 10.32), brachycephaly.

Face

Mild retrognathia, short ear, unossified nasal bone (Fig. 10.32)

Hand

Hypoplastic 5th digit.

Pelvis

- Wide iliac angle.

1st trimester soft markers of trisomy 21 are described in Figures 10.33 and 10.35.

Fetal Echocardiography

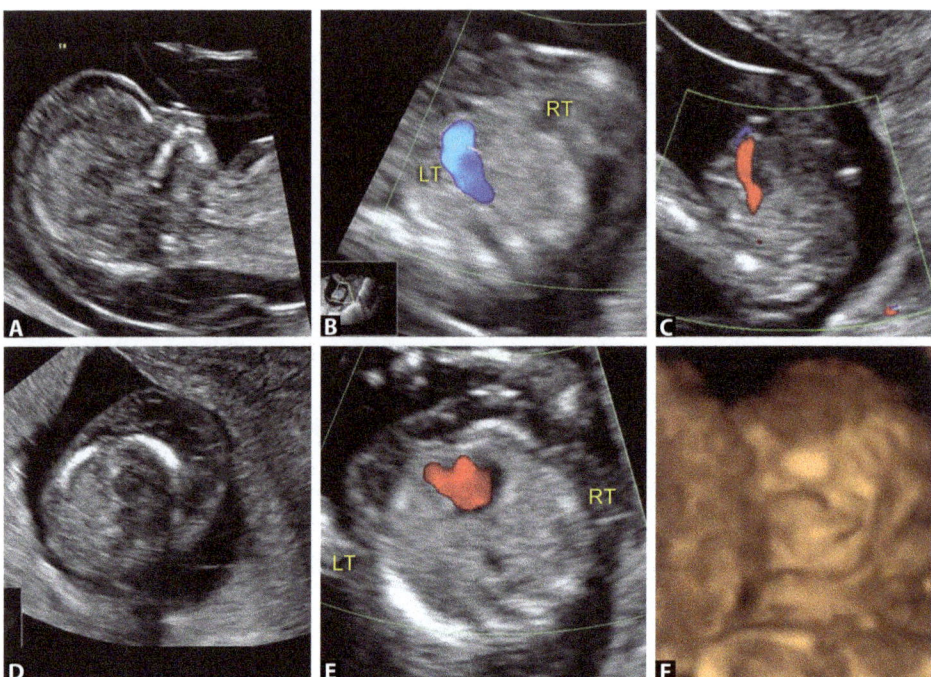

Figs 10.28A to F: Fetus with aortic atresia color Doppler. (A) Hydrops with absent nasal bone; (B) 4-chamber view showing pulmonary artery in blue. Arch of aorta is not seen; (C) Single umbilical artery; (D) Cystic hygroma; (E) 4-chamber view in colors; (F) 3-Dimensions of face showing cleft lip

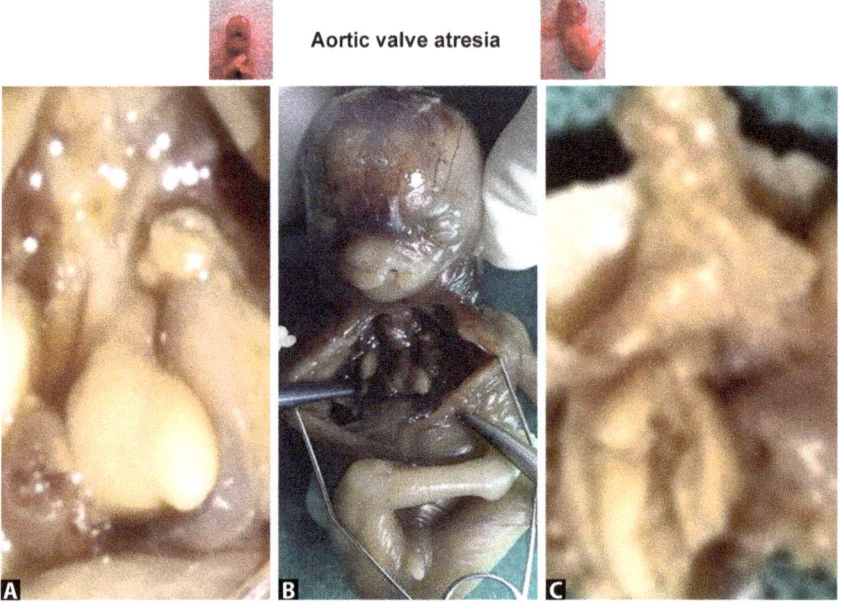

Figs 10.29A to C: Autopsy of 12 weeks fetus showing aortic valve atresia

Genetics and Congenital Heart Disease

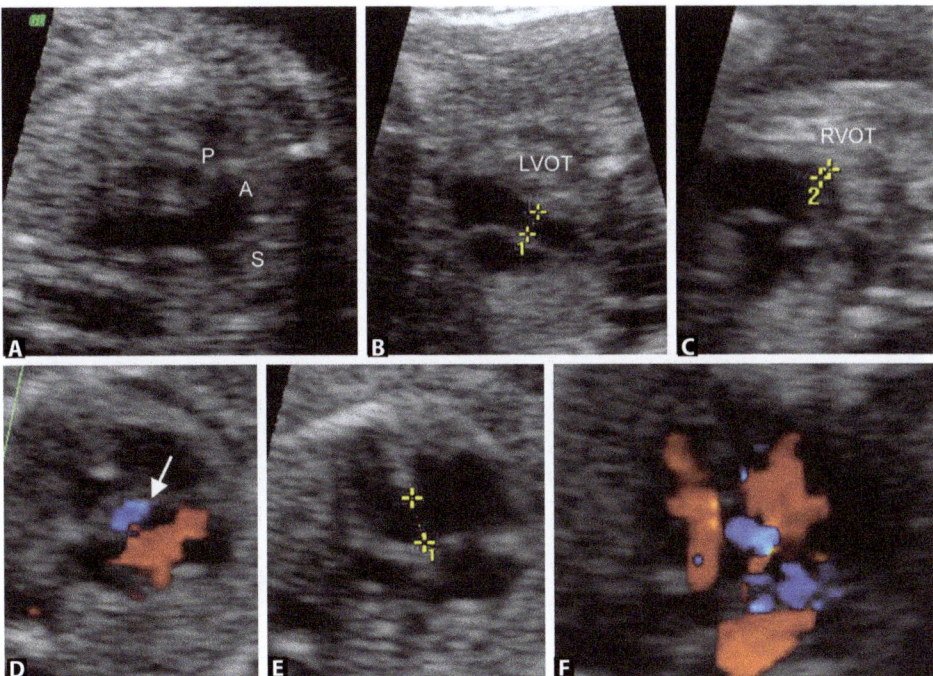

Figs 10.30A to F: Fetal echo of 20 weeks fetus with Down's syndrome. (A) 3 vessel view showing small pulmonary artery; (B) LVOT view showing normal ascending aorta; (C) RVOT view showing pulmonary atresia; (D) ASD; (E) VSD on 2D (F) VSD on color

22q11 DELETION

This is seen in fetuses with deletion abnormality in chromosome 22. The most common microdeletion occurs at 22q11. 22q11 microdeletion occurs in 1:5000 births. Deletion occurs in the long arm of chromosome 22 resulting in a few disorders. These encompass DiGeorge syndrome, velocardiofacial syndrome (Shprintzen) conotruncal face anomaly syndrome, CATCH 22, Cayler syndrome and Opitz G/ABB syndrome. Cardiac anomalies include: conotruncal anomalies, TGA, DORV, TOF, VSD interrupted arch, tricuspid atresia and double arch. Extracardiac anomalies include: absent thymus, velopharyngeal insufficiency, cleft soft palate, CNS, renal, GIT, skeletal anomalies. In conotruncal anomalies, CVS or amnio should be offered to diagnose 22q11 deletion by FISH.

TRISOMY 22 (FIG. 10.34) OR TETRASOMY 22 (CAT EYE SYNDROME)

This is seen in fetuses with 3 or 4 copies in 22nd chromosome. The cardiovascular anomalies include total anomalous pulmonary venous return, TOF, VSD, persistent LSVC, IVC interruption and tricuspid atresia. Extracardiac manifestations include mild mental deficiency, iris coloboma, preauricular tags, anal and renal malformations.

INVASIVE PROCEDURES IN CARDIAC ANOMALY CASES FOR ANEUPLOIDY EXCLUSION

Every patient has a risk of carrying a fetus with aneuploidy based on her age (Table 10.1) irrespective of sonological finding/

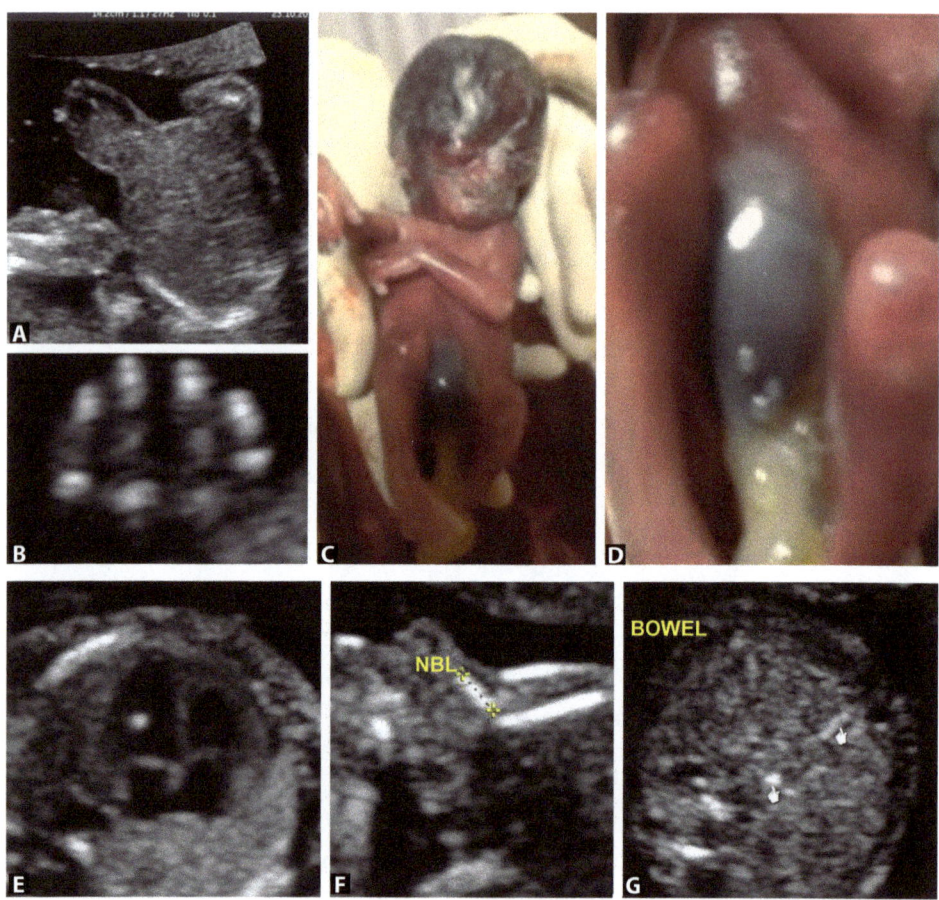

Figs 10.31A to G: 14 week T21 fetus. (A) Omphalocele with liver; (B) Polydactyly; (C and D) Abortus with omphalocele with liver; (E) Echogenic foci in cardiac left ventricle; (F) Short nasal bone (<5th percentile) NBL; (G) Grade 2 echogenic bowel

serum screening findings. Patients who have been diagnosed with a cardiac anomaly with or without extracardiac anomalies qualify for invasive diagnostic procedures (Flowcharts 10.1 and 10.2) like amniocentesis or chorion villous sampling, which help in aneuploidy exclusion. In addition, they may fit into the below mentioned criteria:

- Maternal age more than 40 years
- Previous child with aneuploidy or known genetic syndrome
- Family history of aneuploidy or known genetic syndrome
- Consanguinity
- Abnormal 1st trimester or 2nd trimester ultrasound findings indicating aneuploidy.
- Abnormal serum screening test in 1st trimester or 2nd trimester.

The abnormal 1st trimester soft markers of aneuploidy along with crown-rump length (CRL), nuchal translucency multiple of media (NT MoM), nasal bone (NB) multiples of median and maternal age derive a risk for aneuploidy.

The abnormal 2nd trimester ultrasound markers or sonographic markers of fetal

Genetics and Congenital Heart Disease

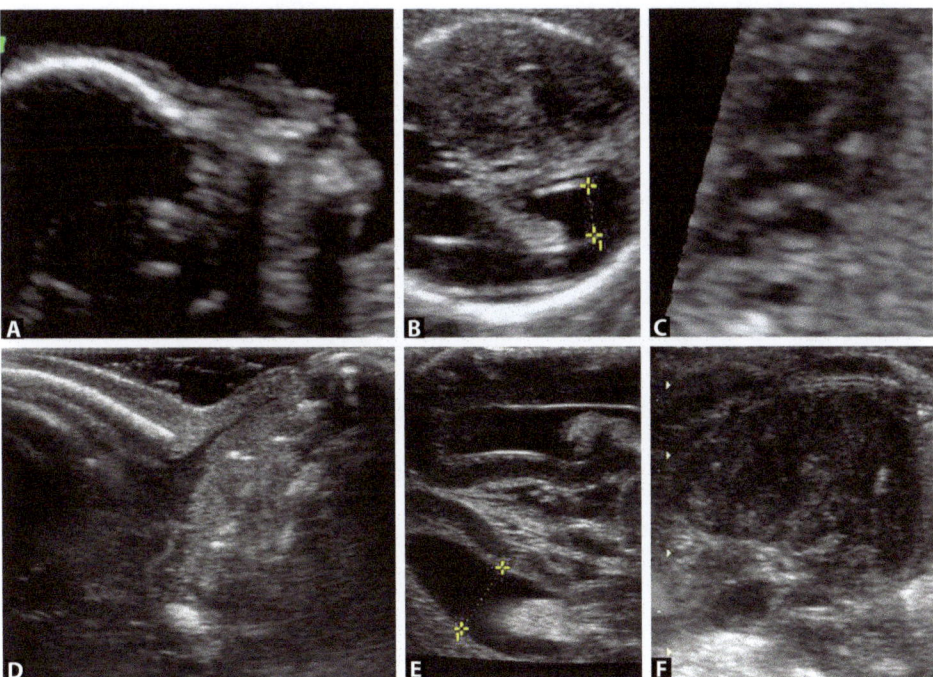

Figs 10.32A to F: T21 fetus. (A) Fetal unossified nasal bone; (B) Fetal ventriculomegaly; (C) Fetal echogenic intracardiac focus; (D) Abortus showing unossified nasal bone; (E) Abortus showing ventriculomegaly; (F) Abortus showing echogenic intracardiac focus

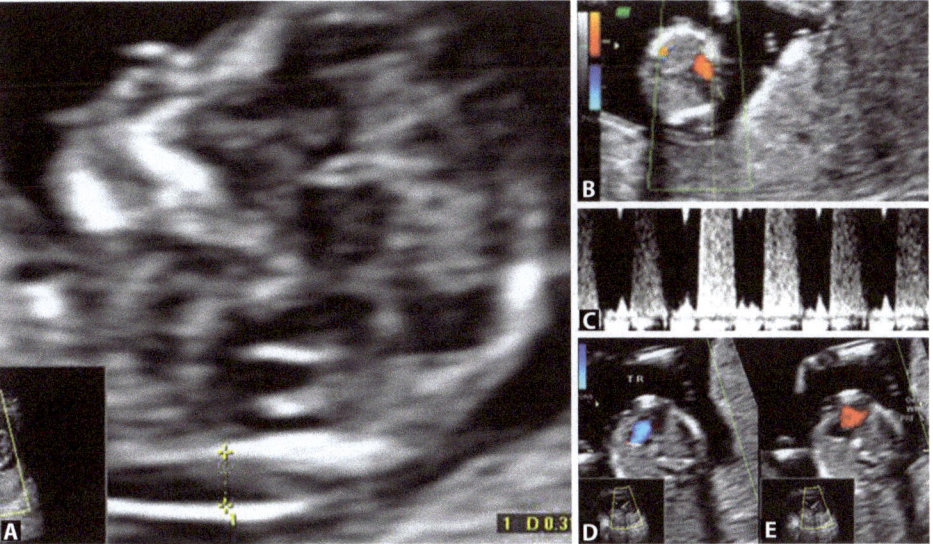

Figs 10.33A to E: Down's fetus showing aneuploidy 1st trimester markers. (A) Fetal sagittal facial view showing absent nasal bone and thickened NT; (B) Tricuspid regurgitation in color Doppler; (C) Tricuspid regurgitation in spectral Doppler; (D and E) Tricuspid regurgitation in color Doppler

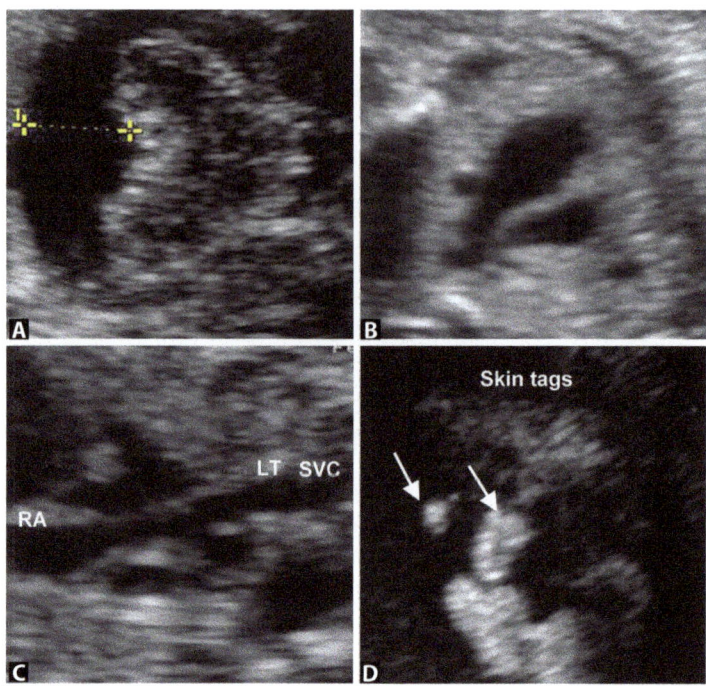

Figs 10.34A to D: Ultrasound of trisomy 22 fetus. (A) Mega cisterna magna; (B) 3 vessel view showing 4 vessels—extra vessel to the left of pulmonary artery is left SVC; (C) Left SVC in long axis; (D) Preauricular skin tags

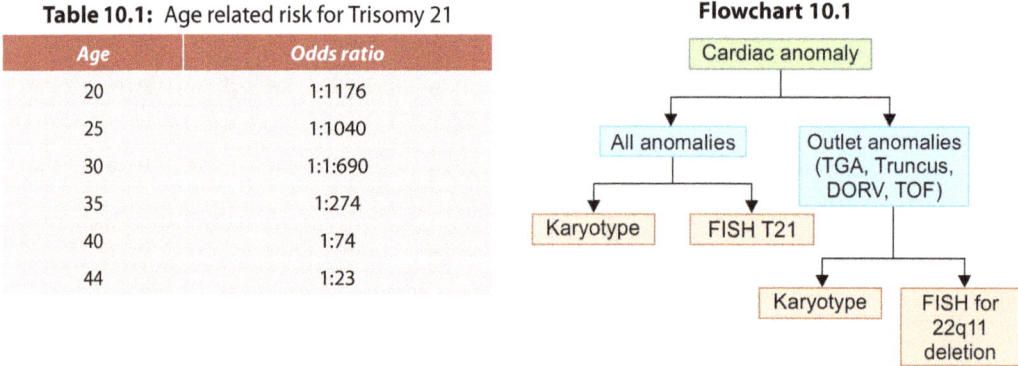

Table 10.1: Age related risk for Trisomy 21

Age	Odds ratio
20	1:1176
25	1:1040
30	1:1:690
35	1:274
40	1:74
44	1:23

Flowchart 10.1

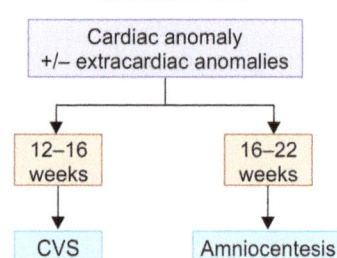

Flowchart 10.2

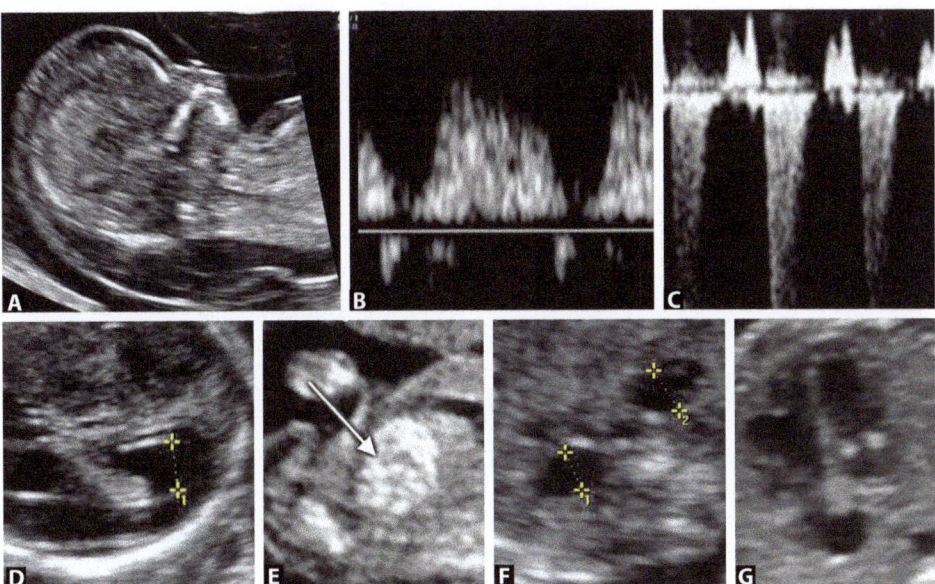

Figs 10.35A to G: Sonographic markers for aneuploidy in 1st and 2nd trimester. (A) 12 weeks fetus showing absent nasal bone and increased nuchal thickness; (B) Ductus venosus showing 'a' wave reversal; (C) Tricuspid valve showing regurgitation; (D) 20 weeks fetus showing dilated cerebral lateral ventricle; (E) Abdomen showing echogenic bowel; (F) Bilateral renal pelvic ectasia; (G) 4-chamber heart view showing echogenic foci in cardiac left ventricle

aneuploidy (SMFA) (Fig. 10.35) have likelihood ratio (LR) (Table 10.2) which is used to alter the first trimester risk or age risk to arrive at a new modified risk for aneuploidy.

The first trimester serum screening (Flowchart 10.3) evaluates MOMs of pregnancy-associated plasma protein A (PAPPA) and human chorionic gonadotropin (hCG). Results indicate low-risk (<1:1000), intermediate risk (1:250–1:1000), high-risk (>1:250) for aneuploidy (Trisomy 21) (Flowcharts 10.4 and 10.5).

The second trimester screening evaluates, MoMs of beta hCG, alpha fetoprotein, unconjugated estradiol and inhibin. Results indicate low-risk, intermediate risk or high risk for neural tube defect and Trisomy 18 and 21.

Combined screening is process by which the NT MoM and first trimester screening MoMs are analyzed to arrive at a combined risk for aneuploidy, which has the highest sensitivity.

Sequential screening is a process by which the first trimester risk is modified

Table 10.2: Likelihood ratio of 2nd trimester sonographic markers of aneuploidy—used to alter background risk

Unossified Nb	6.5
ARSA	3.9
Ventriculomegaly	3.8
Thick NF	3.7
Echogenic bowel	1.6
Pyelectasis	1
EIF	0.9
Short humerus	0.7
Short femur	0.6

Abbreviations: NB, nasal bone; ARSA, abnormal right subclavian artery; NF, nuchal fold; EIF, echogenic intracardiac focus

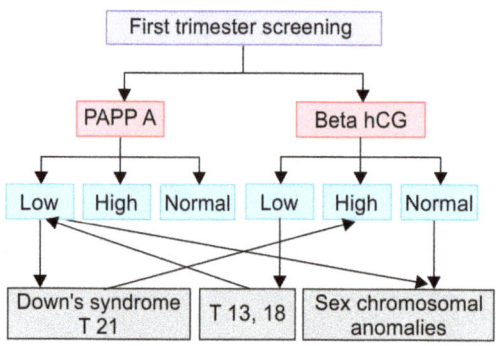

Flowchart 10.3

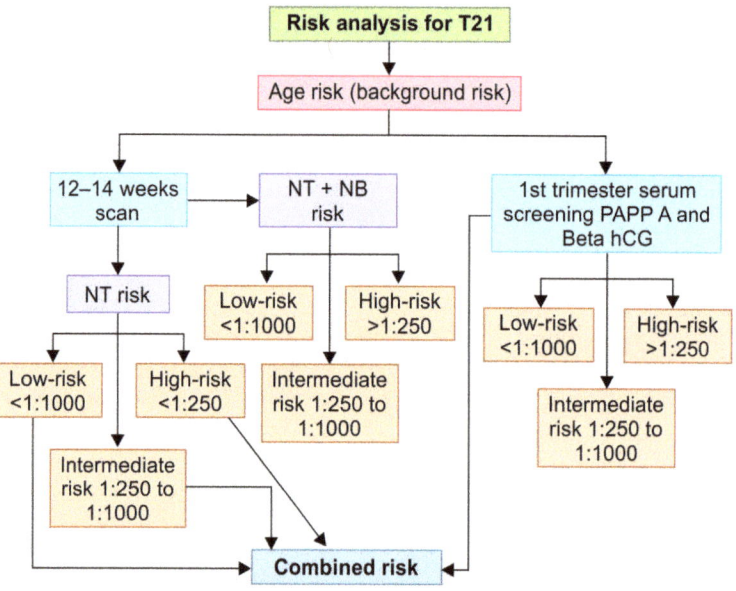

Flowchart 10.4

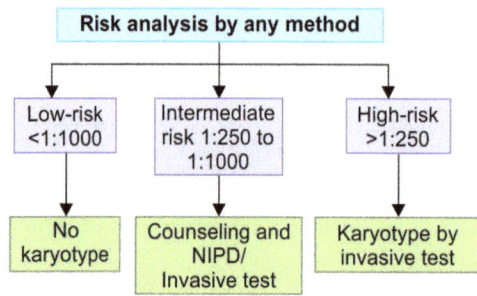

Flowchart 10.5

Abbreviation: NIPD, noninvasive prenatal diagnosis

using 2nd trimester ultrasound markers and 2nd trimester serum screening to arrive at a modified risk for aneuploidy.

By whichever way, a risk may be calculated if the risk is intermediate or high, counseling is done and with informed consent, either CVS or amniocentesis can be performed.

Chorion Villous Sampling (CVS)

This is a procedure where under asepsis and local anesthesia and continuous ultrasound guidance, using 18G heparinized LP needle, chorion villi are aspirated from the placenta and collected into a CVS broth (fluid medium) (Fig. 10.36) and sent for FISH and karyotype.

This is done between 14 weeks and 17 weeks of gestational age.

Amniocentesis

This is a procedure where under asepsis and continuous ultrasound guidance, using 21G LP needle, 20 mL of amniotic fluid (Figs 10.37 and 10.38) is aspirated and collected in a syringe and sent for FISH and karyotype. This is done between 17 to 22 weeks. The prerequisites for the above procedures are:
- Intermediate risk or high-risk for aneuploidy
- Informed consent with form G and form D (formalities)
- Counseling regarding procedure, results, risks, cost, outcome, etc.
- Maternal glycemic status.
- Maternal susceptibility for hemorrhage.
- Maternal blood group (for RH negative mother with RH positive husbands, anti-D injection required after procedure).

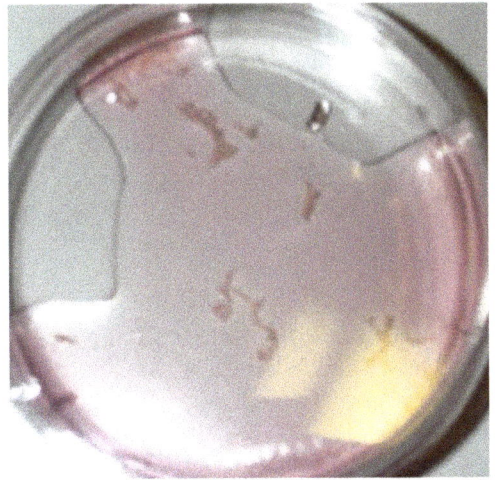

Fig. 10.36: Chronic villi sampling

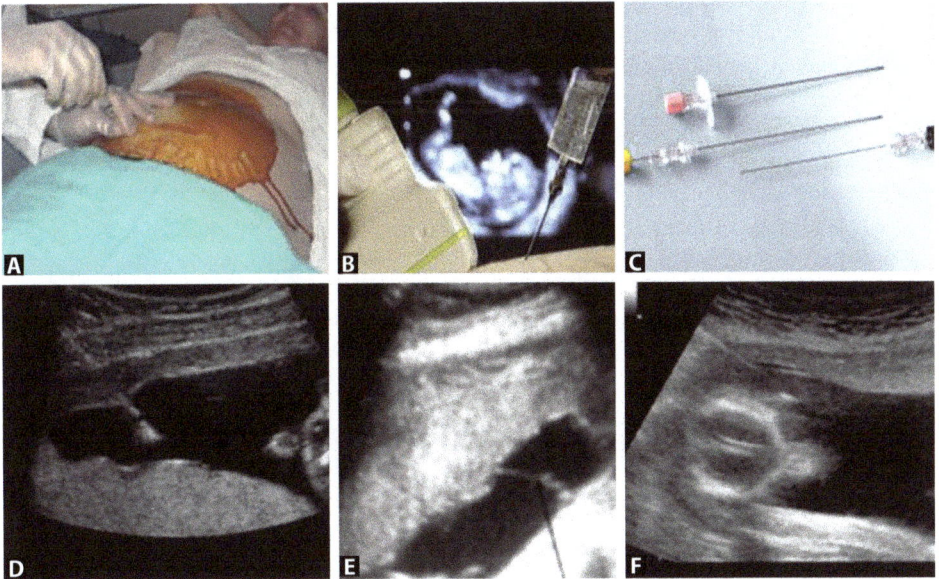

Figs 10.37A to F: Amniocentesis techniques. (A) Sterile abdominal preparation; (B) Amnio needle and syringe; (C) Amnio needles—21 gauge; (D) Amnio needle entering the amniotic sac through myometrium; (E) Amnio needle entering amniotic sac through placenta; (F) Amnio needle touching fetal part

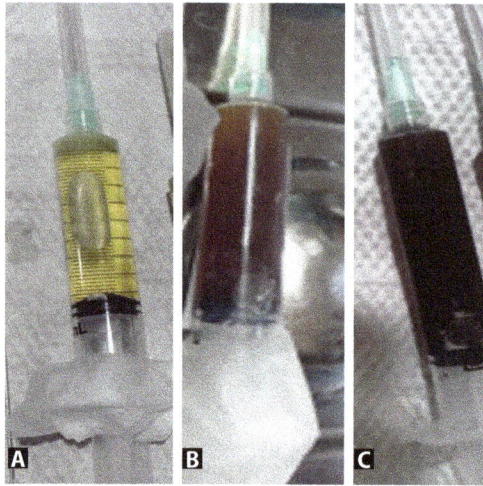

Figs 10.38A to C: (A) Clear fluid; (B and C) Amniotic fluid in a case of prior subchorionic hematoma

Post-procedure rest for 2 days is optimal. Risks of the procedure include miscarriage (<0.5%), infection, leaking PV and bleeding PV. Check scans are done 4 days after procedure to look for above complications. FISH reports are available in 2–4 days. Karyotype requires culturing of amniocytes and can take up to 2–3 weeks time. Failure of culture results in non availability of karyotype and requires repetition of procedure.

A normal FISH and karyotype report ensures 100% absence of the aneuploidy in question. An abnormal FISH and karyotype warrants further counseling and action.

CVS is preferred for single gene defect analysis.

CONCLUSION

It is very important to have a thorough knowledge about the extracardiac abnormalities which can occur in association with various cardiac anomalies. Having this knowledge, it is imperative to look for such association by using proper technique and equipment.

When such associations are encountered, it will help to clarify the disorder into a known genetic syndrome or chromosomal abnormality or otherwise, for the sake of further assessment by invasive or noninvasive methods to arrive at a genetic diagnosis. With the complete diagnosis in hand, counseling regarding termination/continuation of pregnancy can become easier. When the pregnancy is continued, based on the cardiac and extracardiac findings, timing, place and method of delivery can be planned in a center which can tackle cardiac and extracardiac issues by proper competent specialists in various systems, which are abnormally involved. The above complete diagnosis, prognosis and counseling can be achieved only with knowledge and expertise in sonography and invasive techniques.

SUGGESTED READING

1. Basson CT, Bachinsky DR, Lin RC, Levi T, Elkins JA, Soults J, et al. Mutations in human cause limb and cardiac malformation in Holt-Oram syndrom. Nature Genetics. 1997;15: 30-5.
2. Boudjemline Y, Fermont L, Le Bidois l, Lyonnet S, Sidi D, Bonnet D. Prevalence of 22q11 deletion in fetuses with conotruncal heart defects: A 6-year prospective study. J Pediatr. 2001;138:520-4.
3. Copel JA, Pilu G, Kleinman CS. Extracardiac anomalies and congenital heart disease. Sem Perinatol. 1993;17:89-105.
4. Copel JA, Pilu G, Kleinmann C. Congenital heart disease and extracardiac anomalies: Associations and indications for fetal echocardiography. Am J Obstet Gynecol. 1986;154:1121-32.
5. Eva Pajkrt E, Weisz B, Firth HV, Chitty LS. Fetal cardiac anomalies and genetic syndromes. Prenat Diagn. 2004;24:1104-15.
6. Freeman SB, Taft LF, Dooley KJ, Allran K, Sherman SL, Hassold TJ, et al. Population-based study of congenital heart defects in Down syndrome. Am J Med Genet. 1998;80: 213-7.

7. Goel A, Weerakkody Y, et al. Heterotaxy syndrome. Radiopedia.org
8. Greenwood RD, Rosenthal A, Parisi L, Fyler DC, Nadas AS. Extracardiac abnormalities in infants with congenital heart disease. Pediatrics. 1975; 55:485-49.
9. Güçer S, Ince T, Kale G, Akçören Z, Ozkutlu S, Talim B, et al. Noncardiac malformations in congenital heart disease: A retrospective analysis of 305 pediatric autopsies. Turk J Pediatr. 2005;47:159-66.
10. Huggon IC, Cook AC, Smeeton NC, Magee AG, Sharland GK. Atrioventricular septal defects diagnosed in fetal life: associated cardiac and extracardiac abnormalities and outcome. J Am Coll Cardiol. 2000;36(2):593-601.
11. Kim HK, Gottliebson W, Hor K, Backeljauw P, Gutmark-Little I, Salisbury SR, et al. Cardiovascular anomalies in Turner syndrome: spectrum, prevalence, and cardiac MRI findings in a pediatric and young adult population. Am J Roentgenol. 2011;196: 454-60.
12. Lalani SR, Shaw C, Wang X, Patel A, Patterson LW, Kolodziejska K, et al. Rare DNA copy number variants in cardiovascular malformations with extracardiac abnormalities. Eur J Hum Genet. 2013;21: 173-81.
13. Lin AE, Perloff JK. Upper limb malformations associated with congenital heart disease. Am J Cardiol. 1985;55:1576-83.
14. Pradat P. Noncardiac malformations at major congenital heart defects. Pediatr Cardiol. 1997; 18:11-18.
15. Song MS, Hu A, Dyamenahalli U, Chitayat D, Winsor EJ, Ryan G, et al. Extracardiac lesions and chromosomal abnormalities associated with major fetal heart defects: comparison of intrauterine, postnatal and postmortem diagnoses. Ultrasound Obstet Gynecol. 2009; 33:552-9.
16. Tennstedt C, Chaoui R, Körner H, Dietel M. Spectrum of congenital heart defects and extracardiac malformations associated with chromosomal abnormalities: results of a seven year necropsy study. Heart. 1999;82: 34-9.
17. van Karnebeek CD, Hennekam RC. Associations between chromosomal anomalies and congenital heart defects. Am J Med Genet. 1999;84:158-66.

Genetic Contribution to the Origin of Congenital Heart Disease

SJ Patil

ABSTRACT

Congenital heart disease (CHD) is one of the most common congenital human malformations with varying birth prevalence in various study years and among different continents. Outcome of the CHD depends on severity of the malformation itself, associated extracardiac malformation and underlying etiology. Etiologically, CHD is highly heterogeneous anomaly; both genetic and/or environmental factors are known to cause CHD. Understanding the etiology helps not only in the management of patients with CHD, but also in prevention and prenatal diagnosis. In this Chapter, we will discuss about various genetic factors contributing to the origin of congenital heart disease and also discuss some of the common genetic causes of syndromic CHD.

INTRODUCTION

Definition

Definition of congenital heart diseases (CHD) given by Mitchell, et al. 1971: Congenital heart disease is defined as a gross structural abnormality of the heart or intrathoracic great vessels that is actually or potentially of functional significance. Abnormalities of systemic veins and systemic arteries, and arrhythmias unassociated with structural heart defects are excluded.

Congenital heart diseases presents with variable severity and different underlying etiology. Prognosis and management of the CHD depends on its severity (severity of the heart lesion itself and/or associated extra-cardiac anomaly) and the underlying etiology in both the prenatally/postnatally diagnosed patients with CHD. Etiology of the CHDs could be genetic or due to interaction of genetic and environmental factors. Genetic etiologies of CHD include chromosomal [gross deletions and duplications—GCA/copy number variants (CNVs)], single genes, epigenetic alterations and somatic mutations. Etiological diagnosis of CHD, especially in prenatal cases helps in the management and accurate genetic counseling.

Multifactorial etiology (gene-gene/gene-environmental interactions) has been considered the most common cause of congenital heart disease especially in patients with isolated sporadic CHD. With recent advancement in genetic tests, pure genetic origins of CHD are increasingly being identified, although modifier genes/environmental factors may act as modifying factors. In addition there are maternal conditions and teratogenic causes of CHD (causing both syndromic CHD and isolated CHD). However, in majority of patients with CHD the cause remains unknown.

Genetic causes of valvular heart disease, aortic lesions (e.g. Marfan syndrome, etc.), arrhythmias and cardiomyopathy will not be discussed here as the pathogenesis and the clinical presentation is considered entirely different. Although, there are some genetic causes causing both structural heart defects and cardiomyopathy. Also some of the cardiomyopathies can be diagnosed prenatally.

Incidence

Incidence of congenital heart disease ranges from 4-8 per 1,000 live births. If we include bicuspid aortic valve (found in 1-2% of general population) and tiny/trivial lesions, incidence increases to 19-75 per 1,000 live births respectively.

In an European study from year 2000-2005, prevalence of the CHD across the various European countries ranged from 5.36 to15.32 per 1,000 and prevalence of non-chromosomal CHD was 7.0 per 1,000 births.

Birth prevalence is also shown to vary among developed and developing countries. High birth prevalence of CHD is seen in Asia (9.3 per 1,000 live births) and lowest in Africa (1.9 per 1,000 live births) in comparison to European (8.2 per 1,000 live births) and North America (6.9 per 1,000 live births). A higher prevalence of CHD in Asia is partly attributed to higher consanguinity rates.

CLASSIFICATION OF CHD IN GENETIC CLINIC

Congenital heart diseases in genetic clinic are classified as syndromic CHD and isolated CHD based on presence or absence of extracardiac anomaly respectively. This classification of syndromic CHD and isolated CHD helps in management/prognosis and prioritizing genetic test in the proband. As many as 20-30% of the postnatally diagnosed CHD are known to be associated with extracardiac anomaly and the percentage increases to 40-66% if the fetuses diagnosed antenatally with CHD are included. This increase in the percentage of CHD with extracardiac malformation among fetuses with CHD suggest, in some of the fetuses with CHD could lead to spontaneous abortions, still births and medical termination of pregnancy. Table 10.3 shows various etiology of CHD.

Table 10.3: Etiology of congenital heart disease

Etiology	Type of abnormality	Clinical presentation	Inheritance
1. Chromosomal	• Aneuploidy—autosome/sex chromosome • Partial aneuploidies—deletion/duplication—GCA/CNVs • Mosaicism	• Multiple malformation syndrome • Isolated CHD (CNVs)	• Sporadic (de novo) • Parental
2. Single gene defects/Oligogenic	• Single gene—deletion, duplication, point mutation, epigenetic alterations • Two or more genes • Non-traditional inheritance—mosaicism, mitochondrial	• Isolated CHD • Multiple malformation syndrome	• Autosomal dominant • Autosomal recessive • X-linked • Maternal (Mitochondrial) • Sporadic
3. Maternal conditions/Teratogen	• Maternal diabetes/abnormal glycemic control, phenylketonuria • Drugs—antiepileptic drugs, retinoic acids, lithium, etc. • Infections—rubella	• Isolated CHD • Syndromic CHD	
4. Unknown cause	• Possible single gene • Possible chromosomal • Environment/gene interaction	• Isolated CHD • Syndromic CHD	• Any of the above

Abbreviations: GCA, gross chromosomal anomaly; CNVs, copy number variations; CHD, congenital heart disease

CHROMOSOMAL CHD

Chromosomal causes of CHD are aneuploidies (full or partial) detectable by standard chromosome analysis (karyotype) [will be referred here as gross chromosomal anomaly (GCA)] or copy number variants (deletions and duplications) detectable by chromosomal microarray analysis (CMA) (molecular karyotype) (will be referred as CNVc). Clinical presentation of the GCA CHD is syndromic where as those with CNVs CHD; clinical presentation could be syndromic or apparently isolated CHD.

Syndromic CHD with extracardiac malformation, especially with facial dysmorphism, and/or associated abnormal neurodevelopment/growth issues are more likely to be due to chromosomal cause (either GCA or CNVs). Clinical phenotype is recognizable in some of the chromosomal CHD—in both full (e.g. trisomy 21, trisomy 18, etc.) and partial aneuploidies (22q11.2 deletion, 7q11.23 deletion, etc.). It is difficult to recognize clinically the underlying CNV in most of the patients based on the clinical phenotype (unlike 22q11/7q11.23 deletion etc.) due to variable penetrance/expression, age dependent evolving phenotype, less common and recent few publications.

There has been a wide variation in the percentage of chromosomal causes of CHD depending upon the study period, study criteria and the technique used to study chromosomes (standard karyotype and/ or molecular cytogenetics). In the pre-chromosomal microarray (CMA) period 6–13% of live born with CHD were due to chromosomal cause. If fetuses are included then the percentage of chromosomal CHD increased to 22–33%. Further with the delineation of 22q11.2 deletion syndrome and introduction of fluorescent in-situ hybridization (FISH) for 22q11.2 deletion in children with CHD, it was found that 22q11.2 deletion account for 5% of all liveborn CHD patients. In most patients 22q11.2 deletion is small in size (<4 Mb) requiring FISH/ MLPA (Multiple ligation dependent probe amplification) test to identify the deletion.

In the recent years with the recommendation of CMA in birth defects, chromosomal CNVs account for 4.3% of isolated CHD and 14.1% of syndromic CHD (excluding GCA and 22q11 microdeletions). Further in selected group of syndromic CHD with features suggestive of chromosomal aberrations, pathogenic CNVs accounted for 30% of the syndromic CHD patients. In addition, percentapes of CNVs causing syndrome CHD will increase beyond 30%, if small CNVs and/ or likely pathogenic CNVs are included.

Aneuploidies (Complete or Partial) Detectable by Standard Chromosome Analysis Causing CHD–Gross Chromosomal Anomaly (GCA)

Prenatal presentation of CHD with GCA could be isolated or associated with extracardiac malformation, increased nuchal thickness, single umbilical artery, hydrops fetalis, and intrauterine growth restriction etc. Postnatal presentation of CHD with GCA is always syndromic phenotype. Syndromic phenotype with CHD-GCA usually present as multiple malformation syndrome, facial dysmorphism and varying effect on cognitive functions. The most common GCAs among CHD includes trisomy 21, trisomy 18, trisomy 13, and monosomy X. Table 10.4 show the list of common GCA with CHD (both complete and partial aneuploidies).

Common Aneuploidies with CHD

Trisomy 21 (Down Syndrome)

Incidence of Down syndrome is 1 in 700 to 1,000 live births. Clinical manifestation include characteristic face (mid-face

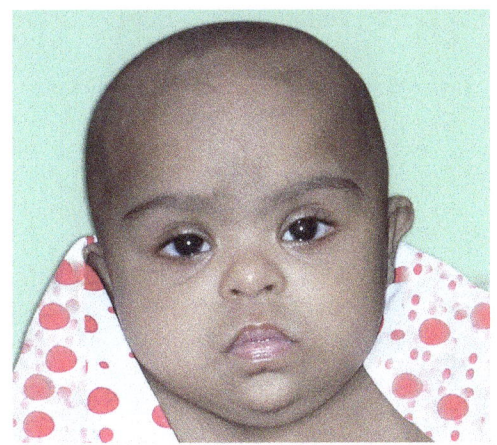

Fig. 10.39: Trisomy 21

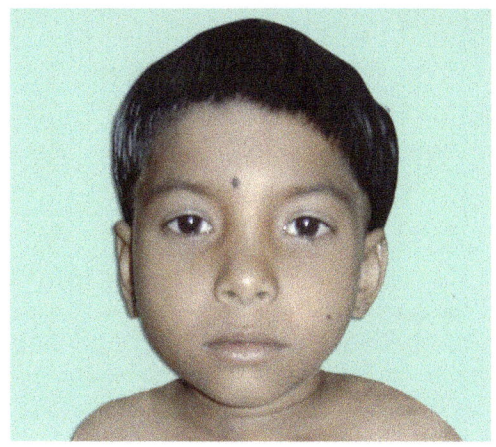

Fig. 10.40: Turner syndrome

hypoplasia, upslant eyes, depressed nasal bridge, small and low set ears, protruding tongue) (Fig. 10.39), intellectual disability, short stature, hypotonia, congenital heart disease and various other physical findings like single palmar crease, sandle gap, fifth finger clinodactyly, etc. About 50% of the children with Down syndrome have CHD. In majority cardiac lesion is atrioventricular canal defect.

Trisomy 13

Trisomy 13 is seen in 1 in 12,000 live births. Common clinical manifestation are microcephaly with or without brain malformation (holoprosencephaly), polydactyly (usually postaxial), microphthalmia, renal malformations, congenital heart disease and bilateral cleft lip and cleft palate. Survival beyond 1 year is unusual especially with life-threatening major malformations.

Trisomy 18

Trisomy 18 occurs in 1 in 6,000 live births. Most common aneuploidy after trisomy 21. Usual presentation includes intrauterine growth retardation, prominent occiput, micrognathia, small palpebral fissures, low set ears, characteristic overlapping fingers, short sternum, rocker bottom feet and congenital heart defect. Most of the patients die by 1 year. Prolonged survival is associated with severe intellectual disability and physical handicap.

Turner Syndrome

Most often diagnosis of Turner syndrome is made when female child presents with short stature and delayed puberty. Other clinical features include webbing of neck, increased carrying angle, CHD, increased pigmented nevi, short fourth metacarpal, renal malformations and hearing problems. Some of them can show typical facial features (Fig. 10.40). Commonest subtype of chromosomal abnormality is 45, X. The incidence is 1 in 2,500 to 1 in 3,000 female live births. Cardiac malformations are seen in 16–23% of the patients. Common cardiac lesions are coarctation of aorta, bicuspid aortic valve and mitral valve prolapse. Even if the initial cardiac evaluation is normal, periodic assessment is necessary to find aortic root dilatation, especially during pregnancy. Hypertension could be due to either cardiac lesion, renal pathology or unrelated to any underlying organ involvement.

Copy Number Variants CHD

Clinically Evident Common Copy Number Variants

- **22q11.2 deletion:** It the most common CNV/microdeletion associated with CHD and variable other clinical features. Incidence of 22q11 deletion ranges from 1 in 4,000 to 1 in 6,000 live births. Most of the cases are sporadic. Around 5–10% are familial cases, inherited as an autosomal dominant disorder. Clinical manifestations in patients with 22q11 deletion are variable, both intrafamilial and interfamilial. Major clinical findings in patients with 22q11 deletion include characteristic face, CHD, immune function abnormalities (80%), cleft palate (44%), hypocalcemia (60%) hypoparathyroidism, and learning difficulties. Characteristic facial features are upslant eyes, puffy eyes, bulbous nasal tip, broad nasal root, hypoplastic alae nasi, small mouth, micrognathia, cup-shaped ears and overfolded helix (Fig. 10.41). Since majority (around 75–80%) of 22q11 deletions have CHD, FISH/MLPA investigation for 22q11 microdeletion is indicated in patients with CHD especially with characteristic facial features and conotruncal heart defects.

- **7q11.23 deletion:** It is the other common CNV presents clinically with recognizable phenotype and is widely known as Williams-Beuren syndrome (WBS). Incidence of WBS is 1 in 20,000 to 1 in 50,000. Majority of the cases are de-novo deletion involving 1.5 Mb genomic DNA. Clinical manifestations include characteristic face, overfriendly behavior, intellectual disability (usually mild), hypercalcemia and congenital heart disease. Characteristic facial features are boggy cheeks, small nose, periorbital fullness, wide mouth, malar hypoplasia, full lips, long philtrum and wide spaced teeth (Fig. 10.42). There are reports of familial autosomal dominant inheritance, usually maternal. Eighty percent of William-Beuren syndrome children have cardiovascular anomalies and the most common congenital heart defects are supravalvular aortic stenosis and peripheral pulmonary stenosis.

Other Copy Number Variants Causing CHD

Copy number variants (CNVs) are defined as segments of DNA either duplicated or deleted of size ranging from few hundred base pairs (usually >1kb) to millions base pairs, usually

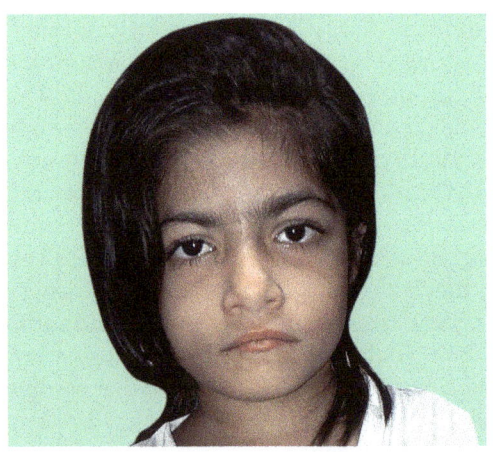

Fig. 10.41: DiGeorge/Velocardiofacial syndrome

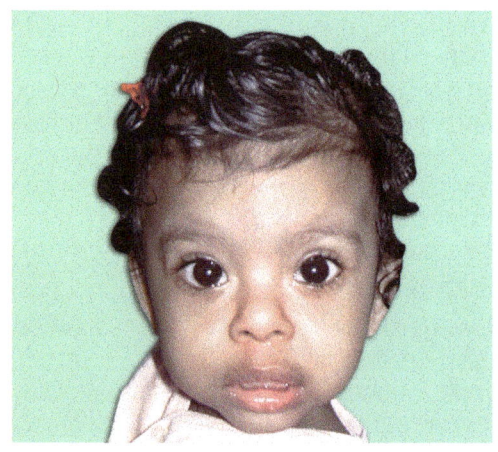

Fig. 10.42: Williams syndrome

resulting in copy number change of genes on a particular chromosome (gain or loss) and are not detectable by standard chromosome analysis. CNVs could be inherited or de-novo (sporadic) and polymorphic (normal variant) or pathogenic. Pathogenic CNVs cause disease phenotype due its gene content—dosage dependent or regulatory sequences (genes and its regulatory sequences involved in the development of heart). Chromosome microarray is a useful test in clinical practice to identify CNVs in both prenatal and postnatal patient samples. Here, it is genome wide analysis of CNVs/microdeletions/microduplications irrespective of clinical phenotype.

Pathogenic CNVs among CHD patients has led to discovery of many new single genes causing CHD. Yet in some of the CNVs precise mechanism of pathogenesis is not clearly understood. Some of the common CNVs reported in both isolated CHD and syndromic CHD are listed in Table 10.4.

CHD and Chromosomal causes at Narayana Institute of Cardiac Sciences (NCIS)

All cardiac defects with extracardiac manifestations patients referred to genetic clinic for genetic evaluation from 2009–2014 were included in the study. Those with isolated cardiac defects were excluded from the study. Extracardiac manifestations should be at-least one of the following—one or more additional major malformation—internal or external organ, abnormal neurodevelopment, three or minor malformations, growth issues (overgrowth or growth restrictions), facial dysmorphism and known diagnosed genetic syndrome. All cases underwent clinical genetic evaluation. Investigations were suggested to patients based on initial clinical diagnosis (suggestive of chromosomal disorder)—chromosome analysis (Standard karyotype), FISH for 22q11.2 microdeletion/7q11.23 microdeletion, etc. (targeted test based on clinical impression), chromosomal microarray (CMA). Limitation of the study: It is a hospital-based study; figures of chromosomal causes of CHD represent common causes. Chromosomal analysis was offered to all patients wherever indicated (Standard chromosome and FISH/or chromosomal microarray). However, not all of them took genetic tests offered.

Results and Discussion

Among 2181 syndromic CHD selected, chromosomal abnormality accounted for about 30% (mainly identified through standard Karyotype and FISH). The most

Table 10.4: Chromosomal disorders with CHD

Chromosomal abnormality	Technique used for identifying	Example
Aneuploidy • Autosomal • Sex chromosome	• Standard karyotype	• Trisomy 21 • Trisomy 18 • Trisomy 13 • Turner syndrome
Partial Aneuploidy • Gross deletions/ duplications	• Standard karyotype	del8p, del4p, del5p15.2, del1p36 del11q23,
Submicroscopic partial/segmental aneuploidy • Microdeletions /microduplications (CNVs)	• FISH/MLPA • Chromosomal microarray	• del/dup22q11.2, del7q11.23 • del1q21.1, dup1q21.1, del20p12.3, del15q11.2, del5q33 del16p12.2, del8p23.1, del9q34.3 dup16p11.2, del3p25.1, del7p12.3

common chromosomal cause among syndromic CHD include: trisomy 21 (23.75%), DGS/VCF (2.9%), and Williams syndrome (1.3%) (FISH proven microdeletion syndrome patients) (Table 10.5). The commonest cardiac malformation in these syndromes is AVSD, conotruncal heart defects and SVAS/PPS respectively. The percentage for DGS/VCF syndrome and Williams syndrome increased from 2.9% to 7.0% and 1.3% to 2.15% if clinically sure diagnosed (author own experience) patients were included respectively (without FISH proven). Our results show higher percentage of chromosomal abnormalities because of selection criteria used for inclusion of syndromic CHD patients and limited use of advanced molecular cytogenetic technique (availability and cost). These results are similar to other studies of selected cohort of syndromic CHDs and chromosomal abnormalities. With the use of chromosome microarray in CHD patients, these figures of chromosomal abnormalities in CHD patients are likely to increase.

SINGLE GENE DISORDER CHD

Earlier studies reported single gene causing CHD account for about 2–5% of all CHD. However a recent study by Zaidi, et al. 2013 show single gene mutations account for 10% of severe sporadic CHD. If we consider isolated CHD with family history of CHD, then the single gene mutations account for about 31% of cases. Inheritance of these mutations may be autosomal dominant, X-linked recessive, and autosomal recessive. The most common mutations are dominant mutations associated with both familial and sporadic CHDs. These dominant mutations in CHDs are associated with incomplete penetrance, variable expression and also can lead to different types of cardiac defect.

Various genes identified as a cause of CHD, play important role as cardiac transcription factors, and as developmental pathways genes of cardia. Developmental pathway genes known to cause CHD are RAS-ERK pathway genes (Noonan syndrome and

Table 10.5: Syndromic CHD and Chromosomal cause at NICS# from 2009–2014 (n = 2181)

Chromosomal cause	Number of cases	Percentage of syndromic CHD (n = 2181)	Commonest cardiac malformation
Down syndrome	518	23.75%	Atrioventricular septal defect
22q11 microdeletion	93 [93 + 63 = 156]	4.26% (7.0%)*	Conotruncal heart defects
7q11.23 microdeletion	28 [28 + 19 = 47]	1.3%(2.15%)*	Supravalvular aortic stenosis/Peripheral pulmonary stenosis
Monosomy X	6	0.3%	Left-sided cardiac lesions
Other chromosomal abnormalities	47 (partial deletions/duplications, translocations, Ring chromosomes, microdeletions, microduplications, trisomy 18, trisomy 13, mosaics, etc.)	2.15%	
Total	662	30.35%	

#Narayana Institute of Cardiac Sciences
* Figures indicate FISH proven patients of deletions and in the bracket indicate both FISH proven deletions and clinically diagnosed patient

related disorders, isolated CHD), cilliopathies (Ellis-van Creveld syndrome, hetrotaxy), and H3K4 methylation pathways genes (Isolated sporadic CHD, Kabuki syndrome, CHARGE syndrome, Schinzel-Giedion syndrome). All the recent studies indicate that single genes account for more CHDs than earlier reports and many more genes need to be discovered.

Clinical presentation in single gene CHD is highly variable. The phenotype could be isolated CHD, CHD with one additional major malformation and CHD with multisystem involvement. Table 10.6 gives the list of some of single genes causing syndromic CHD and isolated CHD. Prognosis and management depends on the severity of CHD and associated extracardiac malformations and neurological involvement.

Common Single Gene Disorder Syndromic CHD

Noonan Syndrome and Related Disorders

Noonan syndrome is one of the commonest cause of syndromic short stature with or without congenital heart disease. Noonan syndrome (NS) is a genetic disorder inherited as an autosomal dominant disorder, first described by Dr Jacqueline Noonan. Incidence of Noonan syndrome ranges from 1 in 1,000 to 1 in 2,500 live births as reported in western literature. Clinical manifestations include characteristic face (hypertelorism with down slant eyes, low set posteriorly rotated ears), congenital heart defect, variable degree of intellectual disability, undescended testis in males, webbed neck, short stature, chest deformity and bleeding tendencies. Abnormal coagulation profile reported in various studies ranges from 20-30%. Commonest abnormality is factor XI deficiency. Other features include feeding difficulties, café-au-lait spots, pigmented nevi, scoliosis, unexplained hepatosplenomegaly, urinary tract malformations, acute leukemia and myeloproliferative disorders.

Congenital heart disease is seen in 50-80% of the cases. Commonest cardiac lesions are pulmonary stenosis and hypertrophic cardiomyopathy (HCM). Pulmonary stenosis was seen in 65% of cases and HCM in 19% of cases with NS. Periodic cardiac evaluation is necessary in cases with initial normal cardiac assessment, to find evolving HCM.

Majority of the cases are sporadic. Inherited as autosomal dominant disorder, risk of recurrence in familial cases is 50%. In sporadic cases, empiric risk of recurrence is 1-5%.

There are Noonan-like conditions described in the literature with marked overlapping features. Underlying genetic cause explains the overlapping manifestations. All the genes causing NS and Noonan-like conditions are the genes of RAS-ERK pathway, a pathway involved in cell proliferation, growth and death.

Various Noonan-like conditions described are Costello syndrome, cardiofaciocutaneous syndrome, LEOPARD syndrome, Noonan syndrome with neurofibromatosis and Noonan-like with multiple gaint-cell lesion syndrome. Mutation screening the RAS-ERK pathway genes can detect mutations in 60-80% of the cases of NS and Noonan-like conditions, suggestive of genetic heterogeneity and other unidentified genes (Fig. 10.43).

CHARGE Syndrome

With the discovery of single gene basis, CHARGE association is now known as CHARGE syndrome. Prevalence of 1 in 10,000. Other than ocular coloboma, choanal atresia, heart defects, growth retardation, genital anomalies and ear anomalies for which acronym stands for, features like hypoplasia of semicircular canals, facial dysmorphism,

Table 10.6: Single genes causing CHD

Type of isolated CHD (phenotype MIM number)	Single gene Isolated* (Inheritance)	Single gene syndromic CHD (Inheritance)♣
Tetralogy of Fallot (#187500)	JAG1, NKX2-5, GATA4, ZFPM2, GDF1, GJA1, FOG2, GATA6, HAND2), NKX2-5, TBX1, ALDH1A2, CFC1, NODAL, TDGF1 (AD$^\theta$)	CHARGE syndrome (CHD7) (AD)
Bicuspid aortic valve (#614823,#109730)	GATA5, NOTCH1, SMAD6(AD), TAB2	Turner syndrome#
Atrioventricular canal defects (#600309,#606217,#606215)	CRELD1 (AD), GJA1(Connexin 43) (AR$^\beta$), GATA4,GATA6,TBX5,AVCR1/ALK2,CFC1,LEFTY2, NODAL (AD)	Orofacial digital syndrome (AR,AD), Ivemark syndrome (AR)
Supravalvular aortic stenosis (#185500)	ELN (AD)	William syndrome (7q11.23 deletion) (AD)#
Atrial (108800) and ventricular septal defects	NKX2-5,TBX5, GATA4 (AD), TLL1(AD) TBX20, CITED2, GATA6, IRX4, NKX2-5, TBX20, ZIC3(XLD$^\gamma$), CFC1, TDGF1(AD), CASZ1, ACTC1	Holt-Oram syndrome (TBX5) (AD) Ellis-van Creveld syndrome (EVC/2) (AR) Kabuki syndrome (KMT2D, KDM6A) (AD/X-linked), Mowat-Wilson syndrome (ZEB2)(AD) Thrombocytopenia absent radius syndrome (R8BM8A)(AR)
Pulmonary stenosis (265550)	PTPN11, JAG1, NOTCH2, GATA4, GATA6, ZIC3, ACVR2B, ELN (AD)	Alagille syndrome (JAG1/ NOTCH2) (AD) Noonan and Noonan-like related syndrome (ERK-RAS Pathway genes) - PTPN11, KRAS, SOS1, RAF1, MEK1, HRAS, NF1, SHOC2, CBL) (AD/AR)
Hypoplastic left heart (#241550)	GJA1, NKX2-5, ZIC3, NOTCH1, NR2F2 (AD), RBFOX2	Oculodentodigital syndrome (GJA1) (AD/AR)
Common truncus/ Conotruncal anomaly	NKX2-6 (AR), NKX2-5, TBX1(AD), CFC1, GDF1, GATA6	22q11 deletion (DGS/VCFS) (AD)#, Renal-hepatic-pancreatic-dysplasia (NEK8) (AR)
Coarctation of aorta	NKX2-5/NKX2.5, LEFTY2	Turner syndrome#, PHACE syndrome@
Ebstein anomaly (224700)	MYH7	
Transposition of great vessels(D-TGA)(#608808)	THRAP2, CFC1, GDF1, MED13L, NKX2-5, ZIC3, ACVR2B, FOXH1, LEFTY2, NODAL, MYH6, ISL1	Less likely to be singe gene CHD syndrome or chromosomal
Patent ductus arteriosus (%607411) (#169100)	GTATA6, TFAP2B, MYH11, PRDM6	Char syndrome (TFAP2B) (AD)
Tricuspid atresia (605067)	NFATC1	

* Single genes associated with isolated CHD can also cause other types of CHD
♣ Syndromes are listed in the row based on common cardiac defects found.
Some of the chromosomal disorders are included in the table with common and typical cardiac lesions associated
@ Underlying gene defect not known, θ AD – Autosomal dominant, β AR – Autosomal recessive, γ XLD – X-linked disorder

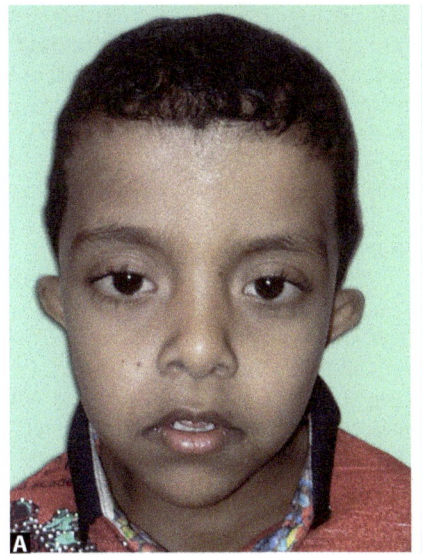
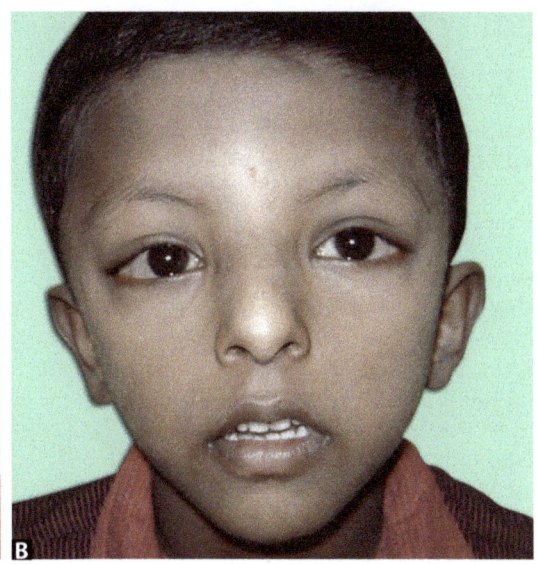

Figs 10.43A and B. Single gene disorders: (A) Noonan syndrome phenotype; (B) Kabuki syndrome

brain stem dysfunction and arhinencephaly have been described. CHD are seen in 50–85% of the cases. Common cardiac lesions are conotruncal heart defects, tetralogy of Fallot being the commonest among conotruncal heart lesions.

CHD7 gene mutations have been identified in 75% of the cases suspected with CHARGE syndrome. Semicircular canal abnormalities seem to be commonest defect seen in *CHD7* gene mutations. Autosomal dominant inheritance with variable expression is known. There are many chromosomal aberrations reported with CHARGE syndrome. *SEMA3E* is the other gene shown to be associated with CHARGE syndrome.

Ellis-van Creveld syndrome

Ellis-van creveld syndrome (EVCS) is an autosomal recessive disorder caused by mutation in the two genes EVC and EVC2. Clinical features are short limbs, postaxial polydactyly, dystrophic nails, missed cleft-lip (partial hare-lip), and CHD. CHD is seen in 60% of the cases with EVCS, commonest cardiac lesion being septal defects.

OTHER CAUSES OF CHD

- **Epigenetic alterations:** Abnormal methylation of certain genes (*NKX2-5, HAND1*), global hypomethylation; **Somatic mutations**—mutations restricted to cardiac tissue causing CHD (*NKX2-5,TBX5,GATA4*).
- **Environmental exposures:** It is expected to contribute for origin of CHD in as many as 13–30% of cases in some specific subtypes of CHDs and to name few of environmental exposures: organic solvents, organochlorine pesticides.
- **Maternal conditions and drugs:** Pre-existing diabetes or gestations diabetes, drugs like anticonvulsants, retinoic acid, substance abuse—caffeine, cocaine alcohol, infections—rubella virus.

SUGGESTED READING

1. Blue GM, Kirk EP, Giannoulatou E, Dunwoodie SL, Ho JW, Hilton DC, et al. Targeted next-generation sequencing identifies pathogenic variants in familial congenital heart disease. Am Coll Cardiol. 2014;64(23):2498-506.
2. Chaoui R, Körner H, Bommer C, Göldner B, Bierlich A, Bollmann R. Prenatal diagnosis of heart defects and associated chromosomal aberrations. Ultraschall Med. 1999;20(5):177-84.
3. Ferencz C, Rubin JD, McCarter RJ, Brenner JI, Neill CA, Perry LW, et al. Congenital heart disease: prevalence at livebirth. The Baltimore-Washington Infant Study. Am J Epidemiol. 1985;121(1):31-6.
4. Geng J, Picker J, Zheng Z, Zhang X, Wang J, Hisama F, et al. Chromosome microarray testing for patients with congenital heart defects reveals novel disease causing loci and high diagnostic yield. BMC Genomics. 2014;17(15):1127.
5. Hoffman JI, Kaplan S, Liberthson RR. Prevalence of congenital heart disease. Am Heart J. 2014;147(3):425-39.
6. Jenkins KJ, Correa A, Feinstein JA, Botto L, Britt AE, Daniels SR, et al. American Heart Association Council on Cardiovascular Disease in the Young. Noninherited risk factors and congenital cardiovascular defects: current knowledge: a scientific statement from the American Heart Association Council on Cardiovascular Disease in the Young: endorsed by the American Academy of Pediatrics. Circulation. 2007;115(23):2995-3014.
7. Mitchell SC, Korones SB, Berendes HW. Congenital heart disease in 56,109 births. Incidence and natural history. Circulation. 1971;43(3):323-32.
8. Tennstedt C, Chauoui R, Korner H, Dietel M. Spectrum of Congenital heart defects and extracardiac manifestations associated with chromosomal abnormalities: results of a seven year necropsy study. Heart. 1999;82(1):34-9.
9. van der Linde D, Konings EE, Slager MA, Witsenburg M, Helbing WA, Takkenberg JJ, et al. Birth prevalence of congenital heart disease worldwide: a systematic review and meta-analysis. J Am Coll Cardiol. 2011;58(21):2241-7.
10. Zaidi S, Choi M, Wakimoto H, Ma L, Jiang J, Overton JD, et al. De novo mutations in histone-modifying genes in congenital heart disease. Nature. 2013;498(7453):220-3.

Genetic Counseling After Diagnosis of Fetal Congenital Heart Disease

Meenakshi Bhat

ABSTRACT

Antenatal diagnosis of a congenital heart defect (CHD) causes great anxiety to the parents and the extended family. Optimal management of the specific defect depends on the extent of cardiac and extra-cardiac involvement. With an increase in knowledge about cardiac development and the multitude of genes underlying every stage of fetal heart formation, it is imperative that in every pregnancy with a CHD, the underlying genetic etiology is sought for and identified. This is important for a family who may wish to know the long-term prognosis in the affected child after repair of the CHD, in planning future pregnancies and in preventing recurrences. Broadly, CHD can be classified as an isolated defect, as part of a genetic syndrome or as caused by teratogens in pregnancy. A detailed family history and clinical assessment will help plan appropriate genetic and metabolic tests. A discussion with the family regarding the genetic etiology and implications, long-term prognosis and prevention of recurrences all constitute genetic counseling. Counseling strategies in common conditions encountered in a cardiology clinic are discussed in this Chapter.

INTRODUCTION

Congenital heart disease (CHD) is the most common serious birth defect and accounts for 0.8–1% of all live births. In several large European studies, genetic syndromes accounted for around 2.4–3.6% of all cases of prenatally detected CHD. CHD has been described in association with nearly 800 genetic syndromes and chromosome aberrations. The three broad etiological categories in which most antenatally detected CHD are likely to belong are: Genetic syndromes, isolated CHD and CHD as a result of a teratogen in pregnancy.

For most families, the diagnosis of a CHD in the fetus may come as a huge shock. For the physician who may approach a defect based on its medical severity, it is important to realize that parents of a fetus with an atrial septal defect may be as distressed as those with hypoplastic left heart syndrome. The questions most commonly asked by the parents are: Why did this happen? What does it mean for the child? Is there a cure or treatment for this? Did it happen because of something the mother did or did not do in pregnancy? How will it affect my child with regard to life-span, career options, marriage and offspring risks? Will this happen again in another pregnancy? What can we do to prevent it from happening again? A detailed discussion regarding these queries forms the basis of genetic counseling.

An approach to genetic counseling in a family with a prenatal diagnosis of CHD begins with elucidation of detailed family history and risk factors. This is followed by appropriate diagnostic testing, discussion of results, prognosis and outcomes as well as recurrence risks.

Family History

Details of other family members with CHD including the type of defect and outcome, known genetic syndromes in the family, parental consanguinity, history of infertility and assisted reproduction, therapeutic medications or surgery in either parent, smoking and alcohol intake, parental height and weight.

Pregnancy

Single or multiple conception, number of previous pregnancies and outcome, maternal diabetes, hypothyroidism or phenylketonuria, infections and fever in first trimester, periconceptional folic acid and other medications in pregnancy with dosage and duration of therapy.

Fetal Ultrasound and ECHO Findings

Increased nuchal translucency, CHD with other cardiac markers (EIF, ARSA, dextrocardia, etc.) and extracardiac anomalies. An anomaly scan should include growth parameters of the fetus and document any asymmetry or situs inversus, frontal and lateral facial profile including clefts, structural brain abnormalities and head size, ocular abnormalities including cataracts, external ear abnormalities on either side, distal limb abnormalities, poly- or oligodactyly, abnormalities of renal size and shape, genital ambiguity and spine shape, measurement of long bones, amniotic fluid quantity for polyhydramnios, oligohydramnios or hydrops. The importance of each of these factors has been discussed in previous chapters. These findings will help determine the most appropriate genetic and biochemical tests in pregnancy.

Genetic Testing

For an affected pregnancy, it is preferable that a fetal sample is taken antenatally rather than after the pregnancy has been discontinued. Testing in pregnancy is done by chorionic villus sampling or CVS (11 weeks of gestation onwards), amniocentesis (from 16 weeks) and very occasionally by fetal cord blood sampling.

Testing for genetic abnormalities can be done by a variety of techniques: Chromosome studies (karyotype) in case of aneuploidies, fluorescence in situ hybridization (FISH) where a microdeletion is suspected and specific DNA tests in single gene conditions. Newer techniques such as array CGH and exome sequencing are used where extended testing is necessary. It is extremely important to preserve a sample for DNA storage from the fetus for future studies where a conclusive diagnosis has not been achieved.

Results are obtained in one to several weeks with most genetic tests. A second meeting is then arranged with the family to explain the results, and to discuss implications and possible intervention. In cases where the cardiac anomaly is detected in late second trimester, intervention may need to precede genetic test results. If the fetus has a chromosomal abnormality, it is necessary to also test both parents to determine if the abnormality has occurred de novo in the fetus or is inherited from a parent. This information also enables the genetic counselor to calculate recurrence risks and suggest appropriate testing in a future pregnancy.

A consultation with the pediatric cardiologist (and surgeon) may help in planning the most appropriate modality of delivery and optimum assessment for surgical intervention after birth. However, if the parents decide to discontinue an affected pregnancy, the counselor will suggest genetic tests and a perinatal autopsy where appropriate to confirm the diagnosis of an underlying genetic condition.

COUNSELING IN COMMON GENETIC SYNDROMES WITH A CONGENITAL HEART DEFECT

Down's Syndrome

With a birth frequency of around 1 in 700, Down syndrome (DS) is the commonest syndrome associated with CHD. About 50% of all DS have CHD with AVSD being the commonest cardiac defect (65%). It is postulated that AVSD in DS occurs as a result of the extra chromosome 21 dosage effects on potentially damaging genetic variants in the VEGF-A gene pathway. Prenatally, DS is usually suspected when a first trimester scan shows increased nuchal translucency, hypoplastic nasal bone, cardiac and other anomalies along with elevated serum screening risks. Invasive testing by CVS or amniocentesis followed by FISH for chromosome 21 markers and a karyotype test is usually done. Newer tests such as multiplex ligation-dependent probe amplification (MLPA), Quantitive fluorescence polymerase (QF-PCR) and non-invasive testing of cell-free fetal DNA (cfDNA) in maternal circulation may also be used in diagnosis. In multiple pregnancies, testing the amniotic sac of the fetus showing features suggestive of DS or a cardiac abnormality may be necessary. Genetic testing determines if DS is caused by Trisomy 21 (95% cases), translocation (3–4%) or mosaic DS (around 1%). Chromosome mosaicism is usually identified by FISH testing.

Genetic Counseling

Counseling in a prenatally suspected case is different from postnatal counseling. In all types of DS, the couple needs to have a discussion with a trained counselor about the spectrum of clinical features seen in DS especially highlighting the universal association with intellectual disability. In India, where support services in child care, education and medical therapy for these affected individuals are few, most parents opt to discontinue an affected pregnancy. For couples who choose to continue, information about place of delivery, evaluation by a neonatologist at birth and planned cardiac intervention must be discussed and arranged.

Trisomy 21 Down's Syndrome

It is the commonest type with three copies of chromosome 21 seen in a karyotype or on FISH (Fig. 10.44). This is usually a sporadic 'one-off' occurrence and parental testing is not warranted. If the mother is aged <40 years in a subsequent pregnancy, recurrence risks are less than 1%. In the next pregnancy, a normal nuchal translucency (NT) scan with first trimester serum screening is usually reassuring to most couples. In very anxious couples at low risk, definitive prenatal tests may be offered after discussion of miscarriage risks related with invasive testing.

Translocation Down's Syndrome

The extra copy of chromosome 21 is attached end on end with an acrocentric chromosome (13, 14, 15, 21, 22). This is also called a Robertsonian translocation. If the fetal karyotype shows a translocation, it is mandatory that both parents' karyotypes are also checked for translocation carrier status. If a parent is a carrier, recurrence risks are increased and definitive prenatal diagnosis should be offered in subsequent pregnancies. In the rare event of a 21:21 translocation where a parent is also a carrier, recurrence risks are 100% in every pregnancy. Assisted reproduction with gamete donation by a non-relative may then be considered.

Mosaic Down's Syndrome

True chromosome mosaicism occurs with a mixed population of cells (usually normal

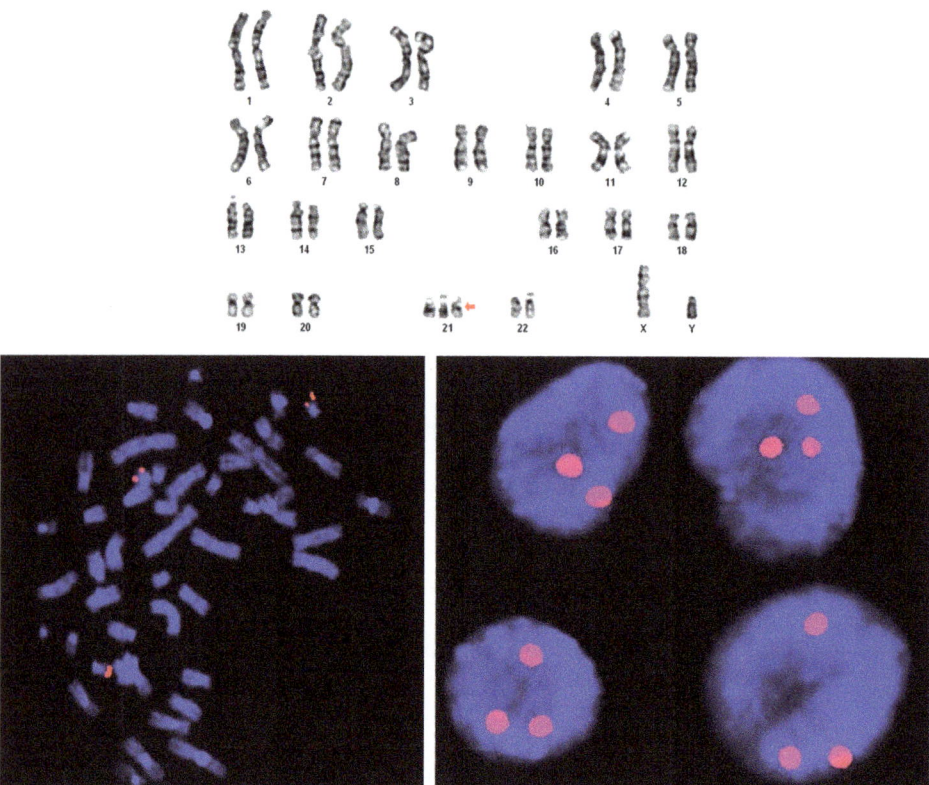

Fig. 10.44: Karyotype and FISH studies in an individual with Down's syndrome showing three copies of chromosome 21
(Images from Centre for Human Genetics, Bengaluru)

and abnormal) and commonly detected by FISH testing. If the prenatal tissue tested is a CVS sample, it is advisable to repeat the investigation in amniotic fluid to rule out confined placental mosaicism. As chromosome mosaicism is the outcome of a post-zygotic cell division error, it is unlikely to recur and parents need not be tested. Counseling should be cautiously optimistic about milder clinical involvement and intellectual disability. The percentage of mosaic affected cells in the fetal sample may not always correlate with the severity or extent of the phenotype.

Chromosome 22q11 Microdeletion Syndrome

Also encompasses the spectrum of velocardiofacial and DiGeorge syndromes. A small percentage of individuals diagnosed with CHARGE syndrome and Cayler asymmetric crying facies syndrome may also have chromosome 22q11 microdeletion. Conotruncal anomalies are seen in 75% of all cases with chromosome 22q11 microdeletion. Conversely, chromosome 22q11 microdeletion should always be tested for in an affected pregnancy with conotruncal CHD

is made. In a large study with over 250 cases of chromosome 22q11 microdeletion, the frequency of cardiac defects was TOF (20%), interrupted aortic arch (13%), VSD (14%) and truncus arteriosus (5.5%). Intellectual difficulty is seen in nearly 90% and overt psychosis or schizophrenia may develop in around 25% from the second decade. Other abnormalities detectable in an antenatal ultrasound include one or more of the following—increased nuchal translucency, dysplastic external ears, cleft palate, thymus dysplasia, renal abnormality, polydactyly, club foot and polyhydramnios.

Genetic Counseling

If the fetus has a conotruncal cardiac anomaly, the couple needs to be counseled about testing for chromosome 22q11 microdeletion. It is important for the couple to know that presence of a microdeletion in the fetus does not predict the severity of clinical findings or intellectual disability after birth. If the test confirms 22q11 microdeletion in the fetus, both parents should be offered testing for the same. In around 10% of cases, one parent (more often the mother) will have the same deletion, but usually with milder clinical involvement. Offspring of affected individuals have a 50% chance of inheriting the 22q11.2 deletion in each pregnancy. In a couple where one parent is affected, definitive prenatal testing by CVS or amniocentesis is recommended in each pregnancy. Testing in Indian laboratories is usually done by FISH using TUPLE or N25 probes. About 85% of individuals have the classical 3 Mb deletion containing around 40 genes. The newer prenatal genetic tests available are by MLPA, chromosomal array CGH and more recently cfDNA.

If both parents have no microdeletion, recurrence in a future pregnancy is around 1% (gonadal mosaicism risk). For low-risk pregnancies, a detailed ultrasound scan in pregnancy including fetal echocardiography from the 16th week onwards is advised.

Cardiac Rhabdomyoma

About 0.016% of pregnancies diagnosed with cardiac tumors, rhabdomyomas account for over 60%. Most originate in the ventricular surface or septum and are usually detected in the 3rd trimester of pregnancy. Rhabdomyomas may be single or multiple and the majority regresses in infancy. About 50% of single rhabdomyomas and nearly all multiple rhabdomyomas are associated with tuberous sclerosis (TS). TS is a rare genetic disorder caused by mutations in one of two genes *TSC1* and *TSC2* and the noncardiac manifestations include cortical and optic hamartomas, intellectual disability and seizures, dermatological and renal abnormalities.

Genetic Counseling

For a couple whose fetus has a cardiac rhabdomyoma, counseling about features of tuberous sclerosis (cognitive disability and autism, dermatological markers and epilepsy) is essential. In the fetus, it is important to check kidneys for angiomyolipomas and a fetal MRI (from 26 weeks gestation) for cortical tubers and subependymal nodules. If any other abnormality suggestive of TS is seen in the fetus, gene testing of TSC1 and 2 is recommended. Identifying a mutation confirms the diagnosis in the fetus. Two-thirds of simplex cases have a TSC2 mutation. Around one-third of cases have an affected parent. Complete evaluation of both parents from head to toe for dermatological signs along with an ophthalmological examination for retinal hamartomas and renal ultrasound for angiomyolipomas is recommended. If a parent is affected (and confirmed by gene testing), the fetus has a 50% chance of inheriting the faulty gene in each subsequent pregnancy. Definitive prenatal diagnosis is by testing a CVS or amniocentesis sample for the familial mutation. If neither parent has a mutation, there is a 1–2% gonadal mosaicism recurrence risk. Tertiary level antenatal scans for cardiac, renal and neurological anomalies are suggested in these cases.

Teratogens

Although, teratogens are not strictly genetic, most teratogens are believed to cause detrimental effects in the developing fetus by adversely affecting important genetic pathways during embryogenesis. The list of therapeutic and environmental agents predisposing to fetal CHD is extensive and only the commonest conditions in practice are discussed here. These include maternal disorders such as perigestational diabetes mellitus and phenylketonuria (PKU), therapeutic medications in pregnancy: Anticonvulsants and vitamin A derivatives, maternal infection in pregnancy including Rubella other TORCH infections.

Maternal Diabetes Mellitus and Obesity

Pregestational and undetected Type II diabetes mellitus (DM) in pregnant women under 7 weeks of pregnancy predisposes to CHD in the fetus. A wide range of defects including laterality and looping abnormalities, conotruncal, septal defects and cardiomyopathy have been described. Prepregnancy evaluation of blood sugar levels and strict glycemic control in early pregnancy is advised in the reduction of these CHDs. Obesity in pregnancy has been the subject of various recent studies. Maternal obesity (BMI >26 kg/m^2) as an independent factor has been associated with a 2–6.5-fold increase in causation of CHD in the fetus.

Maternal Phenylketonuria

With very few exceptions, most adult cases of phenylketonuria (PKU) in India are undiagnosed and untreated. The resulting intellectual disability precludes most affected women from getting married or bearing children. In published literature, the risk of CHD is increased six-fold in mothers with high phenylalanine (PA) levels with the commonest heart defects being TOF, VSD and PDA. Management includes strict control of levels of PA <360 mg/dL periconceptionally either by special diet or the use of sapropterin, a new oral medication.

Anticonvulsant Therapy

Around 1% of all women in the childbearing age group are estimated to be on anticonvulsant therapy. Polytherapy is reported to have greater teratogenic effects than monotherapy. In a planned pregnancy, gradual reduction of the number and dosage of medications is advised under medical guidance. Carbamezepine is the preferred medication with least risk of teratogenesis. The risk of adverse fetal outcomes is greater with maternal convulsions in pregnancy than with polytherapy and therefore medications should not be altered rapidly during a pregnancy. Medications such as hydantoin and valproate have a higher association with fetal CHD. Periconceptional folic acid should be advised in all women on anticonvulsant therapy for prevention of CHD and neural tube defects.

Vitamin A Derivatives

Usually prescribed for dermatological conditions, topical preparations are unlikely to have significant teratogenic effects. Oral intake is likely to cause an embryopathy with craniofacial and limb defects and CHD including outflow tract anomalies, pulmonary stenosis and VSDs. It is important to emphasize that oral vitamin A derivatives are strictly contraindicated in early pregnancy and are also known to remain in the maternal circulation at significant levels several months after discontinuation of therapy.

Maternal Rubella Infection

Congenital rubella infection causes CHD (PDA, branch and main pulmonary artery stenosis and VSD), cataracts, hearing loss and intellectual disability. Prepregnancy evaluation of a woman for rubella immune status and immunization before pregnancy is very effective. Recurrences are possible if the next pregnancy occurs in quick succession.

Maternal Hyperthermia

Any febrile illness in the first trimester that causes maternal hyperthermia increases the risk of CHD two-fold. Any type of CHD can occur and research studies done have not yet established if the CHD occurs as an effect of the febrile illness alone or the combined effects of underlying infection and medications used for treatment.

Prepregnancy Counseling and Teratogens

Detailed prepregnancy assessment about all therapeutic and recreational agents taken by the mother, dental hygiene, hemoglobin values, urinary infection, rubella immunization, information about previously affected pregnancies, evaluation of blood sugar levels and assessment of glycemic control, other metabolic conditions such as hypothyroidism, hyperphenylalaninemia and obesity management is important. The difficulty with optimal prepregnancy management is the fact that most pregnancies are unplanned. Even in the US, it is estimated that 50% of pregnancies are unplanned. One way of addressing, this issue may be to offer prepregnancy evaluation in all women just after marriage, so that they are aware of optimal care in pregnancy. Prescription of periconceptional folic acid and multivitamins in all women planning a pregnancy helps in reducing the incidence of non-syndromic CHD in the fetus. The prepregnancy appointment may also provide an opportunity to educate the couple about the antenatal scans and other screening tests available in pregnancy.

GENETIC COUNSELING IN NONSYNDROMIC ISOLATED CHD

It is important to emphasize that a single type of cardiac defect may be caused by mutations in one of several different genes (e.g. as with TOF). This is known as a heterogeneous condition. Conversely, many different types of heart defects may be caused by genetic mutations in a single gene (e.g. *NKX2-5*). Table 10.6 shows some of the single genes associated with specific congenital heart lesions. For a prenatally detected specific CHD, if other systemic associations are excluded, the geneticist may plan appropriate tests to confirm the fault in a specific gene. With the availability of newer genetic investigations that test several genes at a time (exome sequencing, panel-based next generation sequencing), the likelihood of identifying a causative mutation is maximized. Finding the underlying genetic cause in a specific cardiac defect enables counseling, cascade screening of relatives, calculating recurrence and planning definitive tests early in a subsequent pregnancy.

Table 10.6: Single gene mutations causing non-syndromic congenital heart defect

Cardiac defect	Chromosome location	Gene symbol	Gene name	Syndromes associated
TOF	22q11.2	TBX-1	T-Box 1	Chromosome 22q11 microdeletion
TOF	20p12	JAG1	Jagged 1	Alagille syndrome
TOF	8p23	GATA4	GATA binding protein 4	
TOF	5q34	NKX2-5	NK2 transcription factor related (locus 5)	
AVSD	5q34	NKX2-5	NK2 transcription factor related (locus 5)	
ASD with conduction defects	5q34	NKX2-5	NK2 transcription factor related (locus 5)	
ASD	8p23	GATA4	GATA binding protein 4	
Aortic valve defect	9q34.3	NOTCH 1	Notch 1	
Supravalvar aortic stenosis	7p11.2	ELN	Elastin	William's syndrome
Hypoplastic left heart syndrome	6q21-23	GJA1	Gap junction protein, alpha 1	
DORV	19p12	GDF1	Growth differentiation factor 1	
TA	8p21	NKX2-6	NK2 transcription factor related (locus 6)	
TGA	12q24	MED13L	Mediator complex subunit 13-like	
TGA	2q21	CFC1	Cryptic family 1	
TGA	19p12	GDF1	Growth differentiation factor 1	

Abbreviations: ToF, tetralogy of Fallot; AVSD, atrioventricular septal defect; ASD, atrial septal defect; DORV, double outlet right ventricle; TA, tricuspid atresia; TGA, transposition of the great arteries.

RECURRENCE RISKS AND COUNSELING FOR ISOLATED CHD

Recurrence risks for an isolated congenital cardiac defect are empirically estimated at 2-3%. When two first degree relatives have CHD (similar or different in both), recurrence in a subsequent pregnancy is around 10%. Counseling includes advice about periconceptional folic acid and tertiary level antenatal ultrasound examination, including nuchal translucency scan (11-<14 weeks), anomaly scan and fetal echocardiography between 16-18 weeks gestation in all future pregnancies.

Folic Acid and Folic Acid Antagonists

Periconceptional folic acid given to the expectant mother has been studied to reduce the occurrence of CHD by approximately 40% with maximum reductions in VSDs and conotruncal defects. The optimal dose of folic acid in the prevention of CHD is not established although 0.8 mg/day has been suggested. In countries such as India where a significant proportion of individuals are strict vegetarians, vitamin B_{12} may be concurrently prescribed. Medications such as folic acid antagonists (e.g. Septran, Methotrexate) in the first trimester and homozygous *MTHFR* C677T mutations (mutations is both copies of the gene) in the mother (and in the fetus) can increase the likelihood of fetal CHD occurrence. It is important to emphasize that Folic acid supplementation does not decrease the risk of recurrence of CHD occurring as a part of a genetic syndrome.

SUGGESTED READING

1. Ackerman C, Locke AE, Feingold E, Reshey B, Espana K, Thusberg J, et al. An excess of deleterious variants in VEGF-A pathway genes in Down-syndrome-associated atrioventricular septal defects. Am J Hum Genet. 2012;91:646-59.
2. Au KS, Williams AT, Roach ES, Batchelor L, Sparagana SP, Delgado MR, et al. Genotype/phenotype correlation in 325 individuals referred for a diagnosis of tuberous sclerosis complex in the United States. Genet Med. 2007;9: 88-100.
3. Bassett AS, McDonald-McGinn DM, Devriendt K, Digilio MC, Goldenberg P, Habel A, et al. International 22q11.2 Deletion Syndrome Consortium. Practical guidelines for managing patients with 22q11.2 deletion syndrome. J Pediatr. 2011;159(2):332-9.
4. Bawle EV. Toward better counseling for down syndrome. Letter to the Editor. Genetics in Medicine. 2012;14 (1):168.
5. Brämswig S, Prinz-Langenohl R, Lamers Y, Tobolski O, Wintergerst E, Berthold HK, et al. Supplementation with a multivitamin containing 800 microgram of folic acid shortens the time to reach the preventive red blood cell folate concentration in healthy women. Int J Vitam Nutr Res. 2009;79: 61-70.
6. Chakravarti A, Kapoor A. Genetics and genomics in cardiovascular gene discovery. Cardiac muscle. Fundamental biology and mechanisms of disease. Edited by: Joseph Hill. Elsevier Inc., 2012;231-59.
7. Czeizel AE, Dudás I, Vereczkey A, Bánhidy F. Folate deficiency and folic acid supplementation: the prevention of neural-tube defects and congenital heart defects. Nutrients. 2013;5:4760-75.
8. Jenkins KJ, Correa A, Feinstein JA, Botto L, Britt AE, Daniels SR, et al. Noninherited risk factors and congenital cardiovascular defects: Current knowledge. A scientific statement from the American Heart Association Council on Cardiovascular Disease in the Young. Circulation. 2007;115:2995-3014.
9. McDonald-McGinn DM, Kohut T, Zackai EH. Deletion 22q11.2 (velo-cardio-facial syndrome/DiGeorge syndrome). In: Cassidy SB, Allanson JE, (Eds). Management of genetic syndromes. 3rd Edition. Hoboken, NJ: Wiley-Blackwell. 2010;263-84.
10. Meberg A, Otterstad JE, Froland G, Lindberg H, Sorland SJ. Outcome of congenital heart defects–a population-based study. Acta Paediatr. 2000;89:1344-51.
11. Stoll C, Clementi M. Prenatal diagnosis of dysmorphic syndromes by routine fetal ultrasound examination across Europe. Ultrasound Obstet Gynecol. 2003;21:543-51.
12. Wang, W, Wang, Y, Gong F. MTHFR C677T polymorphism and risk of congenital heart defects: Evidence from 129 case-control and TDT studies. PLoS One. 2013;8:e58041.
13. Winter and Baraitser, London Dysmorphology Database, 2013.

CHAPTER 11

Management of Pregnancy after Prenatal Diagnosis of Congenital Heart Disease

Sunita Maheshwari

ABSTRACT

Management of the mother and fetus after a diagnosis of CHD is made prenatally depends on the nature of the disease and its likely outcome. It involves extensive counseling by an inter disciplinary caring team. Future counseling for subsequent pregnancies assumes importance as well and should include discussion on preconceptual folic acid and a detailed fetal echo at 16-20 weeks. This Chapter discusses in detail both dealing with the current pregnancy as well as planning for future ones.

INTRODUCTION

Pregnancy is meant to be a joyous time. When a doctor needs to break the news that the unborn child has congenital heart disease (CHD), apart from the medical counseling, family counseling and support is of the essence as well. This chapter is divided into 2 sections: (1) management of the mother and baby after a diagnosis of CHD is made prenatally and (2) the counseling that is needed thereafter.

Management of the Mother and Baby

Management of the Pregnancy

In general, mothers to be are advised to continue their normal routine for the rest of the pregnancy, i.e. good nutrition, multivitamins with folic acid, iron, daily exercise and to stay hydrated and rested. It is ideal if full-term can be reached, so that the baby has the optimal chance of growth predelivery.

There are certain instances where maternal delivery of medications may be required, e.g. a baby with a cardiac anomaly and associated supraventricular tachycardia where the mother may need to be administered an antiarrhythmic agent such as flecainide or sotalol in order for transplacental delivery to occur to the fetus. Similarly, in cases where a fetal procedure is planned, e.g. in cases of critical aortic stenosis where in a transplacental valvuloplasty is attempted, the mothers space then needs to be breached. In such cases, a multidisciplinary collaborative team is necessary.

In certain situations, if the CHD is not compatible with life or if life involves several complicated procedures postdelivery with uncertain outcomes, the family may elect to terminate the pregnancy. Under the Indian Act, medical termination is permitted up to 20 weeks of gestation. Such lesions could include hypoplastic left heart syndrome (HLHS), complex single ventricle situations, pulmonary atresia ventricular septal defect (VSD) with multiple collaterals, severe Ebsteins with hydrops fetalis, etc.

In terms of delivery options, when there is a fetus with CHD, it is preferable to deliver the baby via normal vaginal delivery. This is done to avoid a cesarean section scar for future pregnancies, in case the baby does not survive postnatally. The second stage of labor can be shortened with a forceps. However, for maternal or fetal indications such as fetal distress or preeclampsia/small pelvis, etc., a cesarean section may be indicated.

Management of the Baby

When a fetus is diagnosed with CHD, follow-up needs to be done at regular intervals to assess whether anything has worsened (e.g. a fetus with Ebsteins developing hydrops fetalis, pulmonary stenosis converting to atresia, HLHS with an evolving coarctation, etc., which could change fetal or postnatal management). Alternatively, on follow-up, things may have improved (e.g. a VSD getting smaller overtime). Of essence is to decide whether the fetus is in impending distress requiring early delivery or whether pregnancy can be continued to term.

Counseling

Family counseling is essential when a baby is diagnosed with CHD.

Who and Why

In the Indian context, the first question that the family has is 'whose fault is this' or 'why did this happen'? It is important to explain to them that it is not the mothers fault, that genes are carried from both sides, and that many times these are de novo issues since approximately 75% of CHD have no identifiable cause or underlying condition. The second question is whether anything done in pregnancy could have caused this. Again, important to ensure that the parents do not feel guilt. The heart, as is well known, develops by 6 weeks of pregnancy. Barring drug/nicotine ingestion or an unpredictable event such as a viral illness that can cause CHD, there is not very much a pregnant woman can do to prevent CHD in her unborn child, and it is certainly not related to the quantity of food or activities done that most mothers worry about as being the cause of the heart disease.

What Will Need to be Done

Once guilt is removed from the discussion, the next question is what needs to be done next, i.e. 'what will happen to my child?' If the diagnosis is made early in pregnancy, i.e. before 20 weeks, the main counseling is related to outcomes of the CHD postnatally. Minor lesions may cause major stress but require no intervention and therefore, essentially only reassurance of the parents is needed. This would include cardiac lesions such as small VSD's, mild valvular stenosis, etc. In certain lesions, the family can be reassured that a onetime surgery is likely to be corrective. Such lesions include VSD's, primum or other atrial septal defect's (ASD), aortopulmonary window (APW), simple coarctation (CoA), tetralogy of Fallot (TOF), transposition of the great arteries (TGA), etc. In other lesions, the family needs to be explained that more than one surgery may be required and this decision will depend on the clinical situation postnatally, e.g. in truncus arteriosus, pulmonary atresia and their variants, atrioventricular canal, Ebsteins, etc. And then there are those lesions where the family needs to be warned that multiple surgeries will definitely be necessary at varying stages of life, potentially as early as soon after birth. These cardiac lesions include some varieties of pulmonary atresia and single ventricle hearts.

One of the problems with prenatal counseling is the wide variety of presentation of various cardiac lesions with the same lesion needing one or more surgeries and having variable prognosis. An example of this quandary is tetralogy of Fallot where it was initially felt that a onetime repair was sufficient but later studies demonstrated the possible need for further intervention later in life. Although, the vast majority of children will be functional long-term after intracardiac repair some will require a pulmonary valve placement at some point in life. Therefore, counseling gets confusing for the parents as there are so many variables and unknowns from fetal life to adulthood. Having said that, it is important for pediatric cardiologists and fetal medicine specialists to explain the lesion and all possible outcomes, so the family can be mentally prepared as well as take an informed decision regarding continuation versus termination.

With increasing survival, interest is increasingly focusing on quality of life and long-term outcomes, especially neurodevelopmental outcomes, which are a major area of concern for parents. Although these are of concern, the outcome cannot necessarily be predicted prenatally, so this is a gray area for counseling for the physicians involved.

Assess for Other Lesions

A detailed level III ultrasound needs to be performed to rule out other congenital lesions such as Down's syndrome, etc. Amniocentesis may be considered if there are other congenital anomalies and a chromosomal anomaly needs to be ruled out. A history of consanguinity and preconceptual folic acid consumption should be taken.

Future Pregnancy Counseling

Role of Folic Acid

Parents need to be advised that for the next pregnancy, they should have multivitamins and folic acid 3 months prior to conception and continuing into pregnancy.

When you start talking about folic acid for pregnant women, most people say 'Yes, I know about that and I took it'. The fact is that everyone knows they have to take folic acid during pregnancy. However, it is a less well-known fact that folic acid (400 mcg) taken 3 months before pregnancy, i.e. preconceptually has been to show reduce the incidence of congenital heart defects in the unborn child.

Folic acid, also known as folate or folacin, is one of the B group of vitamins. Research suggests that it is hard for women to get enough folic acid by simply eating a balanced diet. Most pregnancies are not pre-planned and little attention is paid to the importance of a proper prenatal diet. The World Health Organization estimates that 43% of all women of reproductive age living in the developing world have iron and folic acid deficiency. The heart develops by 6 weeks of pregnancy, at a stage when a woman does not even know she is pregnant. Thus folic acid started during pregnancy is too late for its protective effect on the heart. The importance of prepregnancy folic acid therefore, needs to be stressed upon the family contemplating their next conception.

Chance of Recurrence in the Next Pregnancy

A detailed fetal echocardiogram at 17-19 weeks of the next pregnancy is also advisable. The normal incidence of CHD is approximately

1%. Once there is a sibling with heart disease, the incidence increases to 2–3%. However, this still implies that 97% the next conception will have a normal fetal heart. Families therefore need to be reassured regarding this as fear exists vis-a-vis future pregnancies. However, left-sided obstructive lesions have higher associations within families. Similarly, autosomal dominant conditions have a 50% chance of recurrence in an offspring. Thus, multiple factors can contribute to a recurrence of CHD making accurate counseling difficult.

Another area that needs family discussion is cost of care involved postnatally and mode and place of delivery. In lesions that may potentially need intervention soon after birth, 'prenatal transport' is advisable, i.e. the mother delivers at a tertiary care center where cardiac facilities and care is available at birth. In situations where intervention is unlikely at birth, e.g. a large VSD, the family can proceed to have delivery at a convenient delivery center near them.

CONCLUSION

A diagnosis of CHD in a fetus is a traumatic experience for a parent. For adequate counseling of the family and management of the pregnancy, it is important that an interdisciplinary team handles the family, ideally consisting of the obstetrician, a pediatric cardiologist and a family social worker, if possible. Interestingly the prenatal diagnosis of congenital heart disease has now allowed a new subspecialty to develop, that of the fetal cardiologist.

KEY MESSAGE

Congenital heart disease in the unborn child requires not just cardiac, pregnancy and genetic counseling, but also social and financial discussions. A multi-team approach is the best approach in this situation.

SUGGESTED READING

1. Ammash NM, Dearani JA, Burkhart HM, Connolly HM. Pulmonary regurgitation after tetralogy of Fallot repair: Clinical features, sequelae, and timing of pulmonary valve replacement. Congenit Heart Dis. 2007;2:386-403.
2. Ferencz C, Rubin JD, Loffredo CA, Magee CM. The epidemiology of congenital heart disease. The Baltimore-Washington Infant Study (1981-1989). Perspectives in Pediatric Cardiology. volume 4. MountKisco, NY: Futura Publishing Co.Inc, 1993.
3. http://ncpcr.gov.in/view_file.php?fid=431
4. http://www.marchofdimes.org/pregnancy/take-folic-acid-before-youre-pregnant.aspx#
5. Loffredo CA, Chokkalingam A, Sill AM, et al. Prevalence of congenital cardiovascular malformations among relatives of infants with hypoplastic left syndrome, coarctation of the aorta, and d-transposition of the great arteries. Am J Med Genet A. 2004;124(3):225-30.
6. McElhinney DB, Marshall AC, Wilkins-Haug LE, et al. Predictors of technical success and postnatal biventricular outcome after in utero aortic valvuloplasty for aortic stenosis with evolving hypoplastic left heart syndrome. Circulation. 2009;120:1482-90.
7. Nollert G, Fischlein T, Bouterwek S, Bohmer C, Klinner W, Reichart B. Long-term survival in patients with repair of tetralogy of Fallot: 36 year follow-up of 490 survivors of the first year after surgical repair. J Am Coll Cardiol. 1997; 30:1374-83.
8. Nora JJ, Nora AH. Genetic and environmental factors in the etiology of congenital heart disease. South Med J. 1976;69(7):919-26.
9. Stoll C, Alembik Y, Roth MP, et al. Risk factors in congenital heart disease. Eur J Epidemiol. 1989; 5(3):382-291.
10. Van Engelen AD, Weijtens O, Brenner JI, Kleinman CS, et al. Management, outcome and follow-up of fetal tachycardia. J Am Coll Cardiol. 1994;24:1371-5.
11. Wernovsky G. Outcomes regarding the central nervous system in children with complex congenital cardiac malformation. Cardiol Young. 2005;15(supl 1):132-33.

CHAPTER 12

Does Prenatal Detection of Heart Disease Improve the Outcome?

Sejal Shah

ABSTRACT

Fetal echo is a diagnostic and a therapeutic tool. In the current era, with advanced imaging facilities and better experience than ever, a lot is being done in the field of fetal cardiac medicine, landing us with an important question if all this is going to make a "difference".

This Chapter is to understand if diagnosis of a heart disease makes a difference in the short- and long-term outcome of heart disease.

INTRODUCTION

Prenatal diagnosis gives an opportunity for parenteral counseling and also provides a 'window' to offer fetal treatment. Parenteral counseling can either lead to change in the perinatal management of the baby or consideration for termination of pregnancy. Fetal treatment may alter the intrauterine course of the disease to a potential favorable outcome. Does this imply that prenatal diagnosis gives a survival advantage to infants born with congenital heart disease (CHD)? Identification of CHD in fetus allows us to intervene early and avoid life-threatening manifestations at birth. Whether better postnatal management of these heart conditions improves outcomes, especially long-term remains debatable.

While understanding the literature available on outcomes of antenatally diagnosed heart disease, following factors and limitations need to be understood.

- Outcomes of CHD diagnosed in antenatal period may be poor compared to those diagnosed in postnatal period as postnatal evaluation would happen on selected babies after excluding spontaneous intrauterine deaths and early neonatal unexplained deaths.
- The prenatal diagnosis on how to proceed with pregnancy would depend significantly on the way counseling is done regarding the long-term outcome of heart disease.
- There is a selection bias as cases that are more likely to be diagnosed prenatally tend to be more severe cases.
- Extracardiac malformations and chromosomal anomalies often accompany cardiac diseases frequently resulting in termination of pregnancy.

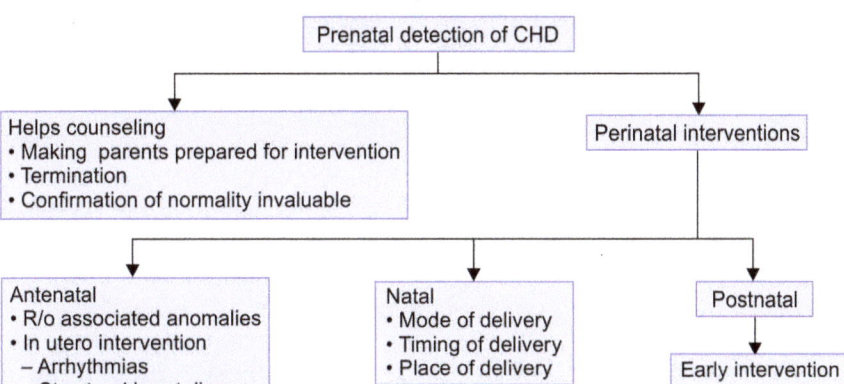

Flowchart 12.1: Role of prenatal detection of CHD

- The sample size in most of the studies has been limited.
- Improvement in neonatal care and general awareness of CHD amongst the pediatricians has helped in aggressive treatment with successful resuscitation of babies with CHD postnatally.

In spite of these limitations, we do understand that the outcome of CHD partly depends on the management done in utero and a successful transition from prenatal to postnatal life. This would depend on the basic anatomical diagnosis of congenital heart disease, associated atrioventricular/semilunar valve regurgitation, ventricular function, arrhythmias, size of ductus and foramen ovale and noncardiac issues.

The Flowchart 12.1 is showing the role of prenatal detection of CHD.

COUNSELING

Preparing Parents for Intervention

Diagnosing a heart defect gives an opportunity to the doctor to explain the parents about the cardiac condition, the possible symptoms at birth, the surgical intervention/s needed and prognosis in terms of quality and quantity of life. This understanding helps parents to come to terms to accepting the cardiac problem and mentally/financially getting ready to receive the baby and doing the best from their side.

Termination

Prenatal diagnosis gives an option of termination in situations where curative surgery postnatally is not feasible. Prenatal diagnosis hence is expected to have profound effect on the incidence of CHD in view of high rate of termination. A population-based study done in 2005 by Khoshnood B, et al. showed an increase in the termination rates after CHD was diagnosed and the most frequent CHD that was terminated was hypoplastic left heart syndrome (HLHS) and univentricular heart.

Reassurance when 'Normal Heart' Confirmed

This is invaluable information for the parents especially when they already have a baby with a heart disease. It is known that many families who have lost a child to CHD have been influenced in their decision to have a next child because of the availability of fetal echo. However, there are situations like 'disproportion between the right and left structures' wherein the natural history is unknown and it raises the possibility of CHD which may evolve further as pregnancy proceeds. Hence, this situation neither provides the assurance of a normal heart nor sufficient information to terminate pregnancy.

PERINATAL INTERVENTIONS

Antenatal Period

To Rule Out Associated Anomalies

It is important to look beyond the heart whenever a cardiac disease is suspected in the fetus. The reason behind this is the fact that there is 5-13% risk of having a chromosomal abnormality in presence of CHD and 25% of babies with complex CHD have extracardiac anomalies. Frequency of association with aneuploidies and/or extracardiac anomalies is highest for atrioventricular septal defect (48%) and lowest for corrected transposition of great arteries.

In utero Interventions

Prenatal treatment: Fetal cardiac intervention (FCI) is considered when either the fetus is at risk for demise due to CHD/arrhythmias OR intervention is expected to alter the evolution of the disease to an extent that the severity of postnatal disease is reduced. This is done if a feasible modality of treatment is available. FCI is expected to give no benefit to the mother, however can have risks to the fetus and/or the mother. Hence, it is considered only if the condition is serious, the potential benefits are higher and this can be achieved in reasonable number of cases.

- *Pharmacological treatment:* Fetal arrhythmias may lead to evolution of heart failure and may also be associated with neurological injury. Fetal echo not only helps us identifying the arrhythmias, defining the likely mechanism, identifying at risk fetus for cardiac failure, but also gives an opportunity to administer targeted treatment in antenatal and postnatal period to improve the outcome. Treatment of fetal arrhythmias has been the first documented prenatal therapy. It consists of maternal medications which transplacentally are delivered to fetus or direct administration through the umbilical vein/intramuscular/intravascular injection which is reserved for refractory cases. Indications for transplacental treatment include:
  - *Tachyarrhythmias:* Tranplacental treatment was first described in 1975 by Eibschitz, et al. for fetal tachyarrhythmia. Sustained fetal supraventricular arrhythmias is the most common indication (AV re-entry/atrial flutter). Digoxin has been the mainstay of treatment. Sotalol, amiodarone and flecainide are also used. Efficacy is more in nonhydropic infants. Early delivery needs to be considered if lungs are matured and there is evidence of hydrops. The outcome of most fetuses is excellent.
  - *Bradyarrhythmias:* Intervention is commonly considered for high degree atrioventricular (AV) block. Autoimmune complete heart block can be treated with dexamethasone to the mother with or without sympathomimetics. Multiple studies have shown that this does not reverse high grade AV block, though it may prevent the progression of first degree AV block to second/third degree AV block. Some studies have shown that dexamethasone with adrenergic agonists in presence of significant bradycardia may improve the overall prognosis of babies with auto immune AV block. However, there is no treatment that consistently reverses or prevents AV block in presence of maternal autoantibodies.

- **Fetal hydrops due to reasons other than arrhythmias:** Though efficacy is unknown, maternal treatment with Digoxin has been described in fetal hydrops due to Ebstein's anomaly, Tetralogy of Fallot with absent pulmonary valve, cardiac tumor, cardiomyopathy, etc.
- **Maternal hypoxia:** It has been used to assess placental function and treat IUGR and to assess pulmonary vasoreactivity in fetuses with HLHS, though benefits are not still clear.

- *Fetal cardiac intervention (FCI):*
  - **Open fetal cardiac intervention:** Challenges faced with open cardiac intervention include severe placental dysfunction, increase in cardiac after load on immature myocardium. Open FCI has been reported in complete AV block (pacemaker implantation) and tricuspid valve (TV) dysplasia with severe tricuspid regurgitation (TV repair), however, it is not considered a viable treatment strategy at present.
  - **Closed FCI:** FCIs are complex procedures with significant fetal morbidity and mortality with multiple issues related to fetal vascular access, fetal lie, variable amount of amniotic fluid and structural complexity.

Balloon aortic valvuloplasty (BAV) was first reported in 1989 in a fetus with aortic stenosis. Since then, FCIs have been done in aortic stenosis, HLHS with restriction of atrial septum, pulmonary atresia/stenosis with intact ventricular septum and AV block.

Balloon Aortic Valvuloplasty

It is considered for fetal aortic stenosis with evolving HLHS to alter the in utero natural history. It has shown improvement in the left heart physiology and growth of aortic and mitral valves but no apparent effect on left ventricular growth per se. Also, prenatal intervention is not a standalone intervention. Need for multiple interventions postnatally still stays. The potential collateral effects of FCI including any adverse neurological consequences are unknown.

Creation of atrial septal defect in hypo plastic left heart syndrome with restrictive atrial septum to arrest the development of abnormal pulmonary vasculopathy seems to have the potential to avoid immediate postnatal deterioration, though more experience is needed to decide postnatal survival benefit.

Pulmonary valve perforation and dilatation in pulmonary atresia with intact interventricular septum has the potential to promote right heart growth and functional development, and hence increasing the chance of having biventricular circulation postnatally.

Fetal epicardial pacing is still experimental in animals. This can be used for fetuses with hydrops secondary to complete heart block or incessant supraventricular tachycardia (where it can be pace terminated).

FCIs are feasible and encouraging; however, we have so far limited experience and much more needs to be learned about FCI's benefits and risks. The high-risks associated with FCI still say that these procedures are 'investigational' in nature and debatable.

Natal Period

Mode of Delivery

Vaginal delivery is satisfactory for most of the CHDs. CS is reserved for complete heart block when it is impossible to assess fetal well-being or in cases where there is a predicted need for early neonatal intervention/availability of a team. If neonatal demise is likely in a situation, perinatal palliative care may be considered and cesarean section should be avoided.

Timing of Delivery

Early delivery is advised in presence of hydrops (due to atrioventricular valve regurgitation, ventricular dysfunction, arrhythmias, complete heart block, cardiac tumors) and in cases of premature ductal or foramen ovale closure.

Place of Delivery

Delivery at a tertiary care center is ideal when early intervention is expected, like in ductal dependent lesion, transposition of great arteries and arrhythmias.

Postnatal Period

Fetal diagnosis of CHD helps us keep PGE1 ready, allows us to intervene soon and keep neonates in stable condition.

OVERALL OUTCOME AND INDIVIDUAL CONGENITAL HEART DISEASE-BASED OUTCOME

One of the initial studies conducted by Copel JA, et al. in 1997 wherein neonates with prenatal diagnosis of CHD were compared with those diagnosed after birth, did not show the expected result of improved survival and shorter initial hospitalization in the overall prenatally diagnosed group. However, survival benefit was seen amongst fetuses amenable to biventricular repair as compared to that requiring univentricular repair.

Later on in 2006, Brown KL, et al. conducted a study to assess whether the route by which neonatal CHD is first detected (antenatal diagnosis, detection in the postnatal ward and presentation after discharge to home) influences outcome after surgery. Though the route to recognition of CHD was not directly related to the outcome measures, it was found that poor presenting condition was most common when CHD was recognized later after the neonate has been discharged home and was least common when recognition was antenatal. Also there was a relationship between poor preoperative condition and worse outcome after cardiac surgery.

Hypoplastic Left Heart Syndrome

Hypoplastic left heart syndrome (HLHS) can be easily diagnosed in fetal life in the basic four chamber view. HLHS is expected to have sudden changes in the hemodynamics at birth leading to severe symptoms soon after delivery. Studies from 1997 to 1999 demonstrated improved preoperative condition of neonates with HLHS after prenatal diagnosis but believed that it may not significantly improve the preoperative mortality or early postoperative outcome amongst neonates managed at tertiary care center. As these studies were conducted several years earlier, they may not reflect the recent advances in optimal management of infants with HLHS. The first time in 2001, a study conducted by Twortzky W, et al. showed improved preoperative clinical status (lower incidence of acidosis, tricuspid regurgitation and ventricular dysfunction) and improved survival after first stage palliation when HLHS was diagnosed prenatally. In 2001, Mahle WT, et al. also showed reduction in early neurological morbidity when HLHS was diagnosed prenatally, however with no reduction in hospital mortality. In 2014, Morris, et al. showed increased neonatal mortality associated with increased distance from the birth center to cardiac surgical center hypothesizing that prenatal diagnosis of HLHS may significantly improve neonatal HLHS survival. The potential impact of prenatal diagnosis on long-term morbidities after Fontan operation, especially the neurocognitive outcome remains unknown; however a positive influence is expected.

Transposition of Great Arteries

Transposition of great arteries (TGA) is a CHD wherein dramatic changes may occur after birth leading to rapid hemodynamic compromise and sometimes death. At the same time, this CHD is amenable to total correction. Arterial switch operation is the operation of choice for TGA, which may sometimes not be feasible if the baby is referred late. Also, TGA is known to have low prevalence of extracardiac malformations and chromosomal anomalies which could have otherwise modify the postnatal outcome.

Study done by Bonnet, et al. in 1999 showed a comparison between preoperative and postoperative morbidity and mortality in neonates with prenatal diagnosis and in neonates with postnatal diagnosis of TGA over a period of 10 years. The results were as follows: (1) Clinical condition at arrival (metabolic acidosis and multiorgan failure) was worse in neonatal group, (2) Preoperative mortality was documented in the neonatal group and was zero in prenatal group, (3) Postoperative morbidity was not different, but the hospital stay was longer in the neonatal group, (4) Postoperative mortality was higher in the neonatal group. Hence, the conclusion was that the prenatal diagnosis of TGA reduces the morbidity and mortality.

Bartlett JM, et al. in 2004 revealed in small study that infants with TGA with intact ventricular septum/with ventricular septal defect with and with prenatal diagnosis differed in respect to perinatal and perioperative variables, but their neurodevelopment at one year of age was similar. Important observations made in the study also included a lower likelihood of birth by spontaneous labor, lower birth weights, lower Apgar 5 scores, higher rate of preoperative endotracheal intubation and surgery at a younger age in children with TGA with prenatal diagnosis as compared to those without prenatal diagnosis. Follow-up studies are necessary to determine later cognitive function as children approach school age.

Pulmonary Atresia with Intact Ventricular Septum

Daubeney PE, et al. in 1998 showed that the probability of survival at 1 year was the same for live born infants whether or not a fetal diagnosis has been made. Also it was noted that there was significant reduction in the live born incidence due to termination of pregnancy.

Coarctation of Aorta

It is a condition difficult to diagnose in fetal life given the number of false positive and false negative diagnoses possibility even in best hands. Coarctation can present postnatally with cardiovascular collapse and acidosis once the ductus arteriosus closes. Earlier studies from 1997-1998 (Copel JA, et al. Eapen RS, et al.) did not show improved survival as a result of antenatal diagnosis. However, in 2002, Franklin O, et al. showed improved survival and preoperative clinical condition when coarctation was diagnosed in antenatal period.

Truncus Arteriosus

Fetal diagnosis showed a younger age at repair, however did not show improved neonatal survival in a study done by Swanson TM, et al. in 2009.

Atrioventricular Septal Defect

Atrioventricular septal defect (AVSD) is a heterogeneous condition which can be diagnosed early in pregnancy with reasonable accuracy. It is often associated with additional cardiac lesions like conotruncal anomaly. In presence of aneuploidy, it is usually an isolated CHD. Associated heterotaxy syndrome is known with AVSD. Significant atrioventricular valve regurgitation can cause hydrops and result in poor prognosis. AVSD with heart block has worse prognosis. Hence, outcome of fetal AVSD depends on the associated lesions—cardiac and extracardiac prompting a detail evaluation.

AVSD diagnosed in utero has been shown to have poor prognosis. A part of this may be as more severe cases are likely to be detected in fetus, high incidence of pregnancy termination and spontaneous intrauterine deaths.

Absent Pulmonary Valve Syndrome

Absent pulmonary valve syndrome (APVS) can be diagnosed prenatally reliably and it is usually suspected by dilated pulmonary arteries. Extracardiac anomalies and major chromosomal anomalies including 22q11 deletion are common with APVS. According to Volpe P, et al. Bronchomalacia was present in majority of cases having cardiomegaly and marked branch pulmonary artery dilatation. Interestingly, the same study showed that all cases of APVS with intact ventricular septum had patent ductus arteriosus, lower branch pulmonary artery dilatation and were not associated with 22q11 deletion in contrast to APVS with tetralogy of Fallot. Prognosis of APVS when diagnosed in fetus is poor due to the fact that more critical ones are detected in fetal life, frequent association with genetic anomalies and common occurrence of bronchomalacia.

CONCLUSION

Prenatal diagnosis is advantageous in duct dependent systemic lesions like hypoplastic left heart syndrome/coarctation of aorta, duct dependent pulmonary lesion like pulmonary atresia, failure of mixing like transposition of great arteries and arrhythmias. Detection of cardiac conditions which can lead to early mortality if not detected and can be cured if treated timely would change the picture of these congenital heart diseases. Hence, prenatal detection of heart disease would improve the outcome in selected cases with complex cardiac malformations and arrhythmias. Fetal echo also enables us to detect heart disease as early as in first trimester and serial observations made subsequently helps us understand the evolution of cardiovascular pathologies seen after birth, thus helping us in better counseling. Prenatal evaluation of the heart has also given an insight into development—natural history of CHD, and hence has allowed us to develop a different bond with parents and also allowed a subspecialty 'Fetal cardiology' to develop.

SUGGESTED READING

1. Bartlett JM, Wypij D, Bellinger DC, Rappaport LA, Heffner LJ, Jonas RA, et al. Effects of prenatal diagnosis on outcomes in D-transposition of the great arteries. Pediatrics. 2004; 113:e335-40.
2. Copel JA, Tan ASA, Kleinman CS. Does a prenatal diagnosis of congenital heart disease alter short-term outcome? Ultrasound Obstet Gynecol. 1997;10:237-41.
3. Franklin O, Burch M, Manning N, Sleeman K, Gould S, Archer N. Prenatal diagnosis coarctation of the aorta improves survival and reduces morbidity. Heart. 2002;87:67-9.
4. Huggon IC, Cook AC, Smeeton NC, Magee AG, Sharland GK. Atrioventricular septal defects diagnosed in fetal life: associated cardiac and extracardiac abnormalities and outcome. J Am Coll Cardiol. 2000;36:593-601.
5. Tworetzky W, McElhinney DB, Mohan Reddy V, Brook MM, Hanley FL, Silverman NH. Improved surgical outcome after fetal diagnosis of hypoplastic heart syndrome. Circulation. 2001;103:1269-73.

Index

Page numbers followed by *f* refer to figure and *t* refer to table

A

Adenovirus 35
Agenesis 158, 161
Airways 6
Alagille syndrome 149, 154, 188
Alpha fetoprotein 148
American Heart Association 111
Amiodarone 112
Amniocentesis 177
 techniques 177*f*
Amniotic fluid 87, 178*f*
Anal atresia 161
Anemia 122
Aneuploidies 182
Anophthalmia 158
Anorectal atresia 165
Antiarrhythmic
 drugs 111, 138
 therapy 111
Anticonvulsant
 syndrome 149
 therapy 196
Aorta 24, 81*f*, 107*f*, 132, 153
 arch of 170*f*
 ascending 47*f*, 132*f*
 coarctation of 35, 51, 63, 63*f*, 64*f*, 80*f*, 158, 188, 209
 descending 14*f*, 15*f*, 47*f*
 overriding 71

Aortic
 arch 13, 14*f*, 27, 47*f*, 49, 64*f*, 132*f*
 size of 27
 flow 107
 root 56*f*
 stenosis
  critical 62, 138, 139, 142*f*
  severe 62*f*
 valve 79, 88
  annulus 49
  atresia 170*f*
  cusps 62*f*
  defect 198
  stenosis 158
Aortopulmonary septum,
 formation of 12*f*
Aorto-septal discontinuity 79
Apert syndrome 52
Arachnoid cyst 165
Arrhythmia 97, 207
 types of 103, 109
Artery
 left pulmonary 28
 normal pulmonary 63*f*
 posterior pulmonary 153
 umbilical 49, 124, 124*f*, 125*f*
Artrioventricular septal defects 51
Ascitis 134*f*
Asplenia 161

Atresia 188
 aortic 163*f*
Atretic
 pulmonary valve 66*f*
 tricuspid valve 65*f*
Atria 7
Atrial
 contraction 99, 126*f*
 ectopic tachycardia 96, 98, 107
 flutter 96, 107, 111
 isomerism 152
 re-entry tachycardia 107
 septal defect 35, 55, 150, 158, 188, 198, 201
 septum 7
  formation 10*f*
Atrioventricular
 block 113
 canal 5*f*, 7, 8*f*
  defect 165, 188
 connection 26
 defect 60*f*
  complete-balanced 58*f*
 dissociation 114*f*
 interval 106, 111
 re-entry tachycardia 107, 107*f*
 septal defect 35, 58, 149, 150, 158, 165, 198, 209
 time interval 107

valve 8f, 30f, 58f, 59f, 128, 129f
   flow 48f
   functions 26
   leaflets 49
   regurgitation 121
   single 60f

B

Balloon
   aortic valvuloplasty 207
   dilatation 142
   pulmonary valvotomy 139
Banana sign 165
Bicuspid aortic valves 52, 188
Biliary atresia 161
Brachiocephalic vein 5
Bradyarrhythmias 206
Bradycardia 96
Branch pulmonary arteries 131

C

Campomelic dysplasia 149, 151
Cardiac
   anomalies 148, 151
   axis 26, 41, 55
   biometry 39, 48
   chambers 26
   defects 165
   embryology 1
   function 26, 134
   malformations 157
   position 26, 55
   rhabdomyoma 195
   rhythm 26, 30
   size 26, 55, 123
   tumors 122
Cardiofaciocutaneous syndrome 187
Cardiothoracic ratio 49
Cardiovascular profile score 49, 133
Carotid arteries 14f
Cat eye syndrome 171
Cavum septum pellucidum 165
Cellular death, abnormal 17
Central nervous system 158, 163, 165, 169
Cephalad sweep 27
Cerebellar hypoplasia 163, 165
CHARGE syndrome 149, 154, 187, 188
Choledochal cyst 161
Chondroectodermal dysplasia 149
Chorioangioma 69
Chorionic villus sampling 149
Choroid plexus cyst 159f, 163, 165
Chromosomal disorders 185t
Chronic villi sampling 177f
Cisterna magna 160f, 165
Cleft
   lip 158, 164, 166f
   palate 164
Clubbed foot 164
Coloboma 158
Complete atrioventricular septal defect 55
Complete heart block 35, 114, 114f
Complex single ventricle situations 201
Conduction system 12
Congenital
   cardiac anomalies 51, 52
   complete heart block 37
   diaphragmatic hernia 158, 161f
   heart defect 19, 157, 193
   heart disease 1, 17, 33, 34, 34t, 35, 36, 39, 85, 96, 147, 180, 181, 181t, 187, 191, 200, 204, 208
   origin of 180
   pathogenesis of 17
   junctional ectopic tachycardia 107
   pulmonary airway malformation 56f
Congestive cardiac failure 120
Conotruncal anomalies 158
Corneal opacity 158
Cornelia de Lange syndrome 149, 151
Coronary sinus 25
Corpus callosum 166f, 167f
   agenesis of 158
Costello syndrome 187
Coxsackie 35
   virus 151
Cyclopia 164
Cyst, renal 157f
Cystic hygroma 164, 170f
Cystic kidney 162f
Cytomegalovirus 35, 151

D

Dandy-Walker malformation 158
Dandy-Walker syndrome 165
Deoxygenated blood 121
Dextrocardia 192
Diabetes mellitus 35, 196
Diaphragmatic hernia 161f, 164, 165
Diffuse transverse arch hypoplasia 88
DiGeorge syndrome 27, 184f, 194
Digoxin 111
Distal pulmonary arteries 6
Double bubble sign 162f
Double outlet right ventricle 35, 78, 158, 198
Down syndrome 171f, 182, 186, 193, 194f
Ductal arch 27, 28, 47f, 131f
   size of 27
   typical Hockeystick appearance of 47f
Ductus arteriosus 14f, 15f, 47f, 74, 131
   diameter 49
Ductus venosus 16f, 49, 54f, 101f, 125f, 134, 175f
Duodenal atresia 161, 162f, 165
Dysplastic brain 165
Dysplastic kidney 161

E

Ebstein's anomaly 67, 69, 69f, 158, 188
Ectomesenchymal tissue, abnormal migration of 17
Edward's syndrome 164
Ejection time 132

Index

Ellis-Van Creveld syndrome 52, 149, 188, 189
Encephalocele 158
End-diastolic ventricular diameter 49
Endocardial cushion defects 158
Endocardial tubes 3f
  fusion of 3f, 4f
Epiblast 2f
  cells 2f
Esophageal atresia 153f, 165
Esophagus 82f
Extracardiac anomalies 157
Extracellular matrix, abnormalities of 17

F

Facial dysmorphism 158
Fallot's tetralogy 74
Fetal
  anemia 69
  aneuploidy 148
  anomalies 148, 149, 166f
  aortic valvotomy 143f
  arrhythmia 89, 95, 96, 97t, 99f
  atrial flutter 108f
  balloon aortic valvotomy 138, 139, 141
  bradyarrhythmias 113
  cardiac
    defects 51
    function 39
    intervention 138, 144
    registry 139
  cardiovascular profile score 134t
  chest wall 143f
  circulation 15f
  congenital heart disease 147, 191
  echocardiography 1, 33, 34, 36, 36t, 37, 38, 85, 86, 92
    timing of 37, 86
  heart 24, 25f, 29, 10f, 120, 132f
    block 144
    failure 120, 122
    physiology of 13
    rate 97, 107
    screening 40
  hemoglobin 16
  hydrops 207
  magnetocardiogram 95, 102
  neuro sonogram 160f
  pericardiocentesis 144, 144f
  pulmonary valve perforation 142
  rhythm 116
  supraventricular tachycardia 107f
  tachyarrhythmia 105, 109, 138, 143
    management of 109, 111
  tachycardia 110
    management of 110
  tumor 69
Fish proven microdeletion syndrome 186
Flecainide 112
Fluorescence in situ hybridization 169f, 182, 192
Folic acid 198
  antagonists 198
  role of 202
Foramen ovale 26, 57f, 127, 139
  form of 26
  normal pulse Doppler of 127f
  stenting of 143
Fossa ovalis 43f

G

Gastrointestinal
  malformations 161
  system 164
  tract 165
    anomaly 162f
Genetic
  syndromes 148
  testing 192
Genital agenesis 162
Genitourinary
  system 164
  tract 165
Goldenhar syndrome 149, 154
Gray scale machine controls 20t
Great arteries 78f, 79f
  complete transposition of 76, 76f, 77f
  congenitally corrected transposition of 77, 78, 79f
  transposition of 46, 149, 198, 209
Great vessels 83f
  transposition of 188

H

Heart 2, 124
  block
    complete 115
    second degree 96, 103
  disease, pathogenesis of 1
  failure 133
  rate 30, 39, 48
  syndrome 142f
Hematoma, subchorionic 178f
Hemi vertebrae 150f
Hemifacial
  microphthalmia 156f
  microsomia 154
  syndrome 149
Hemorrhage 121
Hepatic venous system, development of 16f
Heterotaxy 152
  syndromes 149
High body mass index 88
Holoprosencephaly 158, 163
Holt-Oram syndrome 52, 61, 149, 188
Horseshoe kidney 162
Hydrocephalus 160f
Hydrops 151
  fetalis 109, 201
Hyperextension 164f
Hypertrophic cardiomyopathy 187
Hypoblast 2f
Hypognathia 164
Hypoplasia 158
  renal 161
Hypoplastic
  left heart syndrome 51, 60, 122, 139, 151, 158, 198, 201, 205, 208
  right heart syndrome 140
Hypospadias 162

I

Inferior vena cava 29, 30f, 47f, 126
Inlet ventricular septal defect 51, 55, 57
Innominate artery 47f
Intact ventricular septum 139, 140, 209
International Society of Ultrasound in Obstetrics and Gynecology 86
Interventricular foramen 11f
Intracardiac blood flow, abnormal 17
Intramuscular injection 141
Intrathoracic stomach 161f
Isovolumic
　contraction time 132
　relaxation time 132
Isthmus
　aortic 131
　diameter 49
Ivemark syndrome 188

J

Jejunal atresia 161, 162f, 165
Jeune's syndrome 149
Joint dislocation 162
Junctional tachycardia 96, 107

K

Kabuki syndrome 187, 188, 189f
Knee genu recurvatum 164f

L

Leopard syndrome 187
Levocardia 53f
Lidocaine 112
Limb anomalies 158
Lithium 52
Lower limbs 165
　anomalies of 162
Lung
　hypoplasia 56f, 158
　parenchyma 6

M

Magnesium infusion 112
Malalignment ventricular septal defect 56f
Malignant fetal arrhythmias 95
Marfan's syndrome 149, 154
Maternal
　diabetes mellitus 196
　digoxin 133
　hyperthermia 197
　hypoxia 207
　infections 35
　phenylketonuria 196
　rubella infection 197
　teratogens exposure 35
Meckel's diverticulum 161
Mega cisterna magna 174f
Meningomyelocele 158, 162
Mesocardia 78f
Mexilitine 112
Microphthalmia 156f, 158
Mitral valve 88, 128, 132f, 134
　annulus 49
Mosaic Down's syndrome 193
Mowat-Wilson syndrome 188
Multiple giant-cell lesion syndrome 187
Multiple malformation syndrome 181
Mumps 52
Muscular interventricular septum 9
Musculoskeletal anomalies 162
Myocardial function, abnormal 129f
Myometrium 177f

N

Nasal bone 172
Neural tube defect 163
Neurofibromatosis 187
Non-syndromic congenital heart defect 198t
Noonan's syndrome 52, 61, 149, 151, 187, 189f
Nuchal edema 151, 164

O

Obesity 196
Oculodentodigital syndrome 188
Olfactory nerve agenesis 158
Omphalocele 163f, 164, 165, 172f
Open fetal cardiac intervention 207
Optic nerve agenesis 158
Orofacial digital syndrome 188
Oxygenated blood 120

P

Parallel great arteries 76
Paroxysmal junctional reciprocating tachycardia 96, 98
Parvovirus 35
Patau syndrome 163
Patent ductus arteriosus 188
Patent foramen ovale 88
Peak aortic systolic velocity 62f
Pelvis 169
Persistent left superior vena cava 149
Phace syndrome 188
Phenylketonuria 196
Phenytoin 52
Placenta 3
Polysplenia 161
Pregnancy 192
　management of 200
Premature atrial
　beats 96
　complexes 104f
　contractions 103
Premature ductal closure 135
Premature ventricular
　beats 96
　complexes 103, 105f
Prenatal Diagnosis and Therapeutics Act 140
Propranolol 112
Proximal pulmonary arteries 7
Pulmonary artery 45f, 47f, 62f, 65f, 67f, 68f, 72f, 78f, 80f, 81f
　bifurcation of 28f
　dilatation 68f

Pulmonary atresia 46, 65, 66f, 67f, 73, 73f, 74f, 139, 140, 165, 209
　ventricular septal defect 201
Pulmonary valve 79
　annulus 49
　syndrome 73, 74f, 75f, 210
Pulmonary vein 30f, 126, 127f
　arterialization of 140
Pulmonary venous
　connection 26, 78f
　system 7
Pyelocaliectasis 164

R

Regurgitation
　aortic 35
　mitral 122, 128f, 134
　pulmonary 74, 135f
Renal cortical cysts 161
Retrognathia 169
Rhabdomyoma 157f
Rubella 35, 52

S

Sacrococcygeal teratoma 90
Schinzel-Giedion syndrome 187
Semilobar holoprosencephaly 166f
Semilunar valves, pulse Doppler of 130f
Septal defects 26, 158
Septoaortic discontinuity 90f
Septum
　formation of 8f
　primum 57f
　　atrial septal defect 51
　　formation of 10f
　secundum, formation of 10f
　transversum 3f
Short rib polydactyly syndrome 149
Single gene
　disorders 189f
　mutations 198t

Sinus
　bradycardia 96, 113
　rhythm, normal 97
　tachycardia 96, 97, 106, 107
Situs
　abdominal 41f, 47f
　abnormality 52
　evaluation of 41f
　inversus 53f, 149, 150, 159f
Sjogren syndrome 35
Skin defects 158
Small pulmonary artery 65f, 67f, 74f, 171f
Smith-Lemli-Opitz syndrome 149, 151
Somatic mutations 189
Sotalol 112
Speckle reduction 22
Spina bifida 156f
Spinal hemi vertebrae 150f
Spiral aortopulmonary septum 12f
Splenic
　agenesis 158
　anomalies 161
Stenosis
　aortic 35, 122, 139
　pulmonary 53f, 67, 122, 165, 187, 188
　subcritical pulmonary 68f
　tracheal 152f
Subclavian artery 81
　abnormal right 175
Superior vena cava 27, 29, 45f, 47f, 107f
Supravalvar aortic stenosis 188, 198
Supraventricular tachycardia 96, 98, 106, 101f, 110
Systemic venous system 5
　development of 6f
Systolic function 133

T

Tachyarrhythmia 133, 206
Tachycardia 96, 107

Teratogens 154, 196
Tetralogy of Fallot 46, 56f, 71, 72f, 79, 80, 81f, 90, 150, 158, 188, 198
Thoracic asphyxiating syndrome 149
Thrombocytopenia absent radius syndrome 149, 150, 188
Thymic anomalies 158
Tissue harmonic imaging 20
Total anomalous pulmonary venous
　connection 71, 152
　drainage 70
Trachea 28
Tracheoesophageal fistula 158
Transabdominal sonography 87
Transplacental therapy 138
Transtricuspid flow 66
Transvaginal sonography 87
Tricuspid
　atresia 64, 65f, 198
　dysplasia 70f
　regurgitation 69f, 70, 134, 135f, 163f, 165, 173f
　valve 69f, 128, 134
　　dysplasia 69
　　Ebstein's anomaly of 122
　　leaflet 57f, 70f
　　normal pulse Doppler of 129f
Triploidy fetus 159f
Trosseau's sign 28f
Truncus arteriosus 158, 209
Tuberous sclerosis 149, 154, 157f, 195
Turner syndrome 52, 61, 183, 183f, 188
Twin transfusion 121

U

Umbilical artery, single 163, 170f
Upper limbs, anomalies of 162
Urethral valves, posterior 167f, 168f

Uteropelvic junction stenosis 161
Uterus bicornis 162

V

VACTERL syndrome 149, 150
Valvotomy 141
Vein of Galen 69, 122
Vein, umbilical 16f, 17, 49, 54f, 125f, 134
Ventricular dysfunction 110
 ejection 107
 outflows 130
 septal defect 149, 150, 158, 188
 septation 9
 septum 48f
 tachycardia 96, 109-111
Ventriculoatrial interval 98, 111
Vertebral anomalies 162
Vessels, abnormal spatial arrangement of 80
Visceral situs 22, 41
Vitelline veins 6

W

Wenkebach rhythm 106f
Williams syndrome 149, 157, 184f, 186, 188

Y

Yolk sac 3